Praise for
Navigating the Alzheimer's Journey: A Compass for Caregiving

"Wow—what a fantastic resource on caregiving and Alzheimer's disease! I wish it had been available when I was navigating the maze of eldercare for my parents. Knowledge is power—don't get caught unprepared. If you have aging loved ones, here's your roadmap and compass!"

Jacqueline Marcell
Author, *Elder Rage*
Radio host for *Coping with Caregiving*

"Carol Bowlby Sifton is a visionary and practical genius when it comes to enhancing the lives of persons with Alzheimer's disease and their caregivers. More than any other practitioner–scholar in North America, Bowlby Sifton combines careful thinking about effective care with rich case studies and a 'how to' approach. Her work over several decades has served as a model of effective commitment, wise caring, and nobility of purpose. *Navigating the Alzheimer's Journey* will appeal to the everyday caregiver who just wants to know what to do and how to do it, to the professionals in every field who focus on persons with dementia, and to researchers interested in studying the enhancement of the lives of the deeply forgetful and those who care for them."

Stephen G. Post, Ph.D., Professor
School of Medicine, Case Western Reserve University
Author, *The Moral Challenge of Alzheimer's Disease*

"Families will find meaningful treasures in these suggestions for navigating the choppy terrain of Alzheimer's care. Carol Bowlby Sifton offers much more than a compass—she illuminates the 'small things' that ultimately contribute to quality of lives in care relationships."

Lisa P. Gwyther, M.S.W., Associate Clinical Professor
Bryan Alzheimer's Disease Research Center
Duke University Medical Center

"Caring for a loved one with Alzheimer's disease ranks high among life's most difficult challenges.… In *Navigating the Alzheimer's Journey*, Carol Bowlby Sifton has provided the compass every caregiver needs. Few people are as experienced in caregiving as she is. And fewer still write with the insight, wisdom, and grace she brings to this invaluable guide. Alzheimer's caregiving is a very rocky road. But with the compass Carol Bowlby Sifton provides, you will always have a strong sense of direction."

Michael Castleman, Co-author
There's Still a Person In There:
The Complete Guide to Treating and Coping with Alzheimer's

"Using personal stories, professional experience, and evidence-based research, Carol Bowlby Sifton has amassed a useful guide for family members caring for a loved one with Alzheimer's disease. This book offers both hope and practical suggestions for navigating one's way along a long and winding road. Although written for families, it will be also be useful to professionals in the fields of health and aging. This book is so rich with ideas and examples that it should not be read once, shelved and forgotten. It should be kept within easy reach for reference again and again."

Daniel Kuhn, M.S.W.
Mather LifeWays Institute on Aging
Author, *Alzheimer's Early Stages*

"Carol Bowlby Sifton's extensive experience with Alzheimer's, both professionally and personally, provides an excellent guide to the steps, skills, and emotional awareness it took me 11 years of caregiving to learn. This book would have been an invaluable resource for me at the beginning of my trek through the Alzheimer's caregiving process."

Judy Bow, family caregiver

"This is a remarkable book written for caregivers of persons with Alzheimer's disease and related disorders as well as health professionals who need to know what it feels like to live through the different stages of these conditions. The evidence presented is up to date and many case histories illustrate the take-home messages. The occupational therapy background of the author allows for a full discussion of the cognitive, functional and behavioral domains of Alzheimer's disease, without losing sight of the person as a whole."

Serge Gauthier, M.D., FRCPC
Director, Alzheimer Disease Research Unit
McGill Centre for Studies in Aging (Canada)

"Carol Bowlby Sifton shares her fundamental understanding of the needs of people with dementia throughout this treasure chest of concrete and practical suggestions. In sharing her personal and professional experiences she captures the complexities of the challenges dementia caregivers face. Her emphasis on respect and dignity is strengthened by frequent reminders to the caregiver to imagine walking in the shoes of the person whose brain is changing due to dementia."

Sally Callahan, Author
My Mother's Voice

Navigating the
Alzheimer's Journey

Navigating the Alzheimer's Journey

A Compass for Caregiving

by Carol Bowlby Sifton

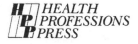
HEALTH
PROFESSIONS
PRESS

Baltimore · London · Winnipeg · Sydney

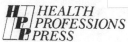

HEALTH PROFESSIONS PRESS

Health Professions Press, Inc.
Post Office Box 10624
Baltimore, Maryland 21285-0624

www.healthpropress.com

Manufactured in the United States of America by Sheridan Books, Fredericksburg, Virginia.

Cover photograph copyright © 2004 by Cathy Stein Greenblat; used here with permission. Originally published in *Alive with Alzheimer's,* University of Chicago Press, 2004.

The stories in this book are based on the author's experiences. Some of the vignettes represent actual people and circumstances. In most of these cases, individuals' names and identifying details have been changed to protect their identities. A few cases use persons' actual names by permission. Other vignettes are composite or fictional accounts that do not represent the lives or experiences of specific individuals, and no implications should be inferred.

Library of Congress Cataloging-in-Publication Data

Bowlby Sifton, Carol.
  Navigating the Alzheimer's journey: a compass for caregiving / by Carol Bowlby Sifton.— 1st ed.
    p.   cm.
  Includes bibliographical references.
  ISBN 1-932529-04-7 (pbk. : alk. paper)
  1. Alzheimer's disease—Patients—Home care.   2. Alzheimer's disease—Patients—Family relationships.   3. Caregivers—Family relationships.   4. Caregivers.   I. Title.

RC523.B678   2004
362.196'831—dc22   2004008988

British Library Cataloguing in Publication data are available from the British Library.

Contents

About the Author

Carol Bowlby Sifton, B.Sc.O.T., O.D.H., is a former family caregiver, an occupational therapist, a clinical consultant, an educator, and an author who has worked extensively with persons with dementia and their caregivers throughout the continuum of care. She is a dementia consultant to numerous long-term care facilities as well as to Veterans Affairs Canada, working in the homes of persons with dementia and their caregivers. Carol also operates Elderactive Occupational Therapy, which specializes in enhancing the quality of life of persons with dementia. She has presented her highly acclaimed interactive workshops throughout North America. In addition, Carol has served as clinical coordinator and assessor for geriatrics at Victoria General Hospital, site of the Queen Elizabeth II Health Sciences Centre in Halifax, Nova Scotia. Furthermore, she has lectured at Dalhousie University's Medical School and School of Occupational Therapy in Halifax and at Mount Saint Vincent University's Family Studies and Gerontology Department, also in Halifax.

Carol is the editor of *Alzheimer's Care Quarterly*, a peer-reviewed journal focusing on quality dementia care that is readily incorporated into the day-to-day activities of professionals across the continuum of care. In addition to this book, *Navigating the Alzheimer's Journey: A Compass for Caregiving*, a companion book by Carol specifically guides professionals who care for people with Alzheimer's disease (visit the Health Professions Press web site, http://www.healthpropress.com, or call toll-free, 888-337-8808, for information). Her earlier book *Therapeutic Activities with Persons Disabled by Alzheimer's Disease and Related Disorders* (Aspen Publishers, 1993) is recognized as a key resource across North America. While serving as national coordinator for the Health Canada/Canadian Association of Occupational Therapists/Alzheimer Canada Dementia Care at Home Project, she wrote *Living at Home with Alzheimer's Disease and Related Dementias* (Canadian Association of Occupational Therapists, 1998), a resource manual for professionals in community care.

Lovingly dedicated to my mother and my best friend,
Muriel Middaugh Sifton,
who through her ever-present love, wisdom,
and nurturing of me and so many others
has been my compass and inspiration,
not only for this book but for my life

Introduction

> I am hoping to break that taboo—of being ashamed of a disease. Why be ashamed of the physical breakdown of brain cells any more than the physical breakdown of other parts of our body? We are not mad, but sick, so please treat us with dignity, do not make fun of us, and do not be ashamed. Maybe I am breaking the ultimate taboo in going public and saying 'I have dementia!' (Boden, 1998, p. xi)

I have been involved in dementia care, as a family caregiver and a professional, since the 1980s. During this time, I have attended many excellent conferences and workshops and have read hundreds of pages from books and journals on dementia. The fantastic growth of information on this topic is exciting and overwhelming. Despite this explosion of information, there has been no change in what is the number one source for learning about caregiving: the day-to-day life experiences of persons with dementia and their caregivers.

As a professional caregiver, I have had the privilege of being with hundreds of persons with dementia and their caregivers, in many settings and in many of dementia's stages. Although each person with dementia and each caregiving situation is unique, I hope that sharing these many caregiving journeys, as well as information from the professional field, may shed some light on your own particular path. I also hope that by knowing one another's story we can grow in understanding together.

To begin, I would like to introduce you to the person who taught me more than anyone else about caregiving: my mother-in-law, Alice Jewel Teeple Bowlby. You will read many more pieces of our caregiving story throughout *Navigating the Alzheimer's Journey: A Compass for Caregiving*.

Alice learned early how to deal with adversity and challenge. As a child, she overcame the crippling effects of polio;
she later trained and practiced as a nurse. Like most of her
generation, she was challenged by the Great Depression and
learned the real value of caring relationships with family and
friends. These life lessons supported Alice in living with dignity and courage through the ravages of Alzheimer's disease
until she died in 1990, just before her 83rd birthday. By the
time of her death, Alzheimer's had robbed Alice of her ability
to care for her home and her personal needs, as well as her
ability to walk, to feed herself, or to tell others about her
needs and wishes. These losses caused Alice and all of our
family tremendous sorrow and often great distress. However,
Alzheimer's did not ever steal the very core of the person we
all knew and loved. When words failed, there was always a
way through touch, smiles, music, family stories, and pictures
to connect with Alice. And Alice always knew who we were. I
am not talking about calling us by name, as that ability left her
very early on. I am talking about the very core of Alice, who
knew that we were her loved ones and recognized the importance that we had in each others' lives.

During the later stages of her disease, my family made the
very difficult decision to move, for work reasons, to California for a year. The nurses at Alice's care facility were always
amazed at how she came alive and responded to our voices
when we called, but this could have just been the excitement
of getting a call from anyone. However, when we returned
home a few weeks before Alice died, her facial and body
expressions and general animation left no doubt that she
knew us. She even knew her teenage grandchildren, whose
appearances had greatly changed since the last time Alice had
seen them. Nathanial, by then age 13, was 10 inches taller;
Miriam, by then age 16, had grown into a young woman.
Alice's greeting to Miriam, who first visited her grandmother

alone, included not only joyful animation but also a muttered "mmm," as if Alice was trying to say her granddaughter's name.

About a month following our return, Alice had a stroke. After almost a week in a deep coma, Alice grasped our hands firmly, looked at us knowingly and lovingly, and drew her last breath. Yes, she knew her family to the very end.

From my own personal experience and from that of others, I have no doubt that persons with dementia continue to have a deep sense of themselves and of their connection with loved ones. Dementia damages brain cells, not a person's humanity or the person's need to continue to be in relationships with others and to be valued and affirmed as a whole person in this present moment. Losing one's memory doesn't mean losing oneself or the people one cares about.

Caregiving takes place within a relationship. Although the effects of dementia lead to changes in relationships, they don't lead to the end of the relationship. The following stories show how two different relationships were shaped by caregiving and the changes that were the result of dementia.

LEITHA AND BOB GLAVIN[1]

The following account is based on a September 1999 visit in the Nova Scotia home of Leitha and Bob Glavin. I have grouped their commentary by related themes, but each person's view was expressed in a separate, private conversation.

Leitha: The most important advice I would give is that you have to walk a mile in the other person's shoes. I have that poem on my fridge, and I read it all the time to remind me. You really have to care, to love

---

[1]An earlier version of this interview appeared in Bowlby Sifton, C. (2000a). Caregiver focus: It's the little things that matter. *Alzheimer's Care Quarterly, 1*(1), 1–4; adapted by permission.

your spouse, to understand what they are going through; that brings understanding and patience. It seems to me it's one thing for a person to know they have heart disease or cancer or something; it is another thing altogether to know that your brain is dying. I think of it like the layers of an onion, dying, one by one.[2] It must be awful. I just want Bob to have as happy and normal a life as possible.

Bob: I just take one day at a time; I try to enjoy life as it is. I go with the flow and try to do the things that I still can do.

If I wasn't busy, I just couldn't get along; they might as well put me out to pasture. I just take my time and plan everything out; it may take me a lot longer, but so what?

I take Lady for long walks. She was really supposed to be Leitha's dog, but I guess she is mine.

During the 2 years prior to this interview, Leitha and Bob had been creatively and bravely living out the reality of Bob's Alzheimer's disease. For more than 4 years prior to Bob's formal diagnosis, they knew something was wrong. Bob noticed that he had more and more trouble planning his carpentry projects. Tasks like fitting molding around a room, which he could previously do easily, started to be difficult. Leitha also noticed uncharacteristic times of irritability. Neither spoke of their concerns until the day Bob couldn't figure out how to hang a door, something he had done many times before. He had to call his son-in-law to help.

Leitha heard about the incident from her daughter, who telephoned, full of concern: "Mom, there has got to be something wrong with Dad; we have to do something." Leitha felt

---

[2]This is Leitha's analogy, not a neurological one.

a knot in the pit of her stomach; her daughter's call confirmed what she already knew in her heart. They went to see their family doctor, who doubted there was a problem. Upon Leitha's insistence, he finally agreed to send Bob to a specialist. The couple had to wait many months but eventually made the 4-hour journey to Halifax to see a geriatrician. After hours of tests and several more trips to Halifax, the geriatrician confirmed that at age 65, Bob had early Alzheimer's disease.

Leitha: I wasn't ready to accept it, but I knew it was true. And I had a good cry. The first decisions were how to cope. We talked about everything from the first day. You have to discuss it and work at it. I found that reading helped, so I would know what to expect. Everything that I have read, Bob has read, and we have shared it with our family. We started right from there to get everything in order—enduring power of attorney and everything. I would recommend the same to others.

At the time of diagnosis, Bob's first words were "I knew something was wrong." After this, Bob asked Leitha what she was going to do. Leitha's response to Bob's question was spontaneous. "We will get through it together, Hon, just like we have everything else." During the interview, she remarked that she still wouldn't have it any other way. From Leitha's caring comments and from watching her and Bob together, it is obvious that the strength of their relationship of more than 40 years is the anchor that steadies them both through this challenging time. "We can still be on the same wavelength," Leitha said. She noted there have been changes, pieces of their relationship that just won't ever be the same, but there has also been growth. She talked about a richer, deeper connection and how Bob has softened, become more expressive with his emotions. Leitha said, "We share lots of hugs, and for the first time, Bob hugs his sons." After a Christmas visit with one son and his family, all were struck that this was the best time they had ever had with Bob.

Bob: I don't know why I am living; I am not worth anything to anybody.

Leitha: Well, you are to me. And don't you ever forget it.

Leitha supports Bob's worth and his dignity in their relationship as well as in the family and community. Although they are both very open about Bob's diagnosis, Leitha is the one who sensitively paves the way with family, neighbors, and the community. She doesn't want him to be embarrassed or ridiculed.

Bob protects his dignity in public in a different way, which is sometimes hard on Leitha, but she understands. He opens conversations with the joking comment, "She is the one who needs the help, not me." Bob was always the provider, the competent organizer. So of course it is very difficult for him to acknowledge that this role is changing, that Leitha is his lifeline—not only for financial and other matters, but also for day-to-day living. For example, they had to call a plumber (for the first time in more than 40 years) because Bob felt that it would "bother his back too much" to be working under the sink. Leitha just said, "That's okay, Hon. We will call the plumber." Another layer off the onion.

Leitha understands that in public pride is at stake and it is easier for Bob to deflect his losses onto Leitha; in private, they are both aware, and they talk and cry and hug and laugh. During one such private moment, they saw an elderly neighbor who has advanced Alzheimer's sitting in a running car while her husband was in the store. Bob was horrified at the potential danger in this situation and made Leitha promise that she would put him in a nursing facility when his disease

had advanced that far. Bob surprised Leitha during Alzheimer's Awareness Month by suggesting that they go to an
open house at a local Alzheimer's care facility. He had seen
the notice in the paper, and he thought it would be good for
both of them to know where he might eventually receive care.

The changes, differences, and losses really hit home to
Leitha and Bob, each in their own way, during a move that
happened just a couple of weeks before the interview.
Although they had been trying to sell their house on the small
island community where Bob was born and they had retired,
nothing had happened for 2 years. In a whirlwind week, however, the house sold, they bought another house, and they
moved. They chose a house together, with Bob acknowledging that it was *their* last house and that he wanted Leitha to
have a house where she would be comfortable on her own.

Leitha: The move was a nightmare—not the work, really,
but it just really hit me then how much Bob had
lost. The truck I had booked to move us turned up
in the afternoon with no loading ramp, and it was
impossible to use. I had to send them away. That
evening, I collapsed in bed at our daughter's [house],
trying to figure out how on earth we were going to
get all of our stuff out the next day. With the help of
good friends and family and lots of phone calls, a
convoy of little pickups was organized and we did it.
What floored me was Bob's response to this crisis.
When I asked him what we were going to do, he
said, "You can figure that out; I've got to get over to
the house and clean the bathroom." Then, it was the
oven. When I arrived, Bob presented me with items
from the fridge to put somewhere. I mean, I couldn't
believe that this was Bob; his strength had always
been taking charge and organizing in a crisis.

Bob: Moving was really hard; I spent more trips up and down the stairs because I would see something somewhere and go to get it and then forget which box it was in or what I was looking for. And so on, like that. I find that I get really tired. I was used to resting every day and I have to get back to that.

As we talked, it was obvious that Leitha understood that Bob had lost the ability to do complicated problem solving; instead, he did the concrete tasks that he could manage. She understood, she grieved, and they carried on.

The new house and neighborhood are "just great," and despite the difficulty, the move has been worth it. After the interview, Leitha and Bob had a month-long, leisurely car trip planned so they could visit family and friends, see the autumn foliage, and spend time together. Although this spirit of joy in what they can share and do and a light-hearted humor pervade, each day is also intermingled with times of genuine sorrow and frustration.

Leitha and Bob are both committed to doing what they can to help others gain from their situation. Early on, Bob asked the geriatrician about donating his brain for research after he passed away. Every year, they make the tiring trip to Halifax for testing. Both have been frustrated with this process, however.

Leitha: I really think they need to ask different types of questions, especially for people in the early stages. There needs to be questions about day-to-day things. And most of all, they need to talk to the caregivers; I mean you just have to be in the home to understand what is really going on. [After the] last tests that Bob had, they told me there was no change and even hinted that maybe the diagnosis wasn't accurate. And here I am at home seeing huge changes. For instance, a few minutes after we get groceries and Bob helps me to put them away, he gets worried that we better go shopping. When I raised this with the doctor, I felt dismissed, as if I couldn't possibly know more than the tests can show. It takes so much out of us both; I am just not sure if we will go back.

Bob: The tests are very hard; I find it very tiring. Sometimes I find it all very hard; mostly it's the little things that are so frustrating. Take today, for instance. I went into town, just really to get a birthday card and a flower for Leitha, and I came home without [them]. It wasn't on my list because it was a surprise, and I completely forgot about it. I find my short-term memory is getting worse all the time.

There are scary times too. The other day, I was talking about something, and I just lost the topic altogether; it was just like somebody had hauled down a window blind in my mind.

Leitha has become not only Bob's lifeline but also a courageous advocate. She has found support in the strength of their relationship, from her faith, from her daughter, from a very good friend, and from the day hospital program and its staff. In other ways, however, she has had to fight for every bit of help, and in some cases, she hasn't found support where she had expected to. Not all family members have been supportive, and some state openly that there is nothing wrong with Bob. They say, "He looks just fine to me," and suggest that the problem is all in Leitha's mind. Another and perhaps more shocking example comes from early on, when they went to a support group meeting and no one turned up, not even the leader. Later, the person apologized saying that there just wasn't anyone in the area with Alzheimer's disease! Since the time of the interview, Leitha has worked with the Alzheimer Society of Nova Scotia to develop a support group. What would Leitha like to see change?

Leitha: There needs to be an end to the stigma of having Alzheimer's disease. What is there to be ashamed of? It is a brain disease. This has to be . . . talked about; there has to be more education. This stigma keeps people from getting help.

I have found the caring and understanding, the human side, missing with some professionals. They may give you a couple of pamphlets and call that counseling. I read them, but not everyone is going to. The caring touch is what counts.

Bob: Lots of people, doctors included, say "It's just old age." This really bothers me.

People down home where I used to live stop and ask me how I am feeling, and I say "fine." They just don't understand, don't want to really, that I'm not sick [in a way they can see; I have a brain disease]. There is so much out there to read, but they won't do it. I find that frustrating, but in the end I realize that this is their problem. . . .

As we ended our discussion, Leitha wholeheartedly agreed with an earlier comment of Bob's: "It is the little things that matter most."

It doesn't cost anything extra or take any more time for both professionals and nonprofessionals to be caring and respectful. This caring component is so essential. If it is missing, no money thrown at the situation is going to matter anyway. What a hopeful message for us all: Something that does not cost a cent can make a huge difference in the lives of people with Alzheimer's disease and their caregivers.

One final anecdote from Leitha and Bob's story reminds us how amazingly skilled persons with Alzheimer's disease can be. Bob had answered a telephone call from one of Leitha's favorite nieces while his wife was out. Bob had recognized the caller's voice but had no idea who she was and was too embarrassed to ask for a name from a person who obviously knew him well. His creative solution was to sit down with Leitha's address book and study every name in it until he found one that matched the voice on the telephone. Later, he was able to convey the message to Leitha. Brilliant problem solving, really—still lots of layers left on the onion.

I thank Leitha and Bob for so openly sharing their triumphs as well as their pain and their challenges. They are an inspiration and had no hesitation in having their names published in the hopes that they may be able to help others, either in person or through the telling of their story.

There are many lessons in Bob and Leitha's story, which I draw upon in the following chapters. Here, I would like to highlight the attitude that Bob and Leitha bring to living day to day with Alzheimer's disease. According to Bob, "I just take one day at a time; I try to enjoy life as it is. I go with the flow and try to do the things that I still can do." Bob seems to value the pleasures and accomplishments of the moment; he is living as fully and richly in the present moment as he can. Leitha echoed this view, saying, "I just want Bob to have as happy and normal a life as possible."

It is my hope that this book will shed further light on ways to celebrate the moment. One of the keys, voiced by Bob, is a reminder of the foundation of any caregiving relationship: "The main thing is that people treat me like a person, just like anyone else."

DEBORAH AND MERV

Deborah and Merv's story (not their real names) provides a strong contrast to Leitha and Bob's. In this case, the caregiver's pain is too private, and the couple's understanding of their situation is quite limited.

Merv is currently a resident of a long-term care facility in the same village where Deborah lives alone in a small apartment. Deborah and Merv tried their best to live a life together and raise two children. They were armed with good intentions while struggling with mental illness, poverty, and a limited understanding of or access to resources for help. Through it all, threads are visible of a love that has held them together for more than 50 years.

Merv had a traumatic childhood, and the scars remain. He had numerous stays in psychiatric hospitals and a longstanding diagnosis of schizophrenia. When I met Merv, it was difficult to sort through his history and determine the accuracy of this diagnosis. Past treatment attempts had included multiple shock treatments and major tranquilizers. It was clear that Merv was disturbed by some of his thought processes. He was obsessed with counting things and had difficulty understanding the space around him (sometimes he refused to leave their small kitchen for an entire day). He also became fixated on certain false ideas—for example, that Deborah was seeing another man whenever she went out. Quick flashes of temper and a refusal to leave the apartment were among the many challenges in his life.

Yet, Merv was a gifted painter who extended his artistic repertoire to include architecture; he even designed the family's home. He capably organized meager finances to provide for the family and was a fabulous cook. His sons say that while they were growing up, it was only through their father's skill that they were able to have a roof over their heads or food on the table.

Sadly, by the time that I met Merv, his many talents were almost entirely obscured by his difficulty with coping on a day-to-day basis. Because he had always had periods of great distress and confusion, certain changes were initially unnoticed by Deborah, his family, and his doctor. For instance, Merv could no longer make an edible meal. He would prepare dishes for supper hours before he needed to and once served sandwiches made from canned dog food. In addition, it was obvious that he was no longer washing himself properly, and his memory was terrible.

Eventually, assessment strongly indicated that Merv had cognitive impairments and perhaps some form of dementia. He was moved to a special program for persons with memory loss. He was almost always reluctant for Deborah to take him to the program, but once there, he greeted staff and others with lots of hugs. Later, he was delighted to see Deborah when she picked him up and greeted her with hugs and kisses. His behavior was a surprise to Deborah and the couple's children because Merv had seldom expressed affection in the past. The family noticed a general softening and a great sense of humor peeking through the memory loss and his lifelong unusual thoughts and behaviors.

These changes in Merv brought Deborah great comfort and hope. It had been a difficult marriage, but this gentle soul had persevered, hoping that her love would change things, that she and Merv would someday be able to enjoy time together. Their children reported that despite the obvious difficulties related to Merv's dementia, this was the happiest period of their parents' married life. Deborah was basking in Merv's increased affection and decreased anger and hostility.

On the down side, Deborah could be described as a "hope junkie." She took these wonderful changes as a sign that even better changes were ahead. For example, she lived in hope that Merv would listen to her reasonable explanations and that he would realize they only had a few years left and should enjoy this time by doing things together. Yet, Merv responded from lifelong patterns of withdrawal, intensified by a fear of failure and the unknown caused by increasing memory problems.

Day program staff spent a great deal of time coaching Deborah in techniques for successfully making requests of Merv. However, Deborah believed that if she repeated her own approach (that of reasoning) often enough, it would work. During a meeting with Deborah and the couple's children, I addressed concerns about Deborah and Merv's poor diet. Merv refused to accept Deborah's offer of preparing a meal, as the kitchen was his territory. Deborah accepted Merv's poor attempts at making meals to avoid hurting his feelings. This was a particular worry because Deborah had diabetes. The family and I worked through a number of ways for Deborah to gently but firmly state that she would prepare the meals. For example, Deborah could *tell* Merv that she was preparing a roast as a treat and *ask* him what time he would like to eat. Deborah enthusiastically accepted such suggestions, and I thought we had made a breakthrough at last. When I asked Deborah to recap what she was going to say to Merv about supper that night, however, she replied, "Would you like me to cook this roast for supper, dear?" Merv would undoubtedly say no, and the problem of poor nutrition would continue.

Eventually, home meal delivery service was provided. This was not discussed with Merv. The children simply told Merv that supper would be delivered shortly. Both Merv and Deborah enjoyed the meals, and Merv made no protests.

In much the same way, we were able to arrange for an assessment by a geriatrician, which confirmed the suspicion that Merv had dementia. Staff worked with the family to put in place as many supports as possible. The couple received home care support to clean the house, bathe Merv, and provide respite for Deborah. Deborah was urged not to leave Merv alone for long periods of time. A generous-hearted nurse patiently answered Deborah's numerous evening distress calls at her home.

We abandoned trying to help Deborah learn other ways of requesting things from Merv. We talked to the couple's children about the likely progression of Merv's dementia and the need to consider how and where their father would receive care when their mother could no longer provide it. We gave them a copy of *A Personal Care Book* (Alzheimer Society, 1993) to fill in details about their father's routines and habits. We explained how this could help to prepare for placement by ensuring that future caregivers knew as much as possible about their father. We also encouraged them to start looking at different long-term care facilities.

The family responded with interest and appreciation to these suggestions, but the whole precarious house of cards came down in one rush. One winter evening before going bowling, Deborah carefully explained to Merv where she was going and when she would be back. That evening, Merv finally acted on his suspicion that Deborah was going to see another man and went out to track her down. Once outside, he could neither find Deborah nor remember how to get back into the apartment, so he wandered about. Fortunately, a neighbor recognized Merv, found the building superintendent to let Merv in, and contacted Deborah. The next day, this person contacted the program staff.

The emergency plan that we had hoped wouldn't be necessary went into high gear. Fortunately, the staff social worker knew of an empty bed in the local Alzheimer's unit. The family was glad for staff support in sharing this news with Merv.

Because the day program's nurse had the closest relationship with Merv, she took on this challenge. The nurse asked Merv for a private chat. She started by saying that she was concerned about Deborah's health. Merv agreed and expressed his genuine concern. He wondered what he could do to help Deborah. The nurse suggested that it would be best if Merv stayed where someone else could take care of things so that Deborah wouldn't worry about him and she could get rest. Merv readily agreed that this was the best idea. After ensuring that he could take his dog with him, Merv went sadly but without protest to his room in the Alzheimer's unit.

Unfortunately, Deborah is dwindling. The loving sparkle in her blue eyes has been replaced by a wistful sadness. Merv is receiving excellent care, but he too is failing physically and cognitively. Yet, despite all of the losses and the pain, Deborah and Merv can still be seen sitting together, holding hands. Deborah gazes with sad adoration at Merv, and he welcomes her visits with glowing smiles and hugs. These moments of caring connection are cherished. After all of the troubled years, Deborah and Merv have finally found moments that they can celebrate together.

GUIDING THE PATH OF CAREGIVING

Although Leitha and Bob captured more·moments of caring connection, both couples found times of shared pleasure and comfort, even amid the stresses and strains of living with dementia.

These two stories represent different aspects of caregiving, partly because of how different the relationships and personalities of those involved were before the onset of dementia. Related to but separate from these differences in personality, the caregivers, Leitha and Deborah, responded differently to the challenges of caregiving.

Leitha decided to learn as much as she could about the changes that Bob was experiencing. She learned how to respond to Bob, as well as how to change the way she spoke to him and the expectations that she had for him. Leitha and Bob, who shared a longstanding close relationship, hoped to get as much out of their time together as possible. Deborah had this same hope, one that she had held for more than 50 years of marriage, yet she seemed to be stuck not only on this hope but also on how she related to Merv. She did not seem able to make allowances for his brain changes, even when given direct and basic examples. Apparently, she could not accept or understand that the major brain changes Merv was experiencing prevented him, for example, from managing all of the steps involved in taking a bath. Deborah persisted in believing that Merv would respond appropriately to reasonable explanations and requests, then was surprised and hurt when he became angry and hostile as a result of his confusion and frustration. Deborah was equally puzzled that Merv readily accepted help with tasks such as bathing at the day program.

As you know, caregiving for someone with dementia is full of challenges, difficulties, and constant confrontation with losses. These come with the territory. Unfortunately neither you nor the person with dementia have any choice or control over how the brain damage progresses. However, you can make choices about how you will respond to these changes. You can choose to grow, change, and learn, or you can choose to remain in old ways of relating. You can choose to live in hope that the person will get better, or you can choose to celebrate the person with all of his or her strengths and losses now, capturing the pleasures to be found in the present moment.

I described Leitha's and Deborah's repsonses to the challenges of caregiving as "different." This word choice is important: Different does not mean better. Both caregivers provided the best care possible, and both based this care on tremendous love and affection for their spouses. Deborah had more difficulty than Leitha in adjusting her love and care to the changes that dementia had made in Merv's abilities. Like most caregivers, she found that dementia changed the rules in their relationship. She was challenged by the lack of precise rules to follow.

Is there a point to sharing and writing about caregiving if there are no rules and every caregiving situation is unique? Yes. Even without fixed rules, there are guidelines based on the common threads of caregiving experiences. *Navigating the Alzheimer's Journey: A Compass for Caregiving* attempts to draw together these common threads and offer suggestions to guide your caregiving path.

I like the term *guide* because according to my 1999 Webster's dictionary, it means "to point out the way." Guiding is pointing out or suggesting the way, not dictating the way. Consider the example of a guidebook on wilderness hikes. The guidebook's information is based on the author's experiences at the time the book is written. It points out paths, beautiful sites, good stopping places, and hazards. It may give an estimate of how long or difficult a hike will be. It may also suggest supplies to carry and preparations to make.

Say that I have never hiked before, much less hiked in this new territory. I would be grateful to have the information in the guidebook. It might give an idea of what to expect and which turns to take. Once on the trail, I might find that conditions have changed since the guidebook was written: Trees might have fallen across a once-clear path, so the guidebook's map helps me to make detours. I use my compass to turn in the right direction and rejoin the path. I also discover that the gentle glen, recommended as a stopping place for lunch and a rest, has become a sodden marsh due to recent heavy rains. So I perch myself on a fallen log and enjoy the splendor of a sea of wildflowers. I can say that the guidebook has served me well. I am not lost, and I will continue on the path. I know that I have the provisions to make the rest of the journey, although it may take me longer than the guidebook predicted. In some places, I may have to make my own decisions and solve problems. Along the way, I also may make some joyous discoveries that are mine alone.

This illustration sums up the purpose of *Navigating the Alzheimer's Journey: A Compass for Caregiving*—to share my experiences and those of others to help point the way on your own caregiving journey. You will find suggestions for taking care of yourself, thoughts on the lived experience of dementia, basic information about Alzheimer's disease and other dementias, tips on communication and environmental accommodations, strategies for helping the person to maintain a familiar lifestyle, and ideas for responding to challenges and planning future care. I hope these suggestions will guide your caregiving journey and help you navigate the obstacles along the way. Even more, I hope you will discover many hidden glens, full of beauty and bloom, which provide hope, joy, and renewal as you walk this challenging path of caregiving.

For the person with dementia,
the most important moment is the present moment.
Tomorrow can scarcely be imagined or anticipated
or understood.
Yesterday is, at best, a dim recollection.
People with dementia live in the moment;
life is most fully experienced in the now.
Our supreme challenge as caregivers
is to embrace this attitude of
living in the moment.
It is here that we find the best opportunity to experience
a measure of joy and fulfillment
during this caregiving journey.

1

Care for the Caregiver

I am still here, trapped beneath this . . . . wet thru wretched
  brain,
through which faint wisps of thoughts, ideas and dreams struggle
  to break free,
while it still defies and defeats my frantic will.
If you leave me or love me less, I am forever lost.
You have taught me how noble a woman's heart can be.
If anywhere else, I shall be on the look out for you;
Meanwhile
look forward
feel free
rejoice in life
cherish the children
guard my memory
and God bless you.

—Howard Quarterman

Mrs. Winona Quarterman found this poem in her husband's
wallet after he had passed away. It had been folded and refolded
many times, but it was clearly in her husband's handwriting.
This very personal thanks and testimony means a great deal

to Mrs. Quarterman, and I am deeply grateful that she has allowed me to share it with you in the hopes that it will provide encouragement during the course of caregiving. Unfortunately, the brain damage that accompanies dementia erodes many abilities, often including loss of the ability to express thanks and appreciation—at least in the usual ways. However, know that each and every person with dementia would echo Howard Quarterman's sentiments, if he or she could.

Providing care for someone with dementia is one of the most challenging jobs in the world. I know that you are a special person because you are taking on this job and working at it to the best of your ability. Many caregivers work so hard at taking care of the person with dementia that they forget about taking care of themselves. This book begins with suggestions and reminders about taking care of a very special person—you. If you don't take care of yourself, it is not likely that anyone else will. If you find it difficult to put yourself first, stop and think about how the person you are caring for would manage if you became ill and couldn't carry on. This isn't a scare tactic. *It is a fact that caregivers of persons with dementia are at much greater risk of having physical illnesses and depression as well as high levels of stress* (Bourgeois, Schulz, & Burgio, 1996; Lindsay, 1994b). Even without meeting you, I know that you are a lifeline for the person with dementia; you know and understand him or her better than anyone else does. Take care of yourself for both of your sakes. Caregiver Sally Callahan put it this way:

> The first thing caregivers should be told, again and again, until they understand it as something necessary to survive, is that the need to care for themselves must be primary. . . . The long, risky road of Alzheimer's caregiving often creates multiple victims. Obviously the patient is victim to the disease, but so can the caregiver and his or her family be victims. This needn't happen. There are ways to be a caregiver

for an Alzheimer's patient that allow the caregiver and his family to remain intact. (2000, p. 190)

There are probably many times when you rightly feel that caregiving is a thankless job. The following is but one example.

 With the same loving, nurturing hands that Jennifer used to draw beauty and life from paper and paint, she helped her husband John care for his brother Ben during the last stages of terminal cancer. The nurturing and gentleness came naturally and easily, but the extra housework was taxing: doing dozens of loads of laundry, making special meals, providing bedside personal care, and hosting friends and family who came to bid farewell. Jennifer's mother-in-law, Felicia, who also needed care as she struggled to cope with Alzheimer's disease, was also living with Jennifer and John. Felicia usually spent her days visiting with her dying son and avoiding the many tasks that swirled around in the busy household.

One day as Felicia was going down the stairs, she met Jennifer, who was coming to collect still another mountain of laundry that stood between them on the landing. Felicia's usual gracious smile suddenly snapped to an expression of angry hostility. She seized Jennifer's tiny, arthritic arms in a vise and angrily spit out, "It is just time that you started to pull your weight around here. I can't be doing everything—dozens of loads of laundry, meals to get, and Ben to take care of. You better show that you are really part of this family and pitch in."

Jennifer was not only astonished and hurt but also felt a flash of anger at this torrent of insult. Just as Jennifer was about to reply in anger and self-defense, which would only be natural, she caught a fleeting look at Felicia's sad and confused eyes. Anger turned to empathy as she glimpsed the damaged brain behind those eyes. Jennifer tearfully told Felicia that she was sorry to have failed her duty and that she would try harder.

As they shared a hug both women dissolved into tears. Felicia calmed down almost immediately. She thanked Jennifer for her renewed effort, saying that she was sorry to have been so cross but that it was getting to be too much for her to take.

I imagine that most of you have stood in Jennifer's shoes, in one way or another. You're trying your best, turning yourself inside out and your life upside down to care for someone with dementia, and you end up on the receiving end of angry and false accusations. Perhaps like Jennifer, you've been told that you aren't doing enough (although doing anything more is unimaginable). Maybe you've received one or more of numerous other unjust accusations:

- You are a thief. I had $100 in my purse and now there isn't any money.
- I know why you are always going out. You are meeting some other man.
- I am not eating that. I know what you are up to. You are trying to poison me so that you will get my money.
- You are just the worst daughter in the world. You never come to visit your poor old mother.

These stinging comments cut to the core and not only hurt you but also make you furious. And so they should. These feelings are completely natural and offer no reason for guilt. The challenge is figuring out how to act on these feelings. *Although all feelings are valid, not all actions are.* If a person with a healthy brain hurls such accusations at you, you may well be justified in returning anger with anger, in standing up for what is true. However, when the person has dementia, it is necessary to count to 10 and step into his or her world to understand where these comments are coming from.

In the preceding vignette, a look into Felicia's eyes gave Jennifer a window into Felicia's damaged brain. Jennifer realized that this was not the healthy, reasonable person she once knew who was speaking to her in this way. Felicia and others with dementia have damaged brains and are trying to make sense of the world. At times, the faulty brain leads to faulty reasoning and faulty logic. Seeing the pile of laundry may have led Felicia to worry about how she was possibly going to get it all done, which led her to turn in fury on Jennifer, the nearest likely cause. Undoubtedly, the distress of being unable to care for her dying son played a part in Felicia's feelings of frustration. Jennifer had the grace and the wisdom to realize that this outpouring was coming from a damaged brain, not from genuine ill will and malice. Although the comments were profoundly painful, she chose to act out of understanding and empathy rather than out of the hurt and anger she rightly felt.

Reacting with empathy is very hard, but what a difference it makes. Suppose that Jennifer followed her natural instinct to make a heated retort about how hard she was working, in order to set the record straight. It is unlikely that Felicia would understand or believe that this was so, leading both she and Jennifer to become still more heated and angry. This would have been a lose-lose situation because the two women would then become even more upset and frustrated.

Instead, Jennifer's response allowed Felicia to feel that she had made her point, which helped Felicia to calm down. The women restored their relationship and expressed feelings with a hug and some tears. To deal with her own feelings, later that night, Jennifer shared her hurt and insight with her husband John.

The damage to the brain is mostly observed as changes in behavior. When a person has a stroke, arthritis, or Parkinson's disease, the paralyzed hand, the gnarled joints, or the tremor makes it obvious that there is a physical problem. The damage caused by dementia is inside the brain, but what people actually see are changes in behavior. Because the damaged brain cannot be seen, it can appear as if the person is trying to be deliberately aggravating. Although this is certainly not the case, it can nonetheless be frustrating. This is made worse by daily and even hourly fluctuations and by the variability in losses from one skill to another. For instance, the person may charmingly answer the door to a perfect stranger and then urinate in the trash can or put the garbage in the refrigerator. Although it is frustrating, remember that the person is trying her or his best to cope with a very damaged brain. **Approximately 80% of the brain damage has already happened by the time that the first symptoms— changes in behavior—appear** (Cummings, 1993).

> *"God grant me the serenity to accept the things I*
> *cannot change, the courage to change the things I can,*
> *and the wisdom to know the difference"* (Reinhold Niebuhr)

We are all only human; we cannot always find the strength and the wisdom to be guided by these words. The sheer exhaustion of caregiving makes it even harder to think before acting on feelings, but this behavior is something to strive for. There is more information on this topic later in the chapter.

CAREGIVING IS CHALLENGING

This is so important to appreciate that it cannot be said often enough: It is not just that you may find caregiving difficult and challenging; it is difficult and challenging, period. Not only that, research has found that providing care for someone with Alzheimer's disease or another dementia is more difficult than providing care for someone with physical problems alone, such as arthritis (Lindsay, 1994b). Providing care for someone with a damaged brain and limited memory and thinking powers is difficult work. Caregiver Sally Callahan commented, "Caregiving for an Alzheimer's patient is a long, exhausting, extremely challenging process. Primary caregiving can overwhelm even the strongest and most dedicated people" (2000, p. 190). This is not the same as saying that the person you are caring for makes caregiving difficult. **Dementia's effect on the brain, not the person, causes the challenges.**

Potential caregivers should not be afraid to voice that full-time caregiving is not for them. Caring for someone with dementia is difficult and demanding. Recognizing that you are not prepared to give this level of care is not a personal failing; it is a realistic understanding of your particular strengths and weaknesses. There are many different ways to provide care. If you are unable to be a full-time caregiver, you can still make the most essential contribution of providing nurturing support as a visitor or helper.

Becoming a caregiver is often gradual and unplanned. The development of dementia is gradual, so spouses, family members, or others may slowly do more for the person without realizing that they are changing roles from companion, spouse, or adult child to caregiver. These changes are especially likely to go unnoticed in the case of a spouse who has always done the household tasks. At some point, however, the line from companion to caregiver is crossed, often when personal care activities become difficult. When this realization comes, caregivers are urged to seek outside advice (see Chapter 10) and begin the assessment and diagnostic process (see Chapter 3). They do not need to travel this road alone. If you have unintentionally become a caregiver, you may feel trapped. Although it can be complicated to get others involved, I urge you to get advice and to carefully consider whether you can or should take on this role.

If you are a caregiver, I have no doubt that you are doing the best you can and giving everything you have to this challenging work. Remember that all of your efforts truly make a difference. Although there is presently no cure for Alzheimer's disease, there is treatment: **The caregiver's care is the best treatment now available for the person with dementia.** The ways in which caregivers talk to, care for, and care about—or treat—persons with dementia has an enormous impact on their quality of life and well-being.

Caregivers can find it very distressing that despite their best efforts, the person does not "get better." We need to rethink what is meant by *get better*. Because dementia is a brain condition for which there is presently no cure, the person cannot get better. However, caregivers can and do help the person to be better—to have better moments, better days, better feelings, and a better quality of life. For example, Jennifer's understanding and nonconfrontational response helped Felicia to calm down; it provided a treatment for Felicia's distress and agitation.

There is much to learn about the art of caregiving, and this does not come by "one-stop shopping." As dementia progresses, caregivers will find their roles and duties changing. **Caregiving is a journey, not a destination; caregiving is a process, not a state of being.** One of the biggest changes is the move from care at home, which involves primarily hands-on caregiving, to full- or part-time care in congregate settings, which involves becoming more of an advocate, facilitator, and communicator.

You know you are not alone in finding caregiving a challenge. The following discussions share some common challenges that other caregivers of persons with dementia have reported (Bourgeois et al., 1996; Lindsay, 1994b). For example, there is no recipe or straightforward method for providing care. "If you have seen one person with dementia you have seen one person with dementia" is commonly mentioned in dementia care settings. Although the brain damage caused by dementia can be described in general terms that provide some guidance, dementia is manifested quite differently from person to person. There is also great variability in the same person between different activities and from day to day and hour to hour, as is illustrated in the following story.

One weekend, when my mother-in-law, Alice, lived in her own, nearby apartment, there was a plumbing crisis. The kitchen drain was plugged and water was running all over the kitchen. It was obvious that grease and other unsuitable materials had been poured down the drain. Because of her nursing background, Alice almost always followed written orders. Thus, her son and I posted a big notice above the sink: DO NOT PUT GREASE DOWN THE SINK. This worked marvelously well, and no grease was put down the drain. Unfortunately, neither was anything else, as Alice would not allow anyone to put anything, including the dishwater, down the sink! The system, which had worked so well for turning on the television and other tasks, wasn't such a raging success this time.

A caregiver's creativity is always on call. A caregiver is the on-the-spot problem solver. I hope that the general guidelines and suggestions presented throughout this book help you meet this challenge.

Another challenging aspect of caregiving is finding someone to relieve you. Caregivers need and want breaks. Paid caregivers, such as home-care helpers, may not have the training or special skills needed to meet the unique challenges of caring for someone with dementia. Although this situation is improving and there are indeed many skilled paid caregivers, there is no guarantee. Some family caregivers report that when they cannot find a paid caregiver who can provide the special care that their loved one needs, it can seem easier not to take the break. Chapter 10 provides suggestions for dealing with this challenge.

Doctors and Other Professionals May Have Limited Understanding of Dementia and Providing Care for Those Who Have It

Joanne's mom, Edna, had always been reclusive and protected her privacy at her old farmhouse on an isolated back road. She could be cranky with visitors, family or otherwise, and preferred her solitary life with her two companions: her overly energetic terrier, Scruffy, and her cigarettes. Joanne had long accepted her mother's choice and had decided to keep in touch by telephone. However, when she took her mother home from a short hospital stay, Joanne was concerned at what she found. The house was not in order, as it usually was. In fact, it was in total disarray. There were cigarette butts everywhere, with burn marks in the carpet and on her mother's clothes. Scruffy obviously had total run of the house, including for bathroom functions. There was very little edible food; most of it was spoiled. Although Edna didn't approve, Joanne cleaned up the best that she could and bought some groceries.

Joanne also telephoned her mother's doctor to express her concern about Edna's deterioration. The doctor maintained that nothing was wrong, that this behavior was just an effect of old age in a person who had always been eccentric. After all, Edna had been able to tell him the date and other information while she was in the hospital.

Joanne was too concerned about her mother's safety to let this go. She contacted a day program and persuaded her mother to go to the program's office for an assessment. Edna reluctantly agreed to make a few visits "just to try it out" and to keep Joanne quiet. At the program, Edna kept to herself and was coolly pleasant. After Edna had been attending for several weeks, staff members were surprised when she remarked that she had really missed them the week before, when she was unable to attend due to a snowstorm. Edna gradually became more open with staff and they were able to put some home supports in place. The staff members were also able to arrange for an assessment by a geriatrician, who diagnosed Edna with probable Alzheimer's disease.

Joanne's concerns were well founded. To have her concerns addressed, she had to endure the anger of her mother (and even other family members) as well as the dismissal of her concerns by Edna's doctor. It had been a difficult process.

Like Joanne, some caregivers find that dementia is not well understood by many health care professionals. This often means that the caregiver has to be the one to provide information and to advocate, not only for him- or herself but also for the person with dementia. Many caregivers find this taxing, especially because this requires assertiveness skills that differ from caregiving skills such as understanding and empathy. Increased public awareness and education for staff are helping to get the message out, but, unfortunately, health care professionals still commonly tell caregivers that nothing can help their situation. This is not true, as you probably already know or will learn from this book and other resources. However, such statements don't help the caregiver's confidence or morale.

Caregivers May Have Had a Strained Relationship with the Person Who Has Dementia

Caregiving becomes especially challenging when the previous relationship was difficult. Nora Keating (1997) described this situation very well by saying that it is difficult to *care for* a person when you don't *care about* the person. Unfortunately,

there are no right answers to this dilemma. If you find yourself in this situation, please seek a skilled counselor to help
you work through your feelings and find a solution. Check
the yellow pages for the local Alzheimer's Association (in the
United States) or Alzheimer Society (in Canada), which
should be able to recommend a counselor or another agency
to help you.

In some cases, the challenge of living with dementia
enables both parties to come to terms with their past or at
least to put past grievances behind them. This may occur
through counseling and/or result from the emotional softening that sometimes comes with dementia. In other cases, the
caregiver is able to work through past feelings independently
or at least put them aside. In still other cases, the relationship
history is so painful that the best response is to involve others
in the person's care. Remember that neither you nor the person with dementia benefits from adding to past difficulties the
challenging situation of providing care for someone with
dementia. Martha Holstein advised,

> We can ignore neither the autonomy of the person with
> AD [Alzheimer's disease] nor caregiver stress. Autonomy
> cannot trump everyone else's needs. Autonomy and stress
> must be viewed through a single lens. While a loving
> caregiver feels stress from witnessing the decline of a
> loved parent, the social emphasis placed on autonomy
> exacerbates that stress. One can almost never do enough.
> (2001, p. 60)

The last line of Martha's advice is critical for caregivers to
hear: "One can almost never do enough." In the end, no one
will benefit from a caregiving situation in which the caregiver is reluctant and resentful.

Alzheimer's Disease and Other
Dementias Are Surrounded by Stigma

A stigma continues to be attached to Alzheimer's disease and other dementias. Again, although education is helping improve this situation, there unfortunately continues to be an uninformed attitude toward dementia and persons who have it. Instead of understanding that it is a brain condition, some people incorrectly consider dementia something that the person or the family can help or should be ashamed of. Tragically, this can lead others to blame persons with dementia for having the symptoms of their condition and believing that if they just tried hard enough, they could do better. This attitude can also make it difficult for caregivers to share concerns and feelings or to get the necessary community support. Caregivers report that they have less contact with some friends and family members after the person develops dementia, as some people don't know how to deal with the situation and stay away. Unfortunately, it is often when people really need extra support that they find out who their true friends are. Please see Chapter 10 for more information on involving others in care.

Community understanding of the caregiver's experience can be limited. Usually the person with dementia has well-preserved social skills, looks "normal," and can present him- or herself very well in brief public appearances. These are wonderful strengths that support the person's self-esteem. However, it can lead others, sometimes even medical professionals, to believe that there is no problem and that the caregiver must be making up all of these problems and changes. This point is shown in the following vignette.

 Audrey was one of eight children in a close-knit family. Although the siblings came together for many family social occasions as their parents aged, it was always Audrey who was there to help them out with daily needs.

After Audrey's mother died, her father started to call even more often, and Audrey noticed that his memory was failing. Even though Audrey lived more than an hour's drive away, she always made the many trips to town to help with real problems (e.g., bills to pay) or imagined ones (e.g., the belief that all of the groceries were gone). Although Audrey genuinely wanted to do her best, the increasing number of telephone calls and trips were beginning to take their toll on her, and she mentioned her concerns to her brothers and sisters. They said that Audrey must be making things up because they had not had any such calls and their father was as sharp as ever when they talked to him. It was only when Audrey began to redirect some of these calls to her brothers and sisters that they began to realize the kinds of difficulties that their father was having.

Caregivers can become isolated because family and friends find coping with dementia caregiving too difficult, as noted in the following quote by caregiver Sally Callahan (2000).

> Friends often don't know what to do, how to help, or what to say to their newly donned Alzheimer caregiver. They can't really understand the wearing nature of caregiving. They may feel that their friend has lost perspective and the ability to enjoy life. . . . So people often just drift away. They call less, until they don't call at all. They pull away from the deep, deep pain that has become so much a fact of life for their former friend. (p. 215)

Sally Callahan described the all-too-common experience of caregivers of persons with dementia as a world with fewer and fewer social contacts—just when social contacts are really needed. Again, this underscores the necessity for caregivers to care for themselves as well as the value of getting support so that relationships and friendships can maintain a more natural balance.

The caregiver may need support because the grieving process is ongoing. A caregiver's relationship with the person with dementia is going to change; there are going to be losses as the condition progresses. Because dementia progresses over a long period of time, these losses will occur over a long period of time. Many caregivers find that with each realization of loss, the grieving process starts again. Please see this chapter's section "Take Time to Grieve" for more information on this topic.

A sense of feeling unappreciated can add to the grief, but remember that the person with dementia often loses the ability to spontaneously show appreciation. In the following passage, Bob shows that he really appreciates the help of his wife, Erika, but he also finds it difficult to accept that he needs this help. Bob explains why he, and certainly others with dementia, may in fact give the person they need the most the hardest time and perhaps the least thanks.

> Sometimes I give Erika a hard time just to be nasty. I guess it's because I'd like to be doing things myself instead of having someone telling me to do this or that. I'm a little boy now. I have a mommy to take care of me. It's not a very good feeling.… My tightest friendship is with Erika. I think we're growing more tightly together. I give her a hard time, but I'm just teasing. She ignores it. I guess I'm letting off steam and frustration. She's awfully good to put up with me. I wouldn't ever do anything that would be detrimental to Erika. I'm lucky to have her. There aren't too many Erikas. (Bob, cited in Snyder, 1999, pp. 85–86)

As a caregiver of someone with dementia, you are working so hard; you especially need a few pats on the back to let you know that what you are doing matters. Unfortunately, the person with dementia may lose the ability to express this appreciation. What you do does make a huge difference and the person you are caring for knows this, but he or she just can't express it. See this chapter's section "Look for Thanks in Ways Other than Words" for some other ways that persons with dementia may express appreciation.

The caregiver may also need support because the person may blame him or her for memory loss and other problems. As discussed earlier in the chapter, such accusations are very difficult and upsetting. Try to remember that these comments are the result of a damaged brain, that this is not the person who you know and love speaking. It is a person with dementia trying to make sense out of a world that seems to have gone seriously off track, where she or he is losing the ability to cope with even ordinary, daily demands. It must be very frightening and a lot easier to blame someone else than to admit that one simply cannot remember something. Please see Chapter 9 for more information on this challenge.

THE ESSENTIAL JOB OF CARING FOR YOURSELF

Perhaps feeling that no one else can care for your loved one in exactly the same way, or as well as you can, is justified. Caregiving becomes a way of life, a habit to which you must adjust in order to survive. While it may be difficult to break out of it, and even more difficult to find acceptable coverage, you *must* for if you don't care for yourself, where will your loved one be? Where will you be? (Callahan, 2000, p. 196)

Because you are a caregiver, you are probably used to putting others' needs ahead of your own. This is especially true when caring for someone with dementia; the effects of brain damage make it difficult for the person to plan for and take care of his or her own needs. It is natural to respond in a nurturing and caring way. In addition, although you may have previously had a mutually supportive relationship (as a spouse, partner, or adult child), dementia makes it difficult for the person to provide the kind of support you are used to or need. This is a tragic loss. Yet, if the relationship before the onset of dementia was not supportive, caregiving may be even more challenging. Please see the section "Caregiving Is Challenging" for suggestions regarding this especially difficult situation.

Caregivers might expect other family members or friends to show extra support or consideration. This is understandable, but if you expect this response, you may be setting yourself up for disappointment. Although some people are expert at offering help and caring support without being asked, most people unfortunately are not.

This leaves one person to look out for you,
the caregiver—and that is you!

I know that this is very difficult to do; however, it is essential. Just as a car cannot run forever without a refueling stop, you cannot go on forever giving and caring without refueling and reenergizing. The way in which you take care of yourself, refuel, and reenergize is individual—it may be just a few minutes working in the garden, a trip to the hairdresser, or a few hours away from caregiving duties—but the need is common to all caregivers. Unfortunately, many caregivers neglect this until they find themselves running on empty. When her time as an Alzheimer's caregiver was finished, Sally Callahan noted the importance of caring for the caregiver:

> The lesson of caring for myself has positioned me for a better, more fulfilling and healthy life. There is part of me that is grateful I was forced to learn it. I survived Alzheimer caregiving, and I am learning to live my life more fully and healthily day by day. (2000, p. 226)

If you find it too difficult to do something just for yourself, stop and imagine how the person that you are caring for will manage if you become too sick or exhausted to carry on. It is a fact that caregivers of persons with dementia have much higher levels of physical health problems—in a Canadian study on health and aging, caregivers had six times the level of other caregivers (Lindsay, 1994b). In addition, 75% of caregivers of persons with dementia are depressed at one time or another. The Canadian study on health and aging reported twice the level of clinical depression for caregivers of persons with dementia as compared with other caregivers. Caregiving is a long journey, and the result of not taking care of yourself may be that you will not be able to finish the journey.

Please take care of the very special person that is you.

The sections that follow offer some suggestions on ways to find support and nurturing for yourself. I wish I could wave a magic wand and tell you how to find the time to do these things; unfortunately, I can't. I can only say that if you make nurturing yourself the priority that it is, you will take time for it. Take a careful look at your day, and make time just for you. Congratulate yourself on making this move toward taking care of yourself; just deciding that you need time for you is a tremendously positive step.

There is always a choice, even if the only choice is how you feel or think about something. Try rethinking which tasks are really essential, and ask yourself some hard questions:

- *Do you really need to do this particular household task just now?* Can it wait until tomorrow or even later? Will anything disastrous result if the vacuuming or dusting is not done now?

- *Is there an easier or faster way to do this?* For example, altering meal preparation may be one way to save time. Although you may pride yourself on your cooking, could you make meals simpler by serving easier-to-prepare foods on some days?

- *Is this something that someone else can do?* The care that you provide is unique, personal, and essential. It is also physically and emotionally exhausting. Unless you find ways to share this care with others, your own health may not allow you to continue to provide this vital care. Think of ways to share care from two perspectives: 1) sharing practical tasks and 2) helping others to develop a personal relationship with the person you are caring for.

Although only certain people can offer the nurturing, personal support that the person with dementia needs, many others can scrub a tub, do laundry, vacuum, or prepare a meal. It may not be possible for you to pay someone to help with housekeeping. What about tapping into the neighbors, friends, or relatives who have said, "If there is anything I can do, just let me know"? This is the time to let them know; they can't know what you need unless you say so. A meal sent over or laundry or vacuuming done can be a big help. Try not to let pride and overindependence stand in your way. For suggestions on involving others, paid and unpaid, please see Chapter 10.

It is truly a sign of strength to understand when you need help and ask for it. Finding others to share in the direct caregiving relationship can be challenging, but it is possible. The first challenge may be for you to let go of your role as sole caregiver. Again, there is probably not another single person who can offer the caring relationship that you do, but there are definitely people who can provide *other* valu-

able caregiving relationships. Some may come to this naturally; others may need guidance from you. Using the All About
Me form (see Appendix A at the end of the book) can help
others get to know the person's routines and needs. The
excellent booklet *You Are One of Us* (Gwyther, 1995) can help
others to learn how to relate to and visit with persons who
have dementia. Here are some suggestions for ways to
encourage others to share in the caregiving relationship,
thereby enriching the person's day and giving you a break:

- With guidance from you, another family member or a
  friend can continue with shared pastimes or develop new
  ones, such as reading the newspaper together, going for
  a walk, making cookies, looking at family photos, listening to music, going for drives, watching videotapes of
  family events or favorite television shows, gardening, or
  any number of other activities that are suggested in
  Chapters 6, 7, and 8.

- Activities with grandchildren or other children, such as
  reading together, can be the basis for a great relationship.

- Friends or associates from hobby, religious, or other
  groups can find ways to be special pals so that the person
  with dementia can still enjoy these activities. The person
  may have lost the initiative and ability to attend these
  events by him- or herself, but if others take the lead, he
  or she often can continue participating for some time.
  For example, a church friend took Alice to Bible study
  every week. Although Alice was unable to go on her own,
  with support from the friend she was able to share in
  readings, offer some surprisingly insightful comments on
  the discussion, and enjoy the fellowship.

- In addition to these informal sources of support, many
  excellent day programs and support groups are available

for persons with dementia. Participating in these can bring positive new dimensions to the person's daily life as well as give you a break. Please see Chapter 10 for more details.

Some other important questions to ask yourself follow:

- *Is this something that you can do with the person you are caring for?* As discussed in Chapters 6, 7, and 8, the person with dementia needs to participate in daily life activities, to be part of the daily routine. You can find suggestions in these chapters for ways to do this.
- *What did you do today that was fun?* All work and no play makes Jill a dull girl and Jack a dull boy. You have the need and the right to have more than just duty in your days. Even 5 minutes of doing something that is fun and brings you pleasure can lift the spirits. Some suggestions follow in the ensuing section.

Take a Moment for You

I hope that this section gives you some ideas of things that you can do every day to take a break from the demands of caregiving. Although it is necessary to get a complete break when you can, this isn't always possible. If you make it a priority—and I am urging you to—you can have mini breaks right at home. If the person you are caring for is resting or busy for a few moments, it is more important to do something for yourself than to sweep the floor, do the laundry, or perform any one of a thousand other tasks. It is time to recharge those batteries.

It helps if you have a special place just for you that is associated with relaxation and rest. In this way, just being there for a moment can provide restoration. Most caregivers do not have the luxury of a separate room reserved for them. If you don't have such a space, think of another place where you can create a sense of psychological privacy, a place that can be yours alone. It is not so much the physical separation that is important but the emotional creation of a space for retreat. This might be a chair in the living room, a rocker in the kitchen or bedroom, or a bench in the garden. It might even be the bathroom, as most people respect the right and the need for privacy in the bathroom. Whatever the location, make it special. Gather simple things that bring you pleasure—a favorite book; a collection of special cards, letters, or mementos; favorite photos; a cozy blanket; a comfortable pillow; potpourri or a scented candle; or a plant. If you can't keep these items in that space, you may want to put them in a portable feel-good basket or box.

Here are some suggested relaxing activities for when you are in your special place:

- Close your eyes and imagine yourself into a treasured past experience. Try to immerse yourself in all of the good feelings and enjoy them again—not to wish you are there now but just for the pure pleasure that the memory brings.

- Celebrate you. Remember a time when you did something special and celebrate again all of the praise that went with it.

- Reread a favorite letter or greeting card.

- Listen to a favorite song. You may not have time to listen to a whole CD, record, or cassette, but a moment with a special song can do wonders. You might keep a personal tape player with headphones in your space just for this purpose.

- Practice relaxation techniques. Relaxation techniques use gentle physical exercises and images to train the mind to relax the body. They can be extremely effective. There are many guided relaxation exercises now available on CD, cassette, or videotape. Although these require more than a moment, with practice something interesting can happen: Your body can become trained to go into relaxation mode with just the start of the recording's sound. Some find that after practice, even sitting comfortably and thinking about the tape or the music on the tape can lead to relaxation.

Although it is best to learn these techniques from an experienced guide or from good-quality recordings, these options may not be available to you. A simple version of engaging in progressive relaxation follows. Make yourself comfortable in a chair, or lie down if you prefer. Loosen any tight clothing and remove shoes and glasses. Put on quiet instrumental music (words are distracting). Close your eyes and focus only on slow, deep breathing. Try to clear your mind of all other thoughts and concentrate only on your breathing. Think that as you breathe in that you are breathing in relaxation and that as you breathe out you are breathing out tension. Begin at your toes and feet and as you breathe in tighten up all of those muscles, then relax as you breathe out. Work your way up your body through all the muscle groups, contracting and relaxing each one three times. At the same time, continue to focus on slow, deep, regular breathing. Finish with contracting all of the muscles in your body and then relaxing your whole body three times. Continue with slow, deep breathing and imagine yourself in a pleasant, quiet location. Focus on that location's pleasant sensory details and, if possible, let yourself drift off to sleep. (Activities such as yoga or tai chi provide another option. They combine physical activity with a meditative focusing of the mind. Although these activities are not for everyone, some people find them very helpful for reducing stress and increasing peace of mind. Many community centers offer short courses in these techniques.)

- Imagine treats that you would like (e.g., a new hat, dinner out, a walk on the beach); write them down and put them in a "Spoil Me" box. This suggestion comes from Sally Callahan (2000), who found that when she did decide to do something for herself, she was often too exhausted to think what she could do. This problem is overcome if suggestions are already in a Spoil Me box.

- Perfect the art of quick power snoozes. I am blessed with this gift from my father, who could sleep on a dime. Many times, a 2-minute snooze is all I need to recharge.

- Reread a favorite poem or passage from a book.

- Have a hot beverage but avoid caffeine, which is stimulating, not relaxing.

- Call a friend.

- Enjoy a plant or flower.

- Read the comics or a page from a humor or joke book. Post favorite cartoons on the refrigerator or another place where they can easily be read for a quick pick-me-up.

- Recall a favorite funny story or joke.

- Look at a photo album.

- Light a candle and watch its warm flame.

- Focus on a lovely picture or on a flower and do long, slow, deep breathing.

- Do a couple of minutes of quick stretching.

- Put on a special outfit that makes you feel great, even if you are not going anywhere.

- Plan something for dinner that you really enjoy.
- Soak your feet in warm water with 2 tablespoons of Epsom salts per gallon of water. If you have a little more time, a warm bath with Epsom salts is very relaxing.
- Rub on a favorite body lotion or hand cream.
- Gently massage your hands and feet.
- Briefly heat a moist hand towel in the microwave and lay it across your forehead and eyes while sitting back in a chair. The moist heat is very relaxing. (The length of time for heating depends on the microwave, but do not exceed 1 minute on the High setting. Be sure to test the temperature with your fingertips before putting the heated towel on your face.)
- Have a favorite healthy snack. A complex carbohydrate with some low-fat protein is a great pick-me-up. For example, have an apple with low-fat cheese or a whole wheat bagel with light cream cheese, a little reduced-fat peanut butter, or sliced turkey. Snacks that are high in fat and sugar should be avoided. Sugary snacks give a quick burst of energy that will bottom out a few hours later as your body adjusts to the extra sugar rush.
- Take a few minutes with a craft, woodworking, or sewing project or other hobby that you find relaxing. Try to have a simple, portable project that you can just pick up for a minute or two as opposed to a large, complex project.
- Engage in a few minutes of brisk physical activity (e.g., shooting a few baskets, hitting practice golf balls, skipping rope), which may release tension and encourage relaxation. Or, take a quick walk. Strive to get fresh air and mild exercise every day. Even a stroll around the house can be helpful if nothing else is possible.
- Pet the cat or dog.

Follow Practices for Healthy Living

Most people are aware of practices for healthy living; the following list is provided for review purposes.

- Eat a balanced, low-fat diet with plenty of fruits and vegetables, lean proteins, and whole grains.
- Get regular exercise, such as walking, at least four times per week.
- Avoid excess caffeine, alcohol, fat, and sugar.
- Get 7–8 hours of sleep per night.
- Drink 7–8 glasses of water per day.
- Balance each day with a combination of work, rest, and play.

The challenge, of course, is following these guidelines when the demands and stresses of caregiving are overwhelming and a quick feel-good experience is needed. Although following the preceding guidelines definitely leads to more energy and better health over the long term, there is great temptation to go for the easy, if temporary, route. Those extra cups of coffee or that chocolate bar can supercharge you through the next few minutes. The trouble is, when these instant energy grabs are not part of a generally healthy lifestyle, you will hit rock bottom even faster. The power surge will only last for a few minutes before you will feel the need for another instant hit.

I know how difficult it is, especially in the midst of caregiving, to maintain these healthy living practices. I went the quick-fix route for years; 40 extra pounds later, I still didn't have the energy I needed. So, I hope that these suggestions sound like "coulds" from someone who has walked this path before rather than annoying "shoulds." Now is the time that you especially need enduring energy, not a quick fix. Try to follow the old adage of short-term pain for long-term gain. For example, cut back on coffee and begin each day with a 5-minute walk. It won't be long before you start to feel the payoffs of more energy and less stress, and these changes in lifestyle will become automatic. Notice that I didn't recommend cutting out the coffee. After cutting back and getting energy from more long-term sources, a cup of coffee and a cookie make a wonderful treat.

Good luck.
This is part of taking care of you, and you are worth it.

CARING FOR YOURSELF WITHIN THE CAREGIVING RELATIONSHIP

In addition to caring for yourself as an individual, it is important to care for yourself within the caregiving relationship. This is essential because you are a partner in a changing relationship.

Share a Special Moment Together

If I Had My Life to Live Over

I'd dare to make more mistakes next time. I'd relax, I would limber up. I would be sillier than I have been this trip. I would take fewer things seriously. I would take more chances. I would climb more mountains and swim more rivers. I would eat more ice cream and less beans. I would perhaps have more actual troubles, but I'd have fewer imaginary ones.

You see, I'm one of those people who live sensibly and sanely hour after hour, day after day. Oh, I've had my moments, and if I had it to do over again, I'd have more of them. In fact, I'd try to have nothing else. Just moments, one after another, instead of living so many years ahead of each day. I've been one of those persons who never goes anywhere without a thermometer, a hot water bottle, a raincoat and a parachute. If I had to do it again, I would travel lighter than I have.

If I had my life to live over, I would start barefoot earlier in the spring and stay that way later in the fall. I would go to more dances. I would ride more merry-go-rounds. I would pick more daisies.

—Nadine Stair (from *If I Had My Life To Live Over I Would Pick More Daisies,* edited by Sandra Haldeman Martz, 1992, p. 1)

Although I started this chapter by acknowledging that caregiving is difficult, I do not want this to lead to an imbalance, to a totally negative view. Caregiving can also be uplifting, rewarding, and joyful. Like the author of the preceding poem, persons with dementia have a remarkable capacity to revel in the moment. It seems that they have had a glimpse into the need to cherish and celebrate the moment. Much joy can be had by joining with the person in celebrating the moment. Take time to pick the daisies or smell the roses and to renew and continue your relationship in whatever ways you can. (See Chapter 2 for a detailed discussion.)

This recommendation is not meant to minimize or suggest that you ignore your grief or the challenges that you face. Rather, it is meant to suggest that you try to keep the challenges balanced by finding joy in day-to-day pleasures. I know from personal experience that when you are in the midst of a painful time, some well-meaning suggestions based on folk wisdom, such as "count your blessings," just don't cut it. There is little to be gained from using a meaningless scale to compare your situation to others who may be worse off. Your pain is your pain and it is real and valid, not to be made light of. I think the real wisdom of "count your blessings" and similar expressions, such as "look at the glass as half full instead of half empty," is found in actually experiencing your blessings, not abstractly counting them. Really smell the roses and revel in them; don't just think about how lovely they are. Getting involved in *really* experiencing the roses (or blessings) can be an actual experince (e.g., touching and smelling real roses, calling to talk to a friend who is a blessing) or a relived experience (e.g., closing your eyes and recalling as vividly as possible the glories of an actual rose or a happy time with your friend). Because it is not always possible to have the firsthand experience, caregivers are invited to relive previous ones, from a rich feeling point of view rather than a more abstract thinking point of view. Experiencing small joys can transport you away from pain to pleasure, even for a few minutes. One caregiver's account of finding joy follows. I thank Dr. Nancy Jeanne Haak, Associate Professor of Speech-Language Pathology at Auburn University in Alabama and a family and professional caregiver, for sharing these thoughts.

> As I sit here trying to sound "eloquent" just an hour or two before December, I reflect upon a number of passages that have brought me solace. One such passage, from the book *Meditations for Women Who Do Too Much* by Anne Wilson Schaef, seems most appropriate tonight. Written by Judith M. Knowlton, it is as follows: *"I discovered I always have choices and sometimes it's only a choice of attitude."*
>
> As each of us thinks of how we would define ourselves, many different labels come to mind. Most of these descriptors reflect the choices we have made in life . . . husband, mother, teacher, chauffeur, cook, housekeeper, nurse, caregiver. When an obstacle such as Alzheimer's disease is set in our pathway (missing us directly but affecting us none-the-less through someone we love), some of us will take up the challenge and choose to assume the role of caregiver. Like explorers from the past, we are determined to set our course despite the cautions from experts and fellow travelers alike. They may forecast a perilous if not impossible journey full of rocks, shoals, fog, and storms. They warn us against risking our health, our fortunes, and perhaps our very future.

As captain or as caregiver, we will inevitably find ourselves tossed about by angry seas, lost in the fog, becalmed,
rudderless, or set adrift. The success of our voyage will
depend on how we meet these challenges, our daily ability
to ride out the storm, to find the wind, to navigate by compass and the stars. My trusty compasses are my diary and
my network of friends and family; they constantly help me
recalibrate my perspective and adjust my attitude. The stars
I steer by are the persons who have been in my care and the
lessons learned from them.

We can choose to lament, be lost and lonely, or we can
choose to seek out the joy in what we do and let it renew
our resolve. Sometimes joy finds us. It may take the form
of a fleeting look of recognition and warm embrace from
our loved one with Alzheimer's. It may take the form of
shared laughter from a silly mistake, shared words from a
familiar prayer, or shared lyrics from an old song sung just
off key. Sometimes joy is present but we are simply too
busy to recognize it. Take the time to see the joy. Maybe it's
in a garden on the way to the doctor's office, in the eyes of
a young child who is unencumbered by recollections of
how things used to be, or in the simple pleasure of enjoying an ice cream sundae when it's not Sunday. Sometimes
joy seems elusive. Seek it out. Look for it in the beauty of
a sunrise after a sleepless night, in the peacefulness of a
sleeping loved one after a fretful evening, or in the closeness of an embrace after a precarious transfer.

Those most likely to survive the voyage are the caregivers who are able to welcome joy aboard whenever it visits. Perhaps the one constant joy is in the opportunity to
begin anew each day in the life of persons with Alzheimer's
disease. We can choose to embrace the person, the days and
the joys within them.

Take a Positive Attitude

Little things—like a single flower blooming in an unexpected place or a loaf of bread that turned out perfectly, as well as things that aren't perfect but wonderful nonetheless—are all things that I have learned to pay attention to and to truly appreciate. Finding beauty helps me handle the pain. (An 88-year-old woman whose son has Alzheimer's, cited in Ballard & Poer, 1999)

This caregiver found comfort and strength by focusing on positives, by taking a positive attitude. What you are doing is difficult, and I am not trying to be a Pollyanna, but I hope that in the midst of the difficulties you can say to yourself, "This is hard, but I can do it." This is sometimes called *positive self-talk*. It can be amazingly powerful. It means replacing negative remarks like "What a dummy" or "I will never get this right" with positive thoughts like "I handled that really well" or "That didn't work, but I'll try something else." Time and time again, caregivers themselves and research about caregivers report that it is not so much the tasks and duties of caregiving that cause caregivers to feel stressed and defeated; rather, it is how they feel about their ability to do these tasks (Bowlby Sifton, 1998). Although the actual duties may not have changed, caregivers who are able to reframe how they think about these duties usually feel less overwhelmed. Caregivers who feel capable and able to manage, who feel positive about their ability to be a caregiver, experience more of the joy of caregiving and less of the burden and stress.

Of course, this is not just a matter of positive thinking. You cannot persuade yourself that you are a capable caregiver if you really don't believe you are. This book and other resources offer many suggestions that I hope will help you to grow in caregiving skills and to learn about dementia. No one is born with caregiving skills or instantly understands how to be a caregiver. It takes work, learning, talking to others, reading, and learning from mistakes made. So, if you don't feel capable now, perhaps you can use these learning opportunities to grow toward. For more on such learning, see this chapter's "Learn as Much as You Can" section as well as Chapter 10.

Unfortunately, learning about caregiving is not one-stop shopping. There is much to learn, and as dementia progresses, caregivers will find their roles and duties changing. As noted previously, caregiving is a journey, not a destination; caregiving is a process, not a state of being. One of the biggest changes is the transition from primarily hands-on caregiving at home to full- or part-time care in congregate settings, where the family caregiver becomes more of an advocate, facilitator, and communicator. Remember, you shouldn't be afraid to say that full-time caregiving is not for you. This is not a personal failing; it is just a realistic understanding of your particular strengths and weaknesses. It is better to come to this realization early and work to make other arrangements.

Look for Thanks in Ways Other than Words

I hope that sharing the following experiences will help you to find similar expressions of thanks in your caregiving relationship. Although these experiences are illustrated by stories involving a particular man, I have been blessed with thanks in different ways from every person with dementia with whom I have spent time.

John Angus, a sensitive and caring man, had earned his living from the land. It was more than a job; it was his life. The challenges of living with dementia meant that he could no longer stay alone on his farm or even work with plants and soil without a lot of help from others. Unfor-

tunately, he was not always in a care situation where his deep need to be connected with the land was understood. This great loss and sorrow, combined with his fading skills in using words, often led to very distressing situations with his caregivers.

Perhaps because I also have deep ties to the land, John Angus and I became special pals. By involving John Angus in a variety of activities that emphasized aspects of normal daily life (e.g., breakfast club, lunch group, sensory stimulation, reminiscence), I was able to support and nurture our relationship. So, even though these activities did not involve plants and growing things, they provided a "normal" environment for our shared connection.

Facial Expressions and Nonverbal Communication

Even though he never once said thanks or called me by name, I have absolutely no doubt that John Angus appreciated every minute of the time we spent together and that he knew me. Whenever I met John Angus— even on occasions when there hadn't been a group and, even more remarkable, after I had been on vacation for 3 weeks—his face came alive with a smile and his entire body echoed this happy greeting. There could hardly be a better way to say thanks.

On one occasion, I was surprised when a nursing colleague told me that John Angus wasn't coming to the group meeting. As I came to the door of his room, she was explaining again that it was coffee time in the kitchen, when Carol brought in old-fashioned things to look at. John Angus looked totally baffled and a little worried. Then he happened to look up and see me in the doorway. His face relaxed to a smile. He stood up from his chair saying, "Oh, so that's it. It is you; you're the one," and he came along happily to have coffee and reminisce with others around the kitchen table.

Persons with dementia may lose the ability to say thanks, to acknowledge our efforts with words. If we are open to them, however, they speak volumes of praise from the eloquent voices of the heart.

Participation and Responses

Because I knew that growing things were so important to John Angus, I arranged a special one-to-one time to do some planting. The first time that I guided John Angus's hands to the soil, his entire physical presence changed and lightened. Tears rolled down his cheeks and he said, "Oh my, this is just heaven, and I had no idea that heaven was so handy to home." On another occasion, after our dining group's meal was finished John Angus said, "Now that was a wonderful dinner. I want you to just take it easy and I will do the dishes. That's what I always did for mother." Although these two responses were dramatic and spoken, there are dozens of ways that persons with dementia say thanks, by responding to a touch with a touch, a smile with a smile, an offer of involvement by participating.

Seeking the Caregiver's Company

When caregiving for someone with dementia, it can often be difficult to get a moment by yourself. The person may follow you and always need to know where you are. This is sometimes called *shadowing*, and it can certainly be challenging. Chapter 9 provides suggestions for coping with this behavior. For now, however, I suggest rethinking the meaning of this behavior: When the person can never let the caregiver out of his or her sight, the person seems to be saying, in a very profound way, "I appreciate you. I realize that you are my lifeline. I need to know where you are." By building reassuring relationships with others (e.g., family members, paid caregivers, day program staff), caregivers may better appreciate the person's compliment and unleash these "golden handcuffs" (i.e., release the person from being so specially linked to one caregiver that the caregiver feels that his or her freedom is restricted).

Trying to Be Helpful

The dishes put away in the cupboard before they are washed, the laundry soaking in the toilet, and the garbage stored in the refrigerator are a few examples of the many challenges that caregivers can experience. Although these episodes certainly are frustrating and should not be encouraged, you might try to turn them around and think about the reasons behind them. Could it be that the person was trying to be helpful and could not quite figure out how to do it? It is my experience that setting up a way for the person to be helpful, to share in the work, decreases failed attempts to be helpful and allows both the caregiver and the person to feel appreciated.

Giving What They Can

One spring morning I had a happy time sharing some springtime sensory delights with John Angus and six or seven other persons with advanced dementia. I remained in the kitchen afterwards, working quickly to prepare for the dining group. I really needed some focused time to prepare so I could give my full attention to the next group. When I heard a knock at the door and looked up to see John Angus through the window, I rather ungraciously thought, "Now what? I just don't have time for this now." When I opened the door, my attitude changed entirely. How humbling and absolutely overwhelming to open the door and be greeted not only by John Angus's beaming face but also by his outstretched arm giving me the tattered but very precious bouquet of mayflowers that his daughter had brought a few days earlier.

Persons with dementia give us what they can. It may not be what we like most, wish for, or expect. However, these gifts are all the more valuable because the person has reached out through the tangle of a damaged brain, and often a battered sense of self, to give. Such gifts flow from a trusting relationship; persons with dementia need to trust that their gift will be honored before feeling free to offer it. For example, Alice couldn't prepare a meal or a snack for those who visited her at the nursing home, but she could—and regularly did—save her afternoon Dixie cup of ice cream. Her purse was a convenient storage place! I invite you to cherish these true gifts of appreciation from the person and to accept them in kind.

Cultivate a Sense of Humor

Take Your Job Seriously; Take Yourself Lightly

The heading of this subsection presents terrific advice from the humorist W. Metcalfe (1996). Caregiving is indeed a serious and demanding job, but taking a lighthearted and playful approach to care frees people from concern about doing things just right. There are so many funny things that happen during this journey of caregiving.

If you can laugh at yourself and with the person you are caring for, it can bring an amazing sense of freedom. Here is an example of when this worked for me.

It had been a wild and woolly morning, but I was finally ready to take Mr. Archibald to his doctor's appointment and out for coffee. Mr. Archibald came out of his room just as I came flying down the hall. When I saw that his shoes were on the wrong feet, it seemed to be the last straw and I inwardly grimaced as I thought of the time it would take to help him change his shoes. However, I put on my best therapeutic face, touched his arm gently and said, "Mr. Archibald, I would like to help you change your shoes; they are on the wrong feet."

Looking puzzled but with hardly a pause, Mr. Archibald replied, "Well, now, there is nary a thing I can do about that. They are the onliest feets I've got, the ones I was born with."

Mr. Archibald's cheerful response entirely dispelled my stress and frustration, and we both enjoyed a great chuckle together as we changed his shoes and went off for a happy afternoon together.

Laughter truly is great medicine. Research shows that laughter increases circulation, improves breathing and digestion, and releases certain feel-good chemicals (endorphins) in the brain (Cousins, 1979; Stone, 1992). What's more, it is free. You don't have to go anywhere to get some, and it is a guaranteed harmless addiction!

It may be hard to find a way to laugh when much of what you experience, as you watch the person you know and love undergo loss after loss, is sadness. This, of course, is exactly why humor and laughter are so important. Here are some suggestions that may help.

Laugh at Your Own Mistakes

Laughing at your own mistakes is hard to do. Although some things that have gone wrong may not have been funny when they occurred, you can probably look back and find some humor in them. This may also help you to be easier on yourself.

In my own caregiving experience, I don't need to go any further than my first day as a paid professional caregiver in a dementia assessment unit. I was fresh out of school, full of enthusiasm and ideas but low on experience. That service provider had never had an occupational therapist, so I couldn't build on anyone else's experience either. It was overwhelming to say the least. I thought, "Well, I will get to know 4 of the 25 clients today, and I will start by reading their charts." The chart reading went very well—so far, so good! Then I went to meet Sally, my first client. At the time, I didn't have too many clues about how to communicate with someone with advanced dementia; therefore, I thought a good approach would be to have Sally show me her room and to try to pick up on some personal cues. When I asked her to show me her room, Sally, who was busy pacing the hall, smiled happily, looked at me with complete bewilderment, and kept on pacing. When a staff member showed us Sally's room, I was surprised to find a gentleman asleep on her bed. Sally wasn't at all upset about this, but for some unknown reason, I decided to suggest that he move to his own room. When I gently woke him to help him move, he smiled pleasantly, said, "I am so sorry," and then lay down to go back to sleep. This continued for a few minutes, with the poor man bobbing up and down. I was persistent, and after several tries, I did manage to rouse this man and move him to his own bed to continue his much-interrupted nap. Of course, by this time, Sally was nowhere in sight!

Laugh with the Person You Are Caring For

 Joe was sitting by the window very involved with his morning paper. As his caregiver walked by, she noticed that he had the paper upside down! She gently asked if he would like her to turn the paper. He replied, "No, it's just fine. Any damn fool can read it right side up, but this takes special talent."

People with dementia continue to have a sense of humor. You have most likely experienced this when the person with dementia skillfully uses humor to protect his or her dignity. Caregivers can use humor in this same way.

In addition, the types of situations that used to amuse the person still do. Make the most of these times and have a good chuckle together. Retell funny stories that have been passed down in the family and the neighborhood. The great thing about these stories is that if you had a good laugh about them in the past, often just thinking about them can bring back the feeling of good humor.

Read Joke Books, Cartoons, Humorous Short Pieces, and the Comics

When you see an amusing cartoon in the daily paper or get a funny card, save it to enjoy again. Post it on the refrigerator or another spot where you will see it often.

Listen to Funny Television or Radio Programs

Cassettes and videotapes provide a great way to fit in some fun when you have a minute to enjoy them. Videotapes of classic comedians, such as Laurel and Hardy, Lucille Ball, Red Skelton, and Carol Burnett, may be enjoyed with the person you are caring for.

Find Healthy Ways to Express Upset Feelings

The following thoughts from caregiver Judy Bow were first shared in the newsletter of the Rush Alzheimer's Disease Center in Chicago, Illinois. They are reprinted here with permission from Judy.

Dark Thoughts

My husband is in the middle stages of Alzheimer's disease. Sometimes I wish that the disease would just hurry up and fin-

ish its job on him. You would be surprised how often this and other unspoken phrases like this have rumbled around in my head. It is easy to feel guilty for having these thoughts. I recently was out for lunch with another woman who cares for her husband with the disease. I am very comfortable with her so I hesitantly told her about these feelings and asked if she ever felt the same. Her face registered immediate recognition and we began to share our internal dialogues. A mutual reaction was, "Oh, my gosh! Do you mean that you think that too?" It was very liberating to be able to discuss this with someone else who not only understands what I'm talking about, but also experiences the same "self talk" that I do.

Our conversation allowed me to release some of my guilt but also gave me the impetus to afford the same liberating feeling to a broader group of caregivers. I have known all along the value of dialogue and sharing of experiences with others in the same boat. I do so in support groups, both locally and on the Internet. However, I couldn't recall ever digging this deeply into the human psyche during conversations in those settings. We certainly discuss our frustrations and challenges but not these dark thoughts that run through our heads. In preparation for writing this article, I asked others to share their feelings of this nature and as a result the floodgates opened. It turns out that most of us experience this type of internal dialogue that sometimes makes us feel just this side of evil.

It isn't evil, of course. It's normal and even therapeutic to periodically acknowledge to oneself the sheer horror that this devastating disease has wreaked on our loved one and our own daily life. To not do so might allow the disease to completely ravage more than just the person with Alzheimer's, which is plenty enough.

At the risk of sounding like George Carlin and his seven bad words, I want to share a random list of these "dark thoughts."

Some of these are my own and others have been contributed by others in a similar situation. Can you relate to any of these?

Why can't she simply die in her sleep or have some sort of unexpected accident?

I hate him, I hate my life, I hate this situation, and I hate the loss of freedom.

Can't she just straighten up those shoulders and walk like a real person? How hard is that?

I could end all of this if I gave one little shove at the top of the stairs.

Would you just shut up? What you are saying makes no sense and doesn't matter!

Are you in there anywhere? I want the old you back.

Why can't I just die—my own death would be a relief.

My family thinks I'm so patient and wonderful—HA! They don't have a clue what runs through my head.

Is he going to die in time for me to have any kind of life or future?

Did "for better or for worse" really mean THIS?

Can she really have become this stupid?

After these thoughts surface in our consciousness, we chide ourselves knowing that it's the disease, not the person, that is causing the problems. Or we remember how much harder it must be for them than for us. And we realize that they would be doing the same thing for us if the situation was reversed.

What is this internal dialogue all about? Certainly it's a phenomenon not unique to caregivers. Positive "self-talk" has always been a useful tool to me. My negative reactions ordinarily eventually are released via discussions, arguments, or decisions involving the other person or persons. However, as caregivers, the dialogue in our head gets louder and tends to remain unresolved because productive communication is not usually possible with the person who has dementia. The indi-

vidual is not capable of understanding or changing his or her behavior anyway. It feels inappropriate, shameful, or embarrassing to share these feelings with friends and family members. But the dark side inevitably creeps into one's mind.

We need to allow the dark thoughts in, even be amused by them sometimes, and, most important, release them by talking with other people who can empathize. It is therapeutic to learn that others have the same kind of thoughts and that they are nothing more than natural outlets for our outrage at the toll that Alzheimer's disease takes on everyone involved. After all, when caregivers step back and reflect, we often recognize that we are the ones who are distraught and our loved ones with Alzheimer's seem relatively happy, strange though it may be. If one's dark thoughts grow darker and become persistent, it is a sign that intensive support such as individual counselling is needed.

So far I have made suggestions about expressing and experiencing happy times. As Judy Bow's frank commentary illustrates, there are also dark thoughts and feelings of anger, frustration, and disappointment. **These feelings are perfectly natural, and caregivers should not feel guilty in any way about having them.** As caregiver Sally Callahan wisely pointed out, "feelings are neither good nor bad, they just are" (2000, p. 203). The challenge comes in figuring out what to do with these feelings. It is not appropriate to blame the person with a damaged brain for generating these feelings in us, to respond to the person with anger and blame. The person is not able to understand this any more than he or she can understand the original cause of the anger. Even more important, it is not the person who is causing the anger; it is caused by the symptoms of dementia.

Yet, caregivers need to express these very real and valid feelings. Some find that being angry at the disease helps to separate the person and his or her symptoms from the disease.

The challenge of expressing difficult feelings is made even more difficult by the fact that society generally makes little place for them. Sally Callahan commented,

> The need to experience and express difficult emotions is often denied to family members by those well meaning friends, spouses, colleagues, and professionals who simply don't know what to say or do. Many feel helpless and at some level afraid that the caregiver's pain may get too close to them. Offers of platitudes and overly simple solutions can make caregivers feel alienated, alone and questioning their sanity and mental health. (2000, p. 201)

Upset feelings that are not expressed cause illness. Emotional health comes about when thoughts, feelings, and actions are in harmony.

It is also important to remember that thoughts and feelings influence behavior, but they do not cause it. An individual can choose how to behave from a wide range of possibilities. The stresses of caregiving can cause an imbalance in thoughts, feelings, and actions. Focusing on thoughts and ignoring feelings can result in stress-related symptoms such as headaches or depression. For example, a caregiver focuses on the thought that her loved one is sick and cannot help the frustrating things that he does. Hence, the caregiver concludes that she should not feel angry when he puts dinner down the garbage disposal. This caregiver is showing signs of depression and needs to understand that it is perfectly legitimate to feel anger and frustration. However, expressing this anger to her loved one through behavior (i.e., behavior motivated by anger) is not legitimate. It is important to find a suitable outlet, however, such as talking to a friend or engaging in physical activity, to express these feelings. **Although all feelings are real and legitimate, it does not necessarily follow that all behaviors are legitimate.**

Conversely, focusing on feelings can cause a caregiver to become excessively emotional. Coping in even ordinary situations may become a challenge, and the caregiver may have difficulty using logic to solve a problem. For example, a caregiver focuses on her feelings of disgust and anger when her husband urinates in the garbage can instead of the toilet. As a result, she's unable to realize that the problem might be solved by removing the garbage can and placing a colored cover on the toilet seat to make it more visible.

Finally, those who focus only on behavior may act impulsively, use poor judgment, and ignore others' feelings. For example, a caregiver is frustrated by the person's repetitive questions. In turn, the caregiver behaves in ways that constantly express this frustration, ignores the emotional needs and feelings behind these questions, and perhaps even ends up blaming the person with dementia—the person with a damaged brain—for having a poor memory.

Here are some suggestions to help to restore a balance of thoughts, feelings, and actions:

- Get in touch with your feelings. The first step to emotional health is letting feelings out and opening up the emotional tap, not turning it off because of guilt or some other reason.

- Find a healthy way to express these feelings. There are numerous ways to do this; experiment and find what works best for you. Some find that physical activity is a good outlet for frustration or anger. This can take many forms, from taking time for a brisk walk or workout to pounding a pillow or a punching bag to my grandmother's solution—scrubbing the floor! Others find comfort in quieter ways, such as keeping a journal or talking to a friend or a trusted professional. Keeping a journal just doesn't seem natural or satisfying to me (which is surprising because I am a writer), so I write my difficult feelings down in letters. Although these letters may never be mailed, it helps me to write my thoughts to an actual person. If you try this method, I also urge you to let a letter sit for several days, especially if it was written in anger, and to reread it several times in a calmer moment before mailing it. Instead of acting on upset and hurt feelings, engaging in a cooling-off period is always a good plan. The folk wisdom of counting to 10 is advice well taken. In addition, although you shouldn't give the person with dementia such a letter, writing to the person you are caring for is a way of expressing feelings.

- Talk with someone else. The listening ear of a good friend or another caregiver who understands what you are going through is invaluable. There are also times when it is important to share your feelings with a professional who can be objective, offer suggestions, and link you with helpful community resources. Your local Alzheimer's Association or Alzheimer Society chapter is a good place to start. The chapter can also link you to an Alzheimer's family support group, providing the opportunity to talk to and share with others in similar situations. Sally Callahan commented on the importance of support groups:

The support groups to which I belonged offered something no one else could—people who *understood what I was living with*. They too were trying to process this foreign behavior by people they love. There were times when I went because I didn't know what else to do with myself. There were times I didn't go because I just couldn't take any more Alzheimer's. But for the most part, in the long run, support groups were the most powerful tool in my bag of tricks. (2000, p. 221)

Take Time to Grieve

"The pain now is part of the happiness then."

In the movie *Shadowlands*, this is the way that author C.S. Lewis expressed his great sorrow as his wife lay dying. Although their time together had been brief, it had been full of joy, making his loss even more painful.

A caregiver who is a family member or friend has a relationship and a shared history with the person. As detailed in Chapter 2, dementia and providing care are bound to change the nature of that relationship. There will also be profound changes in the person who the caregiver has known and loved. These are very real and painful losses. To make things more difficult, the losses happen over a period of years. Caregivers find that with each realization of a change—for example, the first time that the person *seems* unable to recognize them—they are confronted with loss. Each time of loss can start another cycle of grieving. Working through grief is not something that happens once but many times over the long course of dementia.

Although there are well-accepted social practices for mourning someone who has died, the need to grieve for someone who is still living is not well understood. Well-meaning people may say things such as "At least he is still alive." Try not to let such comments undermine your genuine need and right to grieve. Until others have walked your path, they may not understand the pain that you feel with every step. Sally Callahan commented:

> Grief is an enormous problem for the Alzheimer's caregiver. The insidious nature of the losses over such an extended period of time is devastating. Living in a society that neither acknowledges nor supports grief makes things worse. Not only is the patient changing before the caregiv-

er's eyes, their relationship is also changing. Professionals use the term "anticipatory grieving." It is a term I strenuously object to because it seems to *lessen* the validity of the losses and grief. . . . I do not view grief as resolvable but rather something to be experienced and embraced so it can be fully integrated and the person left behind can move on.... Grief is not pleasant. Grief is not easy. But grief is necessary. (2000, pp. 204–205)

As noted, **grieving is a process, not a one-time event** (Ballard, 1993; Kübler-Ross, 1969; Kuhn, 2001). Whatever the loss, there are stages to grief. Experience shows that there is no short cut, that there is no way around—only moving through, growing with each stage. The common stages of grief are denial, anger, sorrow, and acceptance. This process is not a straight line, not a matter of getting through the stages and coming out on the other side once and for all, whole and healed. There are often steps back into earlier stages—for example, the stage of anger or denial. Unfortunately, this is particularly so when grieving for the losses that come with dementia. These losses take place over years, not even months or days. I wish this wasn't so. Based on my work with others and on personal experience, I can assure you that although there may often be two steps forward and one step back, the only thing to do is follow the process. If you allow yourself to do this, you will eventually come out on the other side to acceptance, still feeling sorrow but being healed from a grief that weighs down every moment of every day. It is also vital to point out that no one necessarily has the innate ability to work through the grief process by him- or herself. Getting the assistance of an experienced counselor is an excellent idea.

Denial is natural, a way of protecting ourselves from the worst news until we can cope with it. You may recognize this in yourself, perhaps as you make excuses for the memory lapses or difficulties (e.g., saying that the person is tired). Although denial protects us for a time, staying stuck in denial is unhealthy. It can cause unrealistic expectations, disappointment in ourselves, and frustration with the person who has dementia. Moving forward from denial signals the time to get outside help, to get the advice of a physician, and to begin the process of assessment and diagnosis. Confronting the reality of the diagnosis is painful, but not as painful (for you or the person you are caring for) as not understanding the reasons for changes and difficulties.

Anger naturally follows the realization that there is a problem, or a change, or a loss. You may find yourself shouting—inwardly or out loud—questions such as "Why me?" "Why my loved one?" and "What did I do to deserve this?" You may also find yourself looking with resentment at others who seem to be better off. These are natural reactions. You have a right to be angry. It is indeed true that life is not fair, that neither you nor the person you are caring for asked for or deserves to be dealing with dementia. I wish I could answer your questions, but I can't. I can only advise you to find a healthy way to express this anger, as suggested in the previous section.

Learning more about the disease can help in dealing with anger and frustration. Knowledge is power, and understanding that this is a brain disease not only helps to reduce anger, it also helps you learn ways of responding to the changes in the person with dementia (see Chapter 10 for more information).

Whatever you do, don't store anger inside and don't blame yourself for feeling angry and cheated. Anger turned inward causes very real damage, such as physical and emotional illness. Expressing anger helps you to move on to the next stage, which is genuine sorrow.

The word *grieving* may first bring to mind feelings of deep regret and sadness. This is the time of true realization of loss, of overwhelming sorrow—bottom-of-the-barrel feelings of sadness. This is the time when you just want to cry your eyes out, so you should. There is much wisdom in the saying that you will feel better after a good cry. Crying releases oceans of stored feelings, and science has shown that tears actually have a curative chemistry.

During this time, so great is your well of sorrow that it is sometimes hard to pull yourself up and carry on. At this stage in my own grieving, it took a tremendous effort to put one foot in front of the other, to carry on with some semblance of normal life—going to work and so forth. This is a dangerous time for you, the caregiver of a person with dementia. If your daily work is caregiving, it may be difficult to motivate yourself. **You may be so overwhelmed and exhausted from caregiving that you do not have the strength or the will to pull yourself out of sorrow. This is not a sign of weakness; rather, it could be a sign that you need help for depression.** As many as 75% of caregivers of persons with dementia may suffer from depression (Bowlby Sifton, 1998). Depression is a very real illness, not a character fault. Depression can be a life-threatening illness, but excellent treatments are now available. If you are experiencing the following symptoms for longer than 3–4 weeks, it is essential that you go to your doctor:

- Feelings of hopelessness and worthlessness that last for hours and days at a time
- Crying spells
- Sleeping too much or too little
- Eating too much or too little
- Excessive weight loss or weight gain
- Loss of interest in usual activities

- Difficulty concentrating
- Loss of energy; feelings of great fatigue
- Thoughts of harming yourself

If you are experiencing these symptoms, don't delay in getting help. If anyone you know has these symptoms, encourage him or her to seek medical help.

Eventually, your tears will dry and you will come to the stage of acceptance. It is hard to describe this stage. There is an understanding that what is, is. This understanding brings a sense of peace; within this peace remain pieces of the other stages but with a different feel. Denial may take the form of regret, of "if only" or wishing it wasn't so. This is a natural feeling, but underneath the feeling, you know it is so. There will be times of anger, but it does not dominate the way that it once did. It is also natural that there will be times of sadness. These are part of what my dear friend calls the "dark threads in the rich tapestry, the weaving that is life." Acceptance comes when these dark threads are blended with lighter and brighter patterns. Acceptance allows you to recall and reminiscence about happier times without being totally overwhelmed by sorrow. Acceptance means that you can see the way forward; you wish things were different, but you will make the best of what now is. Acceptance also means that you can begin to reinvest in living life not only with the reality of dementia but also in other relationships and interests.

I wish each of you the courage to work through your grief until you can find beauty and peace in the new pattern, until you can come to the place that C.S. Lewis did in *Shadowlands*, when after his wife's death he said, "The pain then is part of the happiness now."

CARE FOR YOURSELF BY GROWING

Growing is another important part of caring for yourself. The ensuing subsections focus on various aspects of this topic.

Be Forgiving of Your Mistakes

It is important to forgive yourself for mistakes because learning from mistakes is a step in moving on. The following poem addresses this issue:

Now that I've done this for three years, there's so much
I would do differently.
I would be more patient.
I would be easier on myself.
I would let go—of old ideas, old expectations,
old ways of doing things.
I would bury shoulda, woulda, oughta, coulda.
I would learn to appreciate the present.
It was when I compared where we are, what we have,
what he can do with the past that I got into trouble.

(Alyce A., cited in Ballard & Poer, 1999)

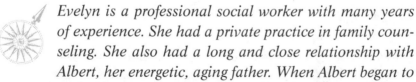

Evelyn is a professional social worker with many years of experience. She had a private practice in family counseling. She also had a long and close relationship with Albert, her energetic, aging father. When Albert began to have difficulty managing the household on his own for physical reasons, Evelyn didn't hesitate to invite him to live with her. Even though Evelyn's home was on the other side of the country, Albert made a happy adjustment to the change and became involved in local activities. Father and daughter traveled and enjoyed many happy years together. After a time, Evelyn began to notice some

changes: Her father seemed to spend increasing time doing very little and had lost interest in reading and his many other activities. Albert tried to be helpful in preparing meals, but this sometimes backfired. One day, Albert became concerned about the strange noises and heat coming from an appliance. He took the precaution of unplugging the breadmaker that was busily kneading bread for dinner guests!

Evelyn began to suspect that her father was developing dementia. She mentioned it to the family doctor, who was willing to conduct an in-home assessment. However, when Evelyn asked Albert about seeing the doctor, he became very angry and said that there was nothing wrong with him. Evelyn mentioned her concerns to her sisters, who lived at some distance, and they dismissed these claims based on the fact that they had perfectly rational, lucid telephone conversations with their father. They felt nothing was wrong, that their dad was as sharp as ever.

When I met Evelyn and Albert, the father–daughter relationship was as hostile as could be imagined. Evelyn thought that she was doing her best—and she was—to make a happy home for her dad. In return, Albert was angry a great deal of the time. For example, on the day that I visited for dinner, Evelyn put forth great effort to make a favorite chocolate dessert for her dad. Albert enjoyed it but remarked that Evelyn never made anything nice like that just for him; she only made such things when guests came. Evelyn retorted that this wasn't true and began to quiz her father with "Don't you remember?" questions. Evelyn also reminded her father that it was hard to keep the chocolate on hand because he always found it and ate it.

Realizing that this conversation was only going downhill, another visitor gracefully intervened. This person changed the topic to the book that Albert had published during his career as a lawyer. Albert cheerfully joined in this conversation and a little while later happily went to bed.

We gathered around a distressed and embarrassed Evelyn and shared in her tears. At this point, I was able to pass on the results of a low-key assessment that I had done while dinner was being prepared. Evelyn was completely shocked. Her dad, a retired tax lawyer, was unable to put the numbers on the face of a clock, spell a word backward, provide the date (or even a close approximation), or answer many other questions about practical things. Albert had been using his social skills to fool just about everyone, including his social worker daughter, about his failing brain.

Evelyn's first reaction was to burst into tears and say that she wanted to be good at this, at caregiving, and that she of all people should know how to be really good at it. During the brief time that I had with her, I tried my best to assure her that no one, even a person with professional training, can instantly understand how to care for someone with dementia. Even with experience, people make mistakes. It did seem to reassure Evelyn to realize that her training, received only 10 years earlier, had included only minimal information about Alzheimer's disease and other dementias.

"Never let a good failure go to waste."

The preceding wise words were spoken by an elderly caregiver. There are no road maps for this caregiving journey that you are taking; there are bound to be wrong turns and mistakes. The wisdom comes in trying to learn from these mistakes rather than getting tangled up in regret or in perfectionism. Expecting perfection is undoubtedly a lifelong trait, and sometimes people who have professional training, like Evelyn, are harder on themselves than caregivers without such training.

No one is perfect, and this is particularly true regarding the challenge of providing care for someone with dementia. You just can't get it right every time. If you keep an open and creative attitude, however, chances are that you will get closer than if you keep searching for the one "right" way. Try to replace the "shoulds" in your thinking with "coulds." It is up to us as caregivers to change our ways; we should not expect the person with dementia to change his or hers. Although a person with dementia certainly can learn, it is much easier for us to learn than the person with a damaged brain.

Seek Support

If the world worked the way it ought to, there would be a rush of people at our side to help us when things go wrong, when we need help. This happens sometimes but not often. When the need is long term and not very specific, as it is with dementia caregiving, it is difficult for most people to understand what to do and how to do it. If there has been an accident, a broken bone, a death, or a serious physical illness, most people understand what to do: send a card, make a telephone call, come for a visit, bring food, and so forth. The people who respond in this way undoubtedly have the same good intentions and thoughts of being helpful when they learn that you are caring for someone with Alzheimer's disease. However, they may have no idea what to do to support and help you.

The only way that other people can know what to do to help is if we let them know. We need to ask for help. There are many challenges here. Perhaps foremost is that you have never asked for help, that you are used to pulling your weight, being independent, not wanting to be a bother. Of course, such assumptions are made on your part; most trusted friends and relatives do not think this way. Nonetheless, it may be easier to ask for help on behalf of the person you are caring for. Regardless of how help is requested, doing so is important: Experience shows that caregivers who have made use of a social support system experience less stress and have an easier adjustment after the person's death (Gwyther, 2001).

What is the worst thing that can happen if you ask for help? The person might say no. This will sting, a bit, but it is not the end of the world. Also, if you think carefully about who to ask to do what and in what way, getting "no" for an answer is unlikely. For more suggestions on asking for help, see Chapter 10.

In addition to people you know, explore your community for other sources of support. The first place to turn is your local Alzheimer's Association or Alzheimer Society chapter. There also is a wide network of support groups in Canada and the United States; see Appendix B at the end of the book for more information. Support groups are usually informal and are made up of people providing care. These people come together to share common concerns, with the guidance of an experienced group leader. Many Alzheimer's Association chapters have education sessions and resource centers as well. Many chapters have a telephone support system for people who cannot attend meetings. There is also a growing number of web-based caregiver resources (again, see Appendix B for suggestions). In areas without Alzheimer's support groups, some people have found attending other support groups, such as Al-Anon or bereavement groups, to be helpful.

Time and time again, caregivers and research report that involvement with spiritual or religious activities is a great source of strength (Post, 2001b). If you have a spiritual or religious background, this may be the first place you turn. If not, spiritual or religious pursuits may be worth exploring. We are all, by nature, spiritual creatures. We all have a need to look outside of ourselves and our situation, to make connections and find strength from something larger and more powerful than ourselves. When coping with Alzheimer's disease or another dementia, this need becomes even greater. The ways in which we experience this connectedness with larger forces outside ourselves is highly individual, however. For some, it may be a formal religious group; for others, it may be quiet meditation and reflection. Sally Callahan commented, "Although I couldn't have heard it myself at the beginning, I urge all involved in the process of Alzheimer's to open their hearts and seek spiritual sustenance and healing" (2000, p. 221).

In addition to attending formal religious services, there are many other ways to find support through spiritual expression. Synagogues, churches, or temples may have informal social, music, or study groups. Some people find that just sitting in the quiet of a sacred building brings peace and comfort.

Conversation with a minister, rabbi, priest, or other caring member of a religious community may be helpful. Such conversations can take place at home as well as in places of worship. Members of your spiritual community can be guided in how to help you by Lisa Gwyther's excellent booklet *You Are One of Us: Successful Clergy/Church Connections to Alzheimer's Families* (1995).

If you are unable to attend services, you may be able to watch or listen to tapes of services or sacred music. There are any number of books or shorter reflection guides that may be a source of understanding and inspiration. For those from a particular religious tradition, reading favorite passages from sacred texts can be comforting.

Prayer and meditation are individual paths to our spiritual selves. They may already be part of your life and a source of strength and support. If not, you may want to explore this possibility. In addition to formal religious centers, the community may offer courses on meditation or activities that have a meditative component (e.g., tai chi, yoga). There are also helpful print and videotape guides to meditation.

Learn as Much as You Can

Knowledge is power.

The more you understand about Alzheimer's disease and other dementias, the more capable and competent you will feel. An important benefit is that you will be better able to stand in the shoes of the person you are caring for, to get a window into the person's damaged brain and understand why the person does certain things. The fact that you are reading or at least glancing at this book shows that you probably understand knowledge is power. Reading a book is not for everyone, however; there are many different ways of learning. Videotapes and other learning resources are suggested throughout this book. Your local Alzheimer's Association or Alzheimer Society chapter is a good resource for locating learning materials as well as for talks and presentations that may be of interest.

Plan for the Future

Although there are no exact time frames or milestones, the person you are caring for will need increasing help as the disease progresses. Although it is not healthy to let worry about the future cloud your present, it also is not healthy to ignore the very real changes that lie ahead. Planning—with the person who has dementia, if possible—for how care will be provided in the future prevents having to respond in a crisis. It also removes a burden from present-day worries. See Chapter 10 for suggestions on care planning.

CONCLUSION

Let me end this chapter by thanking you, on behalf of all persons with dementia, for your loving and dedicated work as a caregiver. I hope that some of the suggestions in this chapter will in some way help to lighten this challenging journey for you. What you do truly makes all the difference in the world for the person's quality of life and well-being; taking care of you is important for both of your sakes. In Chapter 2, you will find some suggestions for living in the moment with the person who you are caring for, which I hope will shed further light on your mutual journey.

2

Living in the Moment

No two days and no two moments are the same. You can't build on experience. You can maybe guess what's going to happen a little while from now—minutes from now, hours from now—we don't know what to expect.

The scariest thing is, I guess, the fact that I have no sense of time. I have not the slightest idea—my brain doesn't—what's ten hours away or what's two hours away.

And if I think that somebody's been, that my wife had been gone a while, I get very antsy. And it may be just a short time that she's been away—it feels like it's forever. (Henderson & Andrews, 1998, p. 47)

MOMENTS OF TERROR
AND MOMENTS TO BE TREASURED[1]

It is in the shelter of each other that the people live.

The preceding Irish proverb, undoubtedly born of generations of confronting the challenge of living in a lovely but often inhospitable landscape, reminds us that true shelter is to

---

[1]Portions of this section previously appeared in Bowlby Sifton, C. (2000d). It is in the shelter of each other that people live. *Alzheimer's Care Quarterly*, 1(1), iv–v; adapted by permission; and in Bowlby Sifton, C. (2001a). Life is what happens when we are making other plans. *Alzheimer's Care Quarterly*, 2(2), iv–vii; adapted by permission.

be found in the company of other people. Nature shows, for example, that trees within a copse survive a harsh climate by supporting each other against the buffeting wind and weather. A lone tree has little chance of survival.

The person struggling to withstand the assaults of Alzheimer's disease or another dementia particularly needs caring support and shelter; he or she needs to be enfolded by positive relationships with others. The following passage describes this struggle for one person with Alzheimer's disease.

> It is like being on an island in the middle of the ocean; I can't see land, I don't know if anyone knows for sure I'm here or if someone will come for me. I don't know where my next meal will come from or where I will sleep tonight. (Bowlby Sifton, 2000d, p. iv)

There could hardly be a more eloquent plea for the surety of shelter to be found in affirming relationships. Hearing this, I was overwhelmed by what an awfully frightening place the world, at that moment, must have been for this person with dementia. The present moment was shot full of terror. None of the usual signposts made sense or brought reassurance. It is small wonder then that this person constantly followed his caregiver, seeking reassurance not only about basic needs (food and shelter) but also about where and who he was.

This poem offers another account of moments of terror.

Openings

It's really scary when you're an old woman.
I'm bereft. I hate being stranded like this,
I want to be in the middle of the town.
But I have no money to speak of,
and I don't know how to get away from here.
I can't open it! The door won't open!

I shall have to grit my teeth and walk like hell.
And it's cold out there without a coat.
How stupid I didn't think of this before.
I've never been in such a situation.
I've missed buses, but this is different.
This door won't open! And that's another!

I didn't expect this predicament. Well, if I'm stuck
I'll just have to ask them for a bed for the night.

(cited in Killick & Cordonnier, 2000)

Living with memory loss can be terrifying. The need for reassurance, for discerning the signposts, is constant. Beyond this special need, dementia damages brain cells—not the person's humanity or need to continue being in relationships with others, to be valued as a worthwhile person in this present moment. It is my absolute belief and experience that despite dementia's ravaging of the brain, persons with dementia, at a very deep and fundamental level, always retain a sense of their own unique self—the core of their being that says "I am me." We all come to understand who we are by our relationships and interactions with others. Persons with dementia particularly need affirming relationships to validate their sense of self.

Cary Henderson described what these relationships mean to him:

> I think that is the one thing that is most difficult about Alzheimer's is loving, continuously and without qualms, without holding anything back—it's a matter of trust. I think probably, though, that anybody who is a caregiver to an Alzheimer's patient, their patience is just going to be continually bothered.
>
> But I think love is the key to all this stuff and love is something that my wife certainly has given to me and the

family has too and there's nothing that I can see to complain about. (Henderson & Andrews, 1998, p. 65)

Supported by the love of his wife and his family, Cary felt not only connected but also content; in this particular moment, he found nothing to complain about. How wonderful! Being in trusting, supportive relationships can and does help to overcome the powerful feelings of loneliness and fear, "of being an island in the middle of the ocean." Trust is key to enabling persons with dementia to feel reassured and supported, to help them overcome fear. Persons with memory loss feel vulnerable and fragile; trusting relationships provide reassurance in moments of fear.

Caregivers face the challenge of creatively bypassing the disease-induced losses in ways of maintaining conventional connectedness—to find ways without words—to reveal and experience relationships on other planes. The challenge is great, especially in a culture in which a person is primarily defined by his or her ability to think and be productive. At the same time, the rewards of making a meaningful connection can be awe inspiring, not only for the person with dementia but for the caregiver.

The move from words and body hugs to heart-speak and eye hugs was incredibly poignant and loving. As the brilliance of my mother's spirit shone through eyes held captive in a ravaged body, I was awe struck, not only that love remained, but that it seemed so much more powerful, almost pure. (Callahan, 2000, p. 243)

Over the years I have had the privilege of making these connections with many persons with dementia. I would like to share one particularly moving experience with you.

If you could meet Pierre in person, I have no doubt that you would agree with me that he is irresistibly charming. The day of our first meeting, I looked down the corridor and saw a frail, bent figure, his gaunt frame contained by a geriatric chair. I offered my hand in greeting and with great difficulty but tremendous dignity, he struggled to rise to return my greeting. Pierre gently took my hand, kissed it with a gallant flourish, and said that he was delighted to make my acquaintance. Pierre had been the loving center of his family for his entire 90 years, and it was clear why! Although he had long since retired from his career as an accountant, Pierre continued to be enthusiastically engaged in living every day to its fullest. Although his step was somewhat unsteady, his feet still moved lightly through his favorite step dances, making use of a partner for balance. Pierre's twinkling eyes let us know that there was always energy for a tease or a joke. Loved and respected, active and enthusiastic, and financially secure, Pierre seemed to have achieved an enviable old age.

There is one more piece of Pierre's story that you should know: He has severe dementia, probable Alzheimer's disease. Over the course of dementia, first his family and then the nursing facility staff found that they were unable to meet the challenges that his severe behavioral symptoms were posing. The most difficult were frequent periods of loud, repetitive clapping and banging and indiscriminate urination and defecation. From this perspective, Pierre's old age may seem more like a great tragedy than something to be envied.

Despite his severe impairments, Pierre was enthusiastic and responsive to sensory stimulation. As he admired and arranged flowers for the dining table, he proudly told me about the things that he had grown in his garden. As he made calculations and arranged papers and documents on his tray, he spoke eloquently, without words, about his managerial skill. He hid the exercise equipment from me and then shook with laughter. Supported by the reassurance of his caregivers, Pierre was once more enabled to affirm the value of his life experiences and, indeed, his own person-hood, which persisted despite the devastation caused by dementia.

Sensory experiences always led to some enlivenment and served to calm Pierre's frequent periods of distress. Over the months, however, Pierre's responsiveness became less animat-ed and less frequent. There came a day, a few months before his death, when Pierre failed to even open his eyes, despite frequent approaches in voice and touch. Because it seemed that Pierre's deterioration had progressed to a stage where he could not be reached, my heart was in my shoes.

Just the same, I continued with our usual good-bye routine. Putting one hand on his shoulder, I took Pierre's hand in mine. I told him that I would see him tomorrow and wished him a good day. At this, his frail fingers came alive again and Pierre grasped my hand. Pierre's sparkling blue eyes opened wide and he lifted his face to mine. Glowing with what could only be called a beatific smile and speaking in a very clear voice, Pierre said, "You have a good heart."

Somehow, my words and actions had made a connection that had enabled Pierre to express himself and experience some personal peace and happiness. While caring for my father as he died of cancer, I had learned that engagement in living continues to the very end. I learned the same lesson about Alzheimer's disease from Pierre. As Yogi Berra said, "It ain't over till its over."

Thank you, Pierre, for the gift of your trust when you were most vulnerable and in need, for allowing me into the shelter of your heart. It is in the shelter of each other that people live. I hope that all persons with dementia and their caregivers are enabled to find shelter with each other as they live with dementia day by day, moment by moment.

Although losing the ability to appreciate time can shoot each moment full of terror, it also gives each moment the capacity to sparkle with freshness and possibilities, to capture joy and excitement like a newly discovered jewel. The following expression of discovery comes from a person with dementia: "When I can't do the big things, I can do the little things. Things are a lot more precious than they were. I go ape on the leaves—I collect them whether I have them or not" (Henderson & Andrews, 1998, p. 77).

In her remarkable book *Who Will I Be When I Die?* Christine Boden reflected on how life has changed, for ill and for good:

> I am more stretched out somehow, more linear, more step by step in my thoughts. I have lost that vibrancy, the buzz of interconnectedness, the excitement and focus I once had. I have lost the passion, the drive that once characterized me. I'm like a slow motion version of my old self—not physically but mentally. It's not all bad, as I have more inner space in this linear mode to listen, to see to appreciate clouds, leaves, flowers. . . . I am less driven and less impatient. (1998, p. 49)

Christine Boden (1998) also pointed out that experiencing something wonderful for the sake of experiencing it—not necessarily remembering it—is a worthwhile activity.

In contrast to the previous comments about the fear and terror that fills some moments, these quotes reflect a theme of moments to be treasured. The author of the following poem reminds the rest of us to slow down and drink in life's beauties.

Glimpses

to see what is beautiful
to hear what is beautiful
they don't know what is beautiful

all these young people
good men, nice boys, fine chaps—
they are too busy to see

it'll be a good bit longer
before you see
what you want to see

but they don't want to see
what in some queer way
they are anxious to see

we see it very rarely
but the difference is
we are trying to see!

(cited in Killick & Cordonnier, 2000)

Expressions of the lived experience of Alzheimer's disease are replete with revelations about an awakened capacity to capture the joy to be found in the moment, to treasure the simple pleasures. If we can free ourselves to join the person in celebrating the moment, we can learn much in this regard.

Alice was always teaching us to appreciate life's joys. For instance, because of her, no one in the family can let the glory of the autumn colors pass by without stopping, even for a moment, to celebrate the splendor of a flaming maple. As I do this now, I can still hear her exclaiming with joy and enthusiasm, as if it was her first-ever sighting, "Oh, my, look at that. Did you ever in all your life see anything so beautiful?" No, Alice, I haven't, and as I look out my window at the crimson and gold that surrounds me, I thank you for opening my heart to the fullness of this moment.

A particular family event also captures the need to be open, to reframe how we think about experiences. Alice was very close to her sister Eula, and this connection remained vital despite separation by distance and memory loss. In addition, Alice really valued family gatherings and celebrations. Knowing how important such events were to Alice, we made every effort for her, as a surprise guest, to attend the celebration for Eula's fiftieth wedding anniversary. Alice was excited when we told her about the trip but even moments later had no recollection about it, the anniversary, or even not having seen Eula in "years and years and years." Given this situation, some friends and family members doubted that all of the effort and expense were worth it. We found it very sad that we had to provide so many clues to help Alice recall her much-loved sister, but we persisted with the planned trip. When the day of the trip arrived, Alice busily got ready, but at least every 5 minutes she asked, "Where is it we are going, dear?" At times, this gentle asking bordered on panic, and she needed a great deal of reassurance from her son during the 5-hour plane and car trip. Even as we approached the door of the hall where the family was gathered, Alice's son kept telling her where they were, why we were there, and who was going to be there. Despite all of these reminders, when Alice and Eula first saw each other, one was just as surprised as the other! Alice was absolutely overcome with delight and surprise at seeing her much-loved sister again. The moment of meeting and recognition was precious, brimming over with joy and celebration.

For Alice, and for us, that moment is what mattered. All of the preparations and the constant questions beforehand were worth it as we celebrated this happy reunion of Alice and Eula. More than a decade later, I still smile, inside and out, as I remember this moment. Of course, we were sad that when the party was over just a few hours later, Alice didn't seem to remember it or understand why she was staying somewhere different. However, we tried not to let this sorrow overwhelm the absolute joy of the moment when the two sisters met.

Many of my experiences with persons with dementia have helped to underscore this same point. As aware as they may be of the sorrows and fears of living with memory loss, this somehow does not overwhelm the joys still to be found in the simple but exquisite pleasures of daily life. Persons with dementia are grand masters at celebrating the precious present. In our move-ahead, future-oriented society, we can all benefit by celebrating the precious present. Thich Nhat Hanh describes this ability in the practice of Buddhism as follows:

> In Buddhism, our effort is to practice mindfulness in each moment—to know what is going on within and around us. When the Buddha was asked, "Sir, what do you and your monks practice?" he replied, "We sit, we walk, and we eat." The questioner continued, "But sir, everyone sits, walks, and eats," and the Buddha told him, "When we sit, we *know* we are sitting. We walk, we *know* we are walking. When we eat, we *know* we are eating." Most of the time, we are lost in the past or carried away by future projects and concerns. When we are mindful, touching deeply the present moment, we can see and listen deeply, and the fruits are always understanding, acceptance, love and the desire to relieve suffering and bring joy. When our beautiful child comes up to us and smiles, we are completely there for her. (1995, p. 14)

Persons with dementia seem to live the folk lesson "If life gives you lemons, make lemonade!" One Thanksgiving, I asked a number of people with dementia living in a specialty ward of a psychiatric hospital what they were thankful for. Here are some of the many answers that they spontaneously gave:

> My family
> My health
> Being here with you

No one said "Nothing" or "What could I possibly have to be thankful for?," which, given their situation, I had expected. These folks were all so challenged by disease symptoms but still found a reason to celebrate life and be thankful. As the following example shows, living in the moment gives persons with dementia a remarkable ability to bloom where they are planted if caregivers are thoughtful gardeners and provide good growing conditions.

 Ruth has advanced dementia, is mostly nonverbal, and requires full assistance with all aspects of her care, including toileting. Most people with Ruth's circumstances would be provided with this care in an institution. However, Ruth's husband Abe, who is very frail and often requires oxygen for emphysema, is determined to keep Ruth at home for as long as possible. It is achingly beautiful to see Abe arrive at the day program with Ruth after their 2-hour trip. First, we hear Abe coming, his labored wheezes announcing his arrival. Then we see Abe, both gnarled hands clutching his cane (still not enough to support his thin frame, which is bent almost double) and gasping for breath. Beaming at his side is Ruth, perfectly turned out, hair done, makeup on, her favorite earrings in place— all of this accomplished by her loving husband.

Initially, Ruth's pleasure at being welcomed by her day program friends distracts her from missing Abe after he departs. However, this only lasts so long; by lunchtime, she is anxiously peering down the hall, looking for her husband. When he returns, there are no words to describe the look of joy, love, and contentment that overwhelms her whole person. With each meeting, it is as if she is seeing Abe for the first time. Abe drinks in this expression of love and returns it, celebrating the moment.

Abe's caregiving journey is by no means total joy. As just one example, after many struggles and mountains of laundry, he's come to understand that Ruth can no longer remember to get to the bathroom on time or even to go when it is suggested. In addition, there is no doubt that he pines for the wife who thrived as a secretary, caregiver for her own parents, and a proud homemaker. Nonetheless, Abe is able to relish Ruth's ongoing expressions of love and affection; he has found that caregiving and daily life are not limited to sorrows and losses.

CAREGIVING TAKES PLACE WITHIN A RELATIONSHIP

As Abe experienced, caregivers are called on to do the lion's share of giving in the caregiving relationship. They must give their time as well as their ability to take care of everyday necessities, to plan for the future, and to problem-solve, and they must give up many personal pleasures and parts of the relationship as it used to be.

Caregiving changes the usual boundaries of a relationship. These boundaries of the relationship have shifted, turned upside down, or vanished entirely, especially the time frame in which the relationship takes place. However, if we can open ourselves to the possibility, then the person with dementia can offer us guidance on—and be our teacher regarding—the many joys to be found by living in and treasuring the moment. **For persons with dementia, the most important moment is the present moment.** Tomorrow can scarcely be imagined or anticipated or understood. Yesterday is, at best, a dim recollection. Persons with dementia live in the moment; life is most fully experienced in the now.

Caregivers are invited to enter into living in and savoring "now" experiences with the person they are caring for. This is our supreme challenge as caregivers: to live in the moment. The person with dementia has a decreased ability to understand and live in our future-oriented world and to adapt and change; it is up to us as caregivers to shift our time orientation. It is up to us to offer a relationship that is built on trust and the essential goodness of the moment. Yet, this situation also offers the best opportunity to experience a measure of joy and fulfillment during our caregiving journey—a point illustrated by the experience of Ruth and Abe.

Ruth was our teacher in so many ways. In our program, staff and participants jointly prepare a community lunch. Over time, participating was increasingly challenging for Ruth, but she could always help stir or mix things. She certainly participated in the all-important social part of the meal, even though she needed a lot of cuing and coaching with regard to eating. One day when I was sitting beside Ruth and providing some gentle direction with her lunch, I noticed her ring. It seemed to be a graduation ring with the number 51 on it. I knew that Ruth had attended business college, so I asked if this was her ring from that school. She said yes, so I asked if she had graduated in 1951. When she again said yes, I commented that I was 3 years old at the time. For a few seconds, Ruth did nothing. Then she turned to me and a slow grin began to light up her face; she looked at me again and really started to giggle. What a contagious giggle, and caught in the humor of me being 3 years old when she graduated from business college, we both collapsed in gales of laughter. When our table mates asked what was so funny, they also caught the joy of the moment; approximately 15 participants and staff totally collapsed with laughter.

We would have been hard pressed to explain to an outsider what was so funny, but it was a wonderful moment for all of us. The expression "I guess you had to be there" sums up the situation. Caregivers who can be there—wherever "there" is—with the person with dementia have much opportunity for joy, much opportunity to celebrate the precious present.

Taking this view of caregiving has implications for all aspects of care: communication, the environment, self-care, and leisure activities. These aspects are detailed in Chapters 4–8.

FINDING A BALANCE

Life is full of odd imbalances and contrasts: parents are over-joyed with their growing child yet miss the special days of babyhood; people eagerly count the minutes to special events, such as a party or the arrival of a friend, yet want the clock to stop when the time comes. Living with dementia further sharpens these contrasting or paradoxical situations: The person wants and needs to be independent yet requires our help more and more; there is an awakened capacity to find joy in the moment yet also the potential for each moment to be full of fear. One person with dementia describes her experience as follows:

> One thing I've noticed is this pulling back. I desperately want to go somewhere. I must go. And then I start pulling away and pulling away. There are too many things that are too scary. If I take myself away from everything I want to do it helps me because I avoid the fear of having to get there. I'm afraid of being in the car and not knowing where I'm going. It's a fear of being stranded. The fear is so strong I can't describe it. It's like I'm saving my life. I don't go any-where when this happens. So I wound myself by trying to protect myself. (Jean, cited in Snyder, 1999, p. 65)

As Lisa Snyder comments in the book from which the pre-ceding passage is taken, Jean's ability to step back and think about her situation is remarkable. "So I wound myself by try-ing to protect myself" is an amazingly insightful comment on the imbalance, the dilemma that confronts many persons with dementia as they try to live with the losses caused by their disease.

As caregivers, we also constantly confront such dilemmas or paradoxical situations. In response, we can only strive for understanding and information to help us arrive at the proper balance for our own caregiving situation. Thinking about these challenges led me to a parallel in my own life experience. After spending almost 35 years of life in various cities, I have moved back to the country. It is sometimes a challenge to maintain a balance between the need for the caring support and interest of neighbors and the need for privacy! As someone once said, "What I really like about living in the country is that everyone knows you. What I really dislike about living in the country is that everyone knows you."

A paraphrase of the preceding folk wisdom can sum up the challenges of being a family caregiver: "What is really good about being a family caregiver is having an intimate, shared relationship history that we can draw on; what is really tough about being a family caregiver is having a shared relationship history that reminds me of how much has been lost and how things will never be the same." For a nonfamily caregiver, the paraphrase might sound like this: "What is really good about being a nonfamily caregiver is that I have no history, so I can appreciate and relate to the person as he or she is now. What is really challenging about being a nonfamily caregiver is not having an understanding of the person's history—his or her likes, dislikes, coping style, strengths, and interests." This point is illustrated in the following example.

 The caregivers at Sunset Manor really enjoyed Mr. Gillespie's merry laugh and teasing ways. Although his attempts to tell an old joke always fell flat, they appreciated his tremendous joie de vivre. They were challenged

and puzzled about a certain behavior, however: He ate well at breakfast and supper, but he wouldn't touch lunch. Unfortunately, Mr. Gillespie had no family nearby who could tell his caregivers more about his life. Finally, one caregiver learned that Mr. Gillespie had worked in the local mill for years. This gave her an inspiration: She blew a whistle at noon, and he eagerly ate the lunch sitting in front of him!

We can only strive for understanding and information to help us arrive at the proper balance for our own caregiving situation. It is my hope that this book contributes to family and nonfamily caregivers coming together to share their understanding of the person's history and current needs, to work together to achieve a balance in these caregiving seesaws or dilemmas. Coming together is vitally important if we are to provide a good quality of life for the person with dementia. This person faces the biggest challenge: wishing to live life to its fullest and to continue as a fully functioning, dignified adult while steadily losing the skills to do so independently and, worst of all, often being unable to tell others about these needs, hopes, and frustrations. I invite you to share in some thoughts that follow about how we can support the person with dementia in not only surviving this challenge but also thriving, with a life full of moments to celebrate.

THOUGHTS ON LIVING IN THE MOMENT
WITH THE PERSON WITH DEMENTIA

Life is what happens while we are making other plans.

Although this expression is part of our folk wisdom in the busy whirl of daily life, most of us seldom take the time to appreciate what it means. Sometimes we need to be startled into realization. This is what happened to Tom when he received a diagnosis of Alzheimer's disease at age 55. In turn, he startled everyone gathered for the preconference session of the 2000 World Alzheimer's Congress when he opened with this statement: "Getting Alzheimer's disease is the best thing that ever happened to me."

Tom went on to explain that he had been so busy throughout his life, establishing a successful business and raising his family, that he had put aside all kinds of plans and dreams until later. After receiving his diagnosis, he decided that "later" had arrived. He turned over his business to his sons and began to work on his personal "someday when I have time" wish list. He decided to capture the joy now and was obviously relishing every moment.

For the most part, those of us living in the Western world are move-ahead, future-oriented people. We are always looking forward to or anticipating something in the future, thinking about how things are going to be. This ranges from the trivial, such as getting our coffee break, to the huge, such as retiring. If we take this view when caring for persons with dementia, it is easy to get bogged down and depressed. In terms of day-to-day abilities, we know that things are only going to get more and more challenging for them and for us. Certainly, as caregivers, we need to plan ahead and prepare. However, we also need to find a balance so that we are not totally preoccupied with the unhappy prospects of steady decline. We need to take a page from Tom's book and celebrate what we have now. Another challenge is to avoid getting stuck in a web of wishing that the person would go back to how he or she used to be. Sadly, at least in terms of practical abilities, this is just not going to happen. We can, however, celebrate the person who is here with us now, appreciating and enhancing the abilities that they do have. Living in either the future or the past is not likely to bring caregivers any particular joy. The greatest potential for experiencing the joy of caregiving is to join the person in celebrating now.

"Michael, don't you ever forget that I am still in here."
As Marie spoke these words, she wagged her finger affec-
tionately at her husband, then ended with a meaningful
tap on her heart. Michael had just moved Marie to a
long-term care facility and both were overwhelmed by emotion.
Marie's parting words were a powerful reminder about what mat-
tered most to her. She wanted Michael to remember that inside
she was still the same person he had loved and lived with for so
many years and that she continued to need to be in a relationship
with him.

Marie's words are echoed in voice and action by all persons with dementia, expressing the universal human need to be connected with others, to feel valued and affirmed as a person. This basic need overrides all practical care needs.

"The person with Alzheimer's disease
has not really lost their personality or their
memory, they have just lost access to it" (Sacks, 1990).

What a wonderful reminder from the inspired humanist and neurologist Oliver Sacks. His book *Awakenings* (also made into a movie) describes his work with people who were locked in a trance state similar to that of advanced Parksinson's disease. He contends that however terrible the ravages of memory and lost skills (which affect the way the person acts in the world—i.e., the external self), the person inside (the internal self) continues. So we return to the central notion that opened this chapter: I have absolutely no doubt that for all persons with dementia, the very core of their being—the center that says "I am me"—persists.

As noted previously, dementia damages brain cells, not the person's humanity, not his or her need to continue being in relationships with others, to be valued and affirmed as a person in this present moment. **Losing one's memory does not mean losing oneself or the people one cares about.** This need for connection is expressed through the whole course of dementia. For instance, John, who loved to read, was blessed with a young volunteer who came to read to him every day when he was immobile and nonverbal in the last stages of dementia. Even though John never opened his eyes or spoke during these visits, every day when the volunteer took his hand and said good-bye, he would tighten his grip on her hand and only reluctantly let go. His body was expressing his heart's desire to continue to be connected with another person.

Bob Glavin, whose story was presented in the Introduction, said that when he meets people on the street, they often comment with surprise, "Well, Bob you seem just the same to me, but I heard that you have Alzheimer's." Bob finds this very frustrating. Shaking his head sadly, he said, "I am still me; I am just the same person. Why does it change who I am because I have a disease? People wouldn't say that if I had cancer or a heart condition."

Christine Boden gave voice to the continuation of her essential self in this way:

> We are each a kaleidoscope of personality, which makes up every facet of who we are. But often we are limited in our range of expression of this multi-faceted person, because of our busyness, the demands and constraints, the expectations of our lives. I believe that God knows us in our entirety, each and every part of the kaleidoscope of who we are. As I unfold before God, as this disease unwraps me, opens up the treasures of what lies within my multifold personality, I can feel safe as each layer is gently opened out.

The fullness of who I once was will be seen in the simplicity of who I am within, surrounded by layer upon layer of memories. These memories form the kaleidoscopic perspectives of all the many expressions of my being over my lifetime. . . .

In each of these aspects of my life, the center of my being was always there within, expressing itself in these many forms of me. This unique essence of 'me' is at my core, and this is what will remain with me to the end. I will be perhaps even more truly 'me' than I have ever been. (1998, p. 49)

It is both our reward and our challenge as caregivers to continue to connect with persons with dementia, to discover creative ways to find access to the inner core of the person, to maintain person-to-person relationships; to express feelings; to share experiences—to capture the moment and celebrate the whole person cloaked by dementia. Michael and Marie, the couple described in the preceding vignette, discovered many such creative connections.

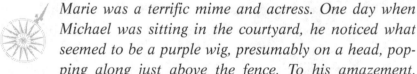

Marie was a terrific mime and actress. One day when Michael was sitting in the courtyard, he noticed what seemed to be a purple wig, presumably on a head, popping along just above the fence. To his amazement, Marie jumped out from behind the fence, underneath the purple wig, full of giggles and delight, which they both shared. Even as Marie's disability increased, they continued to share such moments, often while Michael helped her with her lunch.

The center point of such moments is finding ways to connect with the person—ways beyond words and memory—to be with them in the present moment. I've experienced that it often is the person with dementia who "tells" us the way if we are able to hear.

Admiral McTaggert was one of the most emotionally challenging persons with dementia that I have worked with. Like his wife and young sons, I found it difficult not to be devastated and immobilized by the tragedy of the losses that he was experiencing. By his early fifties, his talents and skill had brought him to the top of his field, and he was an admiral in the Navy. He had received many citations, trophies, and awards, including ones from ordinary seamen who had served under him. Everyone was astonished when this distinguished career sailor began to lose important files, miss meetings, and snap angrily at his staff. His wife also noticed changes, and after much insistence, he finally saw his doctor. The physician recommended a leave of absence for rest and recovery from stress. However, it was immediately apparent when he returned to work that rest had not taken the problem away. After months of specialists' appointments, Admiral McTaggert was diagnosed with Alzheimer's disease.

When I met him almost a year later, I was struck by his commanding presence and charm but also by the severity of his losses. His speech consisted mostly of a string of unrelated social phrases, and he was unable to dress or shave himself. I conducted a home visit to try to help Admiral McTaggert and his wife work out a supportive and safe daily routine. The admiral was welcoming and gracious as he showed me around his house and yard. However, he was so distracted and restless after this that it seemed impossible to involve him in his morning routine to do an assessment. He kept walking around and around the house, opening one door after another. I was unable to understand what he was looking for and kept making wrong suggestions. Unsure how to help or interrupt this search, I followed Admiral McTaggert to the basement. As he opened a door at the far side, he shouted with an enthusiasm that begged me to follow. The search had ended: He had found his den, the walls and shelves

covered with plaques, trophies, and awards from his years of distinguished naval service. I followed his tour of the room, commenting on each award as he glowed with pride. He nodded and looked at me knowingly as if to say, "See, this is who I am; now you know about me." I was honored to have such a personal introduction. After this time of connection, Admiral McTaggert was only too happy to continue with the assessment.

Caregivers can use the intimate knowledge they have of the person, as well as the suggestions in the following chapters of this book, to foster these meaningful connections. It is also vital for caregivers to share their insights and knowledge with other caregivers. This can be accomplished by using Appendix A (All About Me) at the end of the book or a similar resource.

Being stuck in the old ways of relating—words, being equal partners in planning things, and so forth—can hamper ongoing relationships with persons with dementia. The good news is that we don't need to stay stuck in these old groves. Most important, the person we have known is still there; he or she is not lost but is having trouble expressing him- or herself in familiar ways. When caregivers are able to break through these barriers, as Michael and Marie did, both again experience the pleasure of a shared connection. Sally Callahan wrote movingly about how her mother showed her the way to a renewed and wonderful relationship:

> Since my journey I have come to believe that as my mother's defenses, which were constructed over a lifetime, weakened and eventually disappeared altogether, my defenses followed suit, at least when I was with her. Relinquishing our defenses left us free to invite and welcome our spirits, to be together through them, on their plane.

. . . It was as though we had scaled a mountain, all but the top of which had been under the cover of clouds. As we reached the top, the brilliance of the sun reflected through us, freeing our spirits. The climb had exhausted our need to protect our fragile selves. Reaching the summit through the decline of my mother's body, her spirit was freed. She made a gift of that spirit to me, soothing and comforting my grief by inviting *my* spirit to touch *hers.* By accepting her invitation, we created and experienced unconditional love. (2000, p. 244)

Have you ever peered through a kaleidoscope? Even a slight shift in the tube reveals a whole new, wonderful pattern of color. Like Sally Callahan, if we can shift our sights, whole different patterns of relating with the person with dementia can be revealed. Perhaps the person with dementia cannot verbalize that he or she really enjoyed the supper you made, but the enthusiasm and satisfaction with which he or she ate expresses thanks and appreciation.

Sometimes the words follow. This is illustrated by a vignette about Ruth. Earlier in this chapter, stories about Ruth showed that she offered her love to Abe by her radiant, smiling welcome.

Ruth returned to the day program after being away for a few weeks. Her warm smile of surprise and delight told Louise, her nurse, that Ruth remembered her. While drawing blood to test Ruth's blood sugar, Louise was absolutely astonished as Ruth emerged from the shroud of speechlessness to say, "I have missed you."

As caregivers, we are called on to balance living in the moment with planning ahead while drawing on the threads of the past. These are all necessary aspects of caregiving.

WAYS FOR CAREGIVERS TO ENTER
THE WORLD OF SOMEONE WITH DEMENTIA

With a heavy heart, Max finally admitted that he could no longer manage the amount of care that his wife, Mae, required. Max also realized that he was more fortunate than many of his fellow caregivers because he had the dedicated support and assistance of his physician in helping to find quality care for his wife. When she went into a care facility, Max completely trusted the nurses to provide care for his wife, but he still visited every day. He found these visits both reassuring and sad. He regretted that he could no longer care for his wife at home and that she no longer seemed to recognize him.

One day when he came to visit, he was alarmed when he could not find Mae in her room or in the facility's living room. He anxiously approached a group of nurses happily chatting with a new resident and asked where he could find his wife. To Max's amazement, the whole crowd burst into laughter. The new resident wiped away her tears of laughter and said, "Why sho' nuff, Max, I's be right here in front uuh' your nose!" Staff members had helped Mae with a "makeover," including a wig, as a surprise for Max. It was such a successful surprise that he didn't recognize her—but she knew him.

The nurses caring for Mae had found a charming way to bring joy to the altered lives of Mae and Max. It seems that they also offered some powerful lessons to Max and all caregivers: a hint of what it might feel like to not recognize someone near and dear when that person seems to be in a different guise. Even more to the point, many possibilities—new, unexpected, and delightful—can grow out of capturing the joy of the moment and seeing the person with dementia in a different way. I invite you to share in the thoughts which follow on ways to capture some of these joys, to live in the moment.

Celebrate You and Accept a Compliment

- You can provide the best care when you recognize and accept that you are only human—bound to make mistakes from time to time.
- Give yourself frequent pats on the back.

Please put these words on your refrigerator as a daily reminder that YOU ARE TERRIFIC! Remember that you are not superhuman; there is always more to learn, and it is understandable and even expected that you will make mistakes. Be forgiving of yourself and try instead to see missteps as opportunities for learning. It is difficult to celebrate the rich moments that you can have with the person if you are busy beating yourself up for mistakes that you have made. You are doing the very best you can at this moment. For suggestions on problem solving and finding new solutions to challenges, see Chapter 9.

Take Good Care of Yourself

- The person needs YOU.
- You must take personal time to "re-create."

Please see Chapter 1 for suggestions on care for the caregiver.

Appreciate the Nonverbal Ways in Which the Person Expresses Thanks

- The person needs to give something to others.
- You need to feel appreciated.

This topic is also covered in Chapter 1. There, a man named Bob is quoted as saying his closest friendship is with his wife, Erika. He notes how he gives Erika a difficult time but that she puts up with it; in turn, Bob realizes how fortunate he is, as "there aren't too many Erikas" (cited in Snyder, 1999, p. 86).

It is easy to grow frustrated and weary, wishing for appreciation when memory loss leads to statements such as "You never talk to me anymore" after you just had an hour-long chat. I invite you to reframe such comments as a statement of how much you are appreciated and missed when you are not there. I also invite you to "listen" for the ways beyond words that the person says "thanks." If we can get unstuck from hoping for and expecting spoken thanks, we can find appreciation and celebrate many such moments. See Chapter 1 for more suggestions on ways to listen for thanks.

Understand that Caregiving Changes the Nature of Relationships

- The person needs to be part of a caring relationship.
- You can try to accept that the relationship has changed and discover creative ways to continue to be connected and maintain trust.

What an overwhelming job—serving as the person's memory, guiding him or her through the many challenges posed by the daily routine, problem-solving on the spot because what worked yesterday is a disaster today, recalling precious past accomplishments to maintain trust and bolster bruised dignity, and planning ahead to meet future needs for both of you. The skills required in caregiving are endless, the hours are long, and the pay is nonexistent.

This job description certainly wouldn't entice you to sign on. Whatever your relationship with the person with dementia—spouse, sibling, adult child, neighbor, or friend—caregiving through the course of dementia wasn't part of the original relationship. As you know only too well, caregiving changes the entire nature of relationships. A spouse grieves for the companion and lover that once was; the sibling misses the closeness of the shared life from childhood; adult children long for the lost times when they were on the receiving end of care. These are all natural, healthy feelings. As noted in Chapter 1, dealing with such feelings and losses becomes even more challenging if the relationship was difficult before caregiving.

Persons with dementia have much more difficulty in changing ways of relating, doing, living, or being than caregivers do. In addition, persons with dementia are struggling with their own grief over deteriorating skills and independence. Adjusting to these changes is very difficult for caregivers, too. Undoubtedly, being able to be with and celebrate the person as he or she is now, neither as the caregiver wishes the person would become nor as the way the person used to be, calls on caregivers to change, stretch, and grow. However, it is in this way that we also have the greatest possibility to experience "The Joy of Caregiving." I only read excerpts from *The Joy of Sex*, but I gathered the gist of the book's message: Letting go of past constraints and future fears heightens the joy of sex. This is good advice for caregiving, too: Letting go creates the possibility of some really amazing rewards to balance the endless, difficult job requirements of caregiving.

Not all relationship changes are negative, either. In fact, many caregivers—such as Leitha Glavin, whose story was presented in the Introduction, or Ann Davidson, in her book *Alzheimer's: A Love Story* (1997)—report deeper, stronger connections as they come to truly value the time that they have with their loved one. In the following quotations, two caregivers share this experience of a deepening relationship.

When I first noticed something was different, I was angry. I thought he was having an affair. When the doctor told us he had Alzheimer's, I was angry and scared as hell. I felt trapped. I was not going to get caught in caring for a man who had never been an ideal husband.

Somehow all of those emotions turned into quiet resignation and then to love. As strange as it may seem, the last four years of our marriage have been the best. I truly love my husband and would not have missed these times, even with all the heartaches of Alzheimer's. (Mrs. W., cited in Ballard & Poer, 1999)

He has given me so much all of my life, and now he can only take. Yet his presence now, as always, provides deep comfort to my soul. Now I give to him in every way I can. I realize that my giving to him is a result of his giving to me: emotional support, love, spiritual direction, wisdom, advice and all that a daughter needs when she is maturing into a young woman. He's a wonderful man, and I like what he has produced in me. (Phyllis Thomas Immanuel, cited in Ballard & Poer, 1999)

The job requirements don't change. However, by changing how you think about caregiving—that is, expectations that you have of the person you are caring for—you can change how you feel about your job as caregiver. Here is one example of such a change in thinking.

 Abe used to be constantly frustrated that Ruth wasn't able to remember to get to the bathroom on time. He kept expecting her to "learn" this and behave as she had always done. We discussed how he needed to remind Ruth to go to the bathroom because of her poor memory. He tried this but was still frustrated—and doing a lot of laundry—because whenever he asked Ruth if she had to go to the bathroom, she said no. After much practice, Abe finally dropped his old expectations of Ruth's abilities. Instead, every 2 hours he gently took her arm, walked with her to the bathroom and stayed with her

(her attention span was so limited she wouldn't stay seated on the toilet unless Abe reminded her). As a result, instead of spending difficult hours changing Ruth's soiled clothes and doing laundry, he and Ruth enjoyed going out for supper to a local restaurant and took pride in Ruth's being dressed in her best clothing.

Free Yourself to Experience the Joy of the Moment and Capture Simple Pleasures

- The person needs to experience joy and pleasure.
- You can experience the joy to be found in the moment by capturing the simple pleasures.

I think my disease is a slow process, and Kurt helps me to enjoy everything there is to enjoy. . . . As long as one is able to maintain a relatively normal relationship in public, what does it matter if you have Alzheimer's? If I can be an ordinary human being, let me be one. (Betty, cited in Snyder, 1999, p. 125)

Then one day I fumbled into the kitchen to prepare a pot of coffee, something caught my eye through the window. It had snowed and I had truly forgotten what a beautiful sight soft, gentle snowfall could be. I eagerly but so slowly dressed and went outside to join my son, who was shoveling our driveway. As I bent down to gather a mass of those radiantly white flakes on my shovel, it seemed as though I could do nothing but marvel at their beauty. Needless to say, he did not share my enthusiasm; to him it was a job, but to me it was an experience.

Later I realized that for a short period of time, God granted me the ability to see a snowfall through the same innocent eyes of the child I once was, so many years ago. I am still here, I thought, and there will be wonders to be held in each new day; they are just different now . . . now my quality of life is feeding the dogs, looking at flowers. My husband says I am more content now than ever before! Love and dignity, those are the keys. This brings you back down to the basics in life, a smile makes you happy. (a woman in her forties with dementia, cited in Post, 2001b, pp. 28–29)

These words remind us, as discussed in the opening sections of this chapter, that by refocusing on the rainbow, instead of the rain, we can experience moments of joy, capture life's simple pleasures.

Appreciate that the Person Is Aware that He or She Is an Adult

- The person needs to be treated as a dignified adult who makes choices and decisions.
- You can find ways for the person to make choices.

As discussed at the beginning of this chapter, there is no doubt that persons with dementia retain their sense of self, their knowledge that they are an adult. An essential part of being an independent adult is making choices and decisions. Adults are used to making thousands of decisions every day: little decisions, such as when to have breakfast, or much bigger decisions, such as whether to move to a new home. Sometimes, when we have too much on our plate, making these decisions weighs heavily on us, but for the most part, we carefully guard our right to be independent and make choices. When dementia hits, making these decisions and choices becomes difficult. I am sure that you are all too familiar with responses such as "I don't know" or "You decide" when you ask "What would you like to do today?" or "What would you like for lunch?" Such responses may seem to indicate that the person no longer can or wants to make choices. This is not quite true. Like all adults, the person needs to make choices, but as dementia progresses, it becomes increasingly difficult to choose from a big range of choices. The range is too overwhelming; there are too many choices. However, making the choice more manageable (e.g., by asking "Would you like a tuna sandwich or a ham sandwich for lunch?") allows the person to make a decision and to feel in control, dignified, and respected. By searching for opportunities to offer choices and personal control in every activity, caregivers often experience greater ease in involving the person in activities.

For instance, although Alice insisted that she was bathing properly, the "nose test" let us know that she was not. She flatly refused when I offered to help her with her bath. However, when I asked if she would like her bath before or after breakfast, she replied, "After would be better."

At first, I was confused about which choices to offer, but in this situation, the choice was not between having a bath or not having a bath. Rather, it was a choice about the timing— something that Alice could in fact control and decide. Chapter 6 provides more details about offering manageable choices, and Chapter 7 gives suggestions for helping with bathing.

Celebrate the Whole Person

- The person needs to be treated as a whole person who has strengths and weaknesses.
- You can find ways to make meaningful connections, to help the person use his or her strengths to compensate for weaknesses.

Acceptance is hard to teach. In order to learn to accept other people's deficiencies, you have to first be able to accept your own. A person with Alzheimer's disease is many more things than just his or her diagnosis. Each person is a whole human being. It's important to be both sympathetic and curious and to have a real interest in discovery about who that person is. You have to be willing to be present with the person with Alzheimer's. (Betty, cited in Snyder, 1999, p. 123)

Dementia does not define the person. It is one aspect of a whole person with a rich personal history that came before the diagnosis, a history that belongs uniquely to that person until the end of his or her life. Caregivers who can reach out—who can see the glass as half full instead of half empty or the delicious doughnut instead of the hole in the middle—can celebrate the further unfolding of the person's life story. In this way, the person feels validated and affirmed as a worthwhile, dignified adult and is enabled to grow and flourish. Here is one story of how a granddaughter continues to connect.

 As she had done all her life, Anne rushed to her grandmother to share her happy news and get advice. Times and circumstances had changed a great deal for both. Anne was now an accomplished, independent professional; Gramma had dementia. Anne never let her Gramma's difficulty with words stand in the way of their relationship. Anne was bursting with joy as she told her Gramma that she was in love and was sure that the young man was going to propose. As always, Gramma celebrated with Anne, and Anne asked for advice. She asked, "What sort of ring do you think I should ask for?" Gramma replied, "Well, dear, I should think that would be up to him." Anne knew that behind the confusion of dementia, the grandmother whom she loved and counted on was still present. Anne was not disappointed by her belief in her grandmother's wisdom and found ways to maintain a connection.

Chapter 3 provides additional information about using the person's continuing abilities; Chapter 4 offers additional material on communication.

Support, Encourage, and Enable
the Person to Continue with a Familiar Lifestyle

- The person needs to be supported by the familiar rhythms of daily life.
- You can use your intimate knowledge of the person's life story and what matters most to him or her to enrich the person's life NOW.

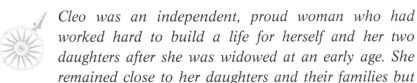 *Cleo was an independent, proud woman who had worked hard to build a life for herself and her two daughters after she was widowed at an early age. She remained close to her daughters and their families but also relished her home and her independence. When her daughter Jill began to notice some uncharacteristic forgetfulness, she gently and sensitively encouraged Cleo to get a checkup. Eventually, Cleo saw a geriatrician and was diagnosed with early-stage Alzheimer's disease. She appreciated the caring kindness with which she received this diagnosis, spoke of Alzheimer's only as her "problem," and carried on with her life. Jill and her family respected Cleo's need to continue in her own home but also kept a careful eye on her safety. Jill initiated gentle discussions about driving; with the advice of her doctor, Cleo eventually agreed that she should stop driving and sell her car. Although Jill had worked sensitively with Cleo, the whole process was naturally very painful. When the car was finally sold and Cleo had a check in her hand, she seemed to be completely befuddled. On the way to the bank, she kept asking Jill where they were going and why and how ever did she get a check for so much money. Jill was astonished at this marked loss of memory and wondered how her mother would manage her banking. Jill persisted, however, as she believed that it was important for her mother to be as involved as possible.*

As soon as Cleo entered her bank, Jill witnessed another astonishing transformation. Cleo walked confidently to the teller with

her check. After greeting the teller and exchanging pleasantries, she said that she wanted to deposit the money in her savings account. When the teller asked her account number Cleo recited it with no problem. When this transaction was complete, Cleo asked to withdraw money from her checking account, for which she also knew the number.

Cleo's story is an example of how familiar routines and settings can enable persons with dementia to continue with daily activities. Caregivers can help individuals with dementia have the best possible moments by understanding and supporting lifelong routines. This topic is detailed in Chapters 3–8.

Understand that We All Need Something to Do

- The person needs to be part of the web of life, to do things that matter.
- You can find ways to bring meaning to the person's day.

I am hungry for the life that is being taken away from me. I am a human being. I still exist. I have a family. I hunger for friendship, happiness, and the touch of a loved hand. What I ask for is that what is left of my life shall have some meaning. Give me something to die for! Help me to be strong and free until my self no longer exists. (J.T., cited in Cohen & Eisdorfer, 1986, p. 21)

As J.T. chronicles his experiences and thoughts on living with dementia, he makes a moving plea for help to continue to be able to do things, to be involved in the web of life. In the following account, Agnes makes the same plea, in actions rather than words.

Agnes, who was in the advanced stages of Alzheimer's disease, seldom sat still. Keeping her safe was a major challenge for her caregivers. Another big challenge was that although Agnes could barely speak, she spent much of her day moaning, shouting, and calling out. Nothing her caregivers tried seemed to meet her needs or lessen her distress.

Then, a summer student came to visit and discovered that the most important thing to Agnes was being able to carry on with her duties as a homemaker. Agnes's new caregiver brought in some unbreakable dishes, dish pans, tea towels, and soap and helped Agnes start washing dishes. To everyone's amazement, Agnes spent several hours carefully washing, drying, and stacking the same dishes, over and over. It was even more amazing that during this time, Agnes didn't call out or pace.

Caregivers continue to help Agnes start washing dishes. She continues to be happy and calm during this activity that is meaningful to her. Now that her need to be active—to be engaged in life—can be met, providing care is no longer such a challenge. Some symptoms of her incurable disease have been treated.

This is but one example of why having something meaningful to do is profoundly important. There is more information on the importance of and ways to support activity in Chapters 6, 7, and 8.

Support the Person's Efforts
to Do the Very Best that He or She Can

- The person needs others to understand what it means to have a damaged brain.

But I know exactly what it is like *not* to have Alzheimer's and to be normal—with a few small slip-ups every now and then, along the lines of 'that always happens to me'. Remember, I used to be free of this disease too!

And I know only too well that this is *not* what it is like now—it's totally foggy in my head, and everything takes lots of effort and control. Without a huge effort, I make slip-ups all the time, but 'normal' people don't need this amount of effort just to keep on track.

I'm OK as long as I am really trying hard, I am well rested and not at all tired. Then I could almost pass for normal. But inside me, it feels as if I am clinging to a precipice by my fingernails. It takes all my effort to stay where I am, and to lose control means 'losing it' totally. (Boden, 1998, p. 57)

- You can learn more about how dementia affects daily life.

But I always feel a bit of life being taken away when I have to back off. If you add it all up, you get a very thin path to use. (Jean, cited in Snyder, 1999, p. 65).

It is one thing to say, "Mom has Alzheimer's"; it is often an altogether different thing to understand what this means about how Mom operates on a day-to-day, moment-to-moment basis. Persons with dementia use every strength, every resource, especially social skills, to try to be as normal as possible. This is indeed a tremendous strength that should be supported. Yet, because we can't see inside the brain and really understand the damage that has taken place, it is easy to be fooled into thinking that persons with dementia are more capable than they really are. This can lead to unrealistic expectations on the caregiver's part and cause frustration for both parties, as shown in the following example.

Susie calls out, "Mom, I'm going to volunteer at church for a little while."
Mom replies, "That's fine, dear."
Susie goes to the church, relieved that her mom is settled happily at home. A short time later, the neighbor arrives with

Susie's mother, who is greatly relieved to see her daughter. Susie's mother tearfully says, "Oh, thank goodness you are here. I had no idea where you were."

Because Susie's mother seemed to understand what was said, Susie assumed that this information would stick. What Susie couldn't see was the severe damage to her mother's brain, which made it impossible for Susie's mother to hold on to this information. She understood and remembered just for that moment; the next moment, it was gone and panic set in. Susie's mother was trying her best to cope, but she didn't have the brain capacity to manage it.

As noted previously, approximately 80% of the brain damage has already happened by the time that the first symptoms of dementia appear (Cummings, 1993). This is a staggering fact, but it does let us know that persons with dementia are trying as hard as they can to use the reduced brain capacity available to them. Caregivers should balance encouragement and support for these efforts with realistic expectations.

It can be especially challenging to understand how the person can pull out all of the stops to do something functional, such as hosting a friend, and then immediately do something dysfunctional. In such circumstances, it is easy to believe that the person is being difficult on purpose. At these times, it is especially important to remember that the person is trying his or her best to function with a damaged brain. Understanding the reasons for these puzzling and frustrating behaviors can help caregivers be more patient and devise creative solutions. Chapter 9 provides more on this approach to problem solving.

Respond to the Emotional Message in What Seems to Be Confused Speech

- The person needs to have his or her feelings understood and to be reassured by trusting relationships.
- You can listen for the feeling in what the person is saying.

Mary has been a long-term care resident for several years. She needs help to get washed and dressed. Mary has many other needs about which she has difficulty telling her care-givers. In one area, however, her need is absolutely clear: She needs to find her husband Joe. She repeatedly asks every person she sees if he or she has seen Joe. Because Joe has been dead for sev-eral years, staff members find this question difficult to answer. Each person answers according to what he or she thinks is right. Some say, "He is dead," which, of course, Mary finds very upsetting and doesn't believe for a minute. Others try to appease her, saying, "Oh, he's busy now; he'll be along later," but this doesn't lessen Mary's distress because he never does come along. As a result, Mary keeps asking and searching, only sure that she really needs Joe.

Finally, Mary's doctor decided to seek a solution to this recur-ring problem. He sat Mary down for a compassionate but logical talk. It went something like this:

"Now, Mary, you know that Joe had a bad heart don't you?"

"Mmhhm," said Mary.

"I gave him a lot of pills and that helped for a while. But after a time, Joe got so sick that we had to take him to the hospital. The ambulance came. Do you remember that Mary?"

"Mm—yes," Mary replied sadly.

"And, Mary, we worked really hard, but we just couldn't save Joe. He died at the hospital."

Mary became tearful, saying," Oh, dear, no one ever told me that before."

The doctor sat and comforted her for a while, and Mary seemed to brighten up just a little. Then the doctor left, feeling quite sat-isfied that he had finally solved this long-standing problem. A few minutes later, someone else walked by and overheard Mary, say-ing, "Hmpf, I guess he doesn't know where Joe is either."

As Mary's caregivers experienced, responding to seemingly confused speech is one of the more difficult parts of living in the moment with the person who has dementia. Every fiber of reason within us, as well as our past relationship with the person, cries out to argue with such obviously incorrect thoughts and statements. Instead, we can strive to realize that the person is making a very powerful "I" statement, letting us know what he or she is experiencing and feeling at that moment.

Every aspect of life for persons with dementia is colored by a memory that gets steadily worse. Initially, they may sometimes be confused about basic information, such as where they live or the name of their spouse or child. As the disease progresses, this confusion becomes increasingly worse, and it is common for them to search for long-dead loved ones, home, the office, or their children. **When this happens, living in the moment means entering into the emotional world, the feeling and need, that is expressed in this searching and longing.** Mary, for instance, undoubtedly missed her husband and his love and companionship. She needed to talk about him, to feel loved and cared for, to be reassured that she could trust those around her to meet her needs. Chapter 4 addresses this topic in depth, but let's consider one more example: searching for one's mother. When do we most want Mom? We want her when we hurt, when we are frightened, when we need someone to trust absolutely, when we need someone to take care of us, and, above all else, when we need someone to love us no matter what. Even as grown adults who may have children, most of us can recall a painful time when we really needed the special care and nurturing that only Mom can offer.

Is there anything more frightening, more painful, more cause for reassurance and loving than struggling to get through each day with the failing memory and deteriorating skills that come with dementia? Caregivers can enter into that emotional moment, that emotional need, by reassuring the person that he or she is loved and cared for, that he or she can trust you. This can be done with words or—even more powerfully—with actions, such as a hug (if appropriate), a touch on the arm, or time spent with the person doing what he or she finds especially pleasurable (e.g., singing a favorite song, getting a snack). Another way of entering the previously described moment and providing reassurance is to talk about the person's mother and agree that he or she must miss her very much.

Entering the moment with the person in this way is quite different from some responses that were suggested or favored in the past. On the one hand, there is the outmoded and unsuccessful Reality Orientation approach (Bowlby, 1993). In this approach, the response is to directly confront the person with the facts, such as saying, "Your mother has been dead for 20 years." Because this is not the person's reality, he or she won't believe you and will be shocked, grief stricken, or furious. For example, even though Mary's doctor presented the news of Joe's death in a compassionate and logical manner, Mary rejected the doctor's reality for her own.

On the other hand, some suggest that it is best to go along with misperceptions by saying something such as "Your mother is busy getting supper; she will come to see you later." You know this will never happen, eventually the person knows it won't happen, and the fear and the need for Mom remains. Neither this sort of deception, nor encouraging the person to live under false hope, nor confronting the person with a harsh reality is living in the moment with the person with dementia. Instead, caregivers are called on to enter into the emotional world—the emotional need that the person is expressing at that moment. For example, the person who is searching for his or her mother needs to be loved, supported, cared for, helped to feel better. In this case, you can best address such needs by providing reassurance that the person is loved and cared for now, by offering verbal and physical reassurance (e.g., hugs). The person may also need to recall and talk about his or her mother. Caregivers can acknowledge the person's longing for his or her mother by saying things like, "Your mother was a wonderful person; you must miss her very much." This approach acknowledges the need without confronting the person directly with the harsh reality that his or her mother is dead.

Understand that the Person Does Use Reasoning

- The person needs to try to make sense out of a confusing world.
- You can let go of trying to talk or reason the person into something.

When I checked Alice's prescription bottles, I realized that she was not taking her pills properly, which of course really concerned me. Being new at caregiving, I presented her with her evening pills, saying that she hadn't been taking them properly. I was flabbergasted when Alice shouted angrily, "I was the registered nurse! Of course I know when to take my pills!" and threw the pills across the room. I retreated from this big mistake. A few days later, I presented her with the gift of a filled pill minder and quietly took away all of the pill bottles.

"You might as well save your breath to cool your porridge."

This thought, voiced by my grandmothers, didn't come to mind when I was dealing with Alice's pills. Now, I often think of it when it comes to trying to persuade, reason with, or sometimes even suggest to a person with dementia that his or her understanding of a particular situation is wrong. There really is no point in doing so; you might as well save your energy. A wise caregiver once said to me, "I won my last argument with Sam before he got Alzheimer's."

The world to someone with memory loss must seem to be constantly changing—confusing, frightening, and totally unpredictable. Because we all need to feel anchored and secure about some things, the person with memory loss uses his or her unique logic (it may not be your logic, but it is still logic) to fasten on to a few constants that must be forever true. For Mary, this constant was that Joe was always there when she needed him. For others, this constant may be a parent or going home. One person's logic may cause him to think that his wife is having an affair. He needs her 24 hours a day and she is not always there; the only possible "reason" for her not being there when he needs her so much is that she is having an affair. Another person's logic may cause her to believe that someone must be taking things because she never misplaced things. As everything else falls about the person in disarray, this one thing must be true. The person is trying his or her best to make sense of what must be a very confusing world. Chapter 9 presents more on responding to these challenges.

Realize that the Person
Can Only Be Who He or She Is at this Very Moment

- The person needs to be accepted for who he or she is now.
- You can learn to appreciate the person's present qualities.

In shaky but still decipherable handwriting, Frank spontaneously wrote "I love Emily" as his sentence on the mental status test. This testimony of love and affection moved me deeply. Here was a man who couldn't begin to tell me his own name, his wife's name, the date, or the answer to any of the standard orientation questions. Obviously, Frank had profound impairments. But in matters of the heart, he clearly had a deep knowledge and awareness. Emily, Frank's wife, had grown able to cherish these heart expressions; they gave her strength during her caregiving days. They also added to her resolve to find ways to care for Frank at home for as long as possible, even though it was very different from how they had both imagined spending their retirement years.

Appreciate that Living Each Day with Dementia Is Difficult

- The person needs others who understand what he or she is going through.
- You can actively imagine, "What if this was me?" and encourage the person to join a support group.

On the one hand, some people are angry about having dementia and aren't interested in spending time with others who have it:

A friend of mine gave me a book on a woman who was writing about Alzheimer's and how gloriously, wonderfully she was handling her disease. I hated that book. I wouldn't consider behaving as well as she did. I guess there are people out there handling this marvelously. But it just isn't me. I want to cry and whine and kick! Not as ladylike, I must admit. There is a little fighting, but mostly it's whining. It's mostly, "Damn it! This is terrible! This shouldn't happen!" Then of course other words come in. There is my goody-goody voice going all the time that says, "There are a lot of things that are terrible, Jean. A lot of people are very sick with terrible things and have real physical pain." You know, this whole story. And then I think, "Stop it! That has nothing to do with me. I have Alzheimer's and I don't like it!"

I'm angry. I'm angry that anybody has it. (Jean, cited in Snyder, 1999, p. 71)

On the other hand, it makes a difference if others understand something about what it is like to have dementia:

It's very different if you know that you are talking with someone who is familiar with the disease; there is a safety net when you talk with people who understand and care about your condition—people who don't step on your feelings or minimize your problem. (Betty, cited in Snyder, 1999, p. 120)

You can never really understand
until you walk a mile in someone else's shoes.

The preceding words are the title to a poem that Leitha Glavin, the wise caregiver whose story was presented in the Introduction, taped to her refrigerator. She keeps it there to remind her what her husband is going through, to try to experience each moment as he lives it with dementia.

Listening to the voices, spoken and unspoken, of persons with dementia can help us to better walk a mile in their shoes. Like all of us, sometimes these voices express joy, sometimes they express fear, sometimes they express sorrow and the need to grieve for the losses they are experiencing. Some of these voices can be found in the books listed in Appendix B. Here is the voice of Betty, asking for understanding:

I think the most urgent issue for everyone is to learn the whole business of acceptance. I've seen too many health care professionals who have never made it to that phase. . . . But they don't really accept the significance of the illness for people. They know the diagnosis, but they don't take the time to find out what it truly means for that person. (Betty, cited in Snyder, 1999, p. 123)

Although it was too long in coming, support groups for persons with dementia are an excellent way for persons in the early stages to find support and understanding in the company of their peers.

There are also some helpful on-line chat groups. Please see the resources in Appendix B at the end of the book for information on finding a support group for persons with dementia.

Realize that Time Can Dissolve and a Trigger Can Cause the Person to Reenter an Old Experience

- The person needs to recall past experiences, savor the good feelings, and have someone who understands the not-so-good ones.
- You can help the person recall past successes and cope with past fears.

Eva was a proud member of the processional and the platform party for graduation from the school program at Sunset Lodge. She sat primly in her chair, head held high, eyes bright and attentive, legs decorously crossed at the ankles. She was quite unrecognizable from the distressed figure that paced the corridors of the special care unit. Because Eva was a retired teacher, school and graduation triggered a return to this familiar way of behaving.

Careful attention to the social and physical environment (see Chapter 5) and structuring the day (see Chapters 6, 7, and 8) can be used to trigger old patterns. Of even more importance, reminders of past experiences (i.e., reminiscing) take the person back to the experience as well as the feelings of accomplishment and worth he or she had at the time. Another example follows.

Myrtle was very upset. She had broken her hip. She was in pain and in a hospital separated from her family and familiar routines. Through a flood of tears, she asked me if I ever wondered why we were put on this earth. Before I could gather a response to this difficult question, she reached over and picked up a small album of family photos and began to flip through the pages. A smile appeared through the tears and she began to tell me who all of these special people were.

For persons with dementia, who often experience failure and frustration, recalling past accomplishments and family or friends can be a great healer. For more details on using reminiscence see Chapter 6.

The word *trigger* was used in the preceding vignettes to describe ways that reminders of past experiences can help the person to recall past successes. However, the term *triggers* is usually used to describe events or circumstances that lead the person with dementia to become distressed or upset. In these cases, the person is recalling past traumatic events. By learning about and avoiding these negative triggers, caregivers can often avoid the distress, as shown in the following example.

 Shower time was very stressful for Jim and his caregivers. He fought against the caregivers, shrieking in terror and desperately flailing all his limbs. When his caregivers learned that Jim's ship had gone down during World War II, they understood why he was so distressed. The rushing water instantly took Jim back to that terrible past event. When caregivers used other bathing methods for Jim (e.g., bathtub, sponge bath), everyone was happier.

Negative triggers can dissolve the years and cause the person to feel as though he or she is back in a past trauma. For Jim, it was the shower water rushing at him. Other examples include being resident in a concentration camp; experiencing sexual or physical abuse; or experiencing a disaster such as a fire, flood, or war. Although the person may live for years without seeming to be troubled by these experiences, memory loss can cause the person to reenter the past trauma. It is vital that family caregivers make the person's story known to other caregivers. In this way, terrible fear, such as what Jim experienced, can be avoided and other less dramatic but still puzzling responses can be understood. In some cases, such as childhood sexual abuse, it is possible that no one knows about the person's experience. If the person becomes fearful and distressed during personal care activities, this might be a clue to a history of abuse.

Stress causes most of us to go back to well-learned ways of coping or responding, even if the methods aren't always ideal. For example, when I am upset or very tired, I seek comfort in favorite—and often unhealthy—foods. I know that this is only a temporary fix, that I need to determine why I am upset, and that I will later regret the bloated feeling and the extra pounds. But these very rational counterarguments sometimes don't cut it, and I go for the hidden stash of chocolate chips anyway.

I believe that few situations are more stressful than losing your memory and your ability to function as an adult. So it is a small wonder that the person with dementia, who can't even produce all of those well-rehearsed counterarguments, sometimes goes back to old behaviors. Here is one example.

Louise had not smoked for 30 years, but when she woke up disoriented in the night she went straight to a hidden pack of cigarettes and lit up. Her caregiver had no success in persuading Louise that she no longer smoked.

Conversely, helping the person to continue with lifelong positive stress relievers, such as walking or playing music, can be a boon.

Appreciate that Nobody Likes to Fail

- The person needs to have successful experiences.
- You can arrange the person's environment to facilitate success.

See Chapters 5–8 for details on these topics.

Understand that the Person May Find Planning and Problem Solving Difficult

- The person may need help with problem solving, but he or she also needs to be consulted for decisions.
- You can assist with problem solving and planning by understanding the person's history, strengths, and weaknesses.

In my early days as a caregiver, I was determined that Alice should and could learn her new address. Several frustrating sessions were spent going over the address, pointing to the street sign outside her window, and looking at the address on the identification card in her wallet. Yet, when I'd ask her to recite her address a few hours later, she couldn't do it. Finally, I got the point and took compensatory steps: We presented her with a lovely necklace that was engraved with her name and address and ensured that her address was available at all possible locations (e.g., posted near the telephone, written down and tucked in various places in her purse).

I had become stuck in thinking there was only one way to solve the problem of Alice not knowing her address. When I kept trying to solve the problem in this way, we were both frustrated. However, when I thought about other approaches that accounted for both her current abilities and lifelong habits and values, I was able to find a successful solution. Chapter 9 provides more details on creative problem solving.

Appreciate that the Person Can Learn

- The person needs to learn in ways other than verbal instruction.
- You can foster other ways of learning (e.g., movement).

The sequel to Alice's address story came a few days later. Alice astonished me when she announced that she was going to the store and then walked, by herself, from her new apartment (in a new city) to the grocery store and back. I had not even been trying to teach this skill, but after a few walks with us, Alice was able to follow this route on her own. Alice had a great deal of trouble verbally reciting her new address, but her motor memory was excellent. This was still true a couple of years later, when Alice was no longer able to stay in her apartment and moved to a nursing home. A month or so after this move, my jaw dropped when Alice appeared at my door. As impaired as she was in some ways, she had learned the two-block route from the nursing home to my house!

Chapter 3 gives more information on using strengths.

Be Patient with Yourself
and the Person Who Has Dementia

- The person needs others to understand that he or she is trying hard to manage and to express needs.
- You can try to understand that the person is not being difficult on purpose.

As Alice's story shows, there will be caregiving challenges because the person has a brain disease that can make doing things difficult.

Formerly a registered nurse, Alice felt back in her element when she entered into a long-term care facility. In fact, she thought she was back at work. She worked hard every day to take care of "her patient" (her roommate), who was a very understanding person. When another nurse had the nerve to give pills to Alice's patient, Alice got angry. A heated argument followed. When the nurse insisted that Alice did not have a patient, Alice hit the nurse. This behavior was quite a contrast to "pleasant nurse Alice," who helped with the medications by pushing the cart and pouring the water.

In the preceding illustration, Alice was back in a nursing setting and was trying her best to use her nursing skills. She needed to feel useful and involved. Caregivers who could understand this need and sought Alice's help experienced fewer challenges in providing care. There is often a solution to challenging behavior if caregivers can reframe how they think about the situation, try to understand the reasons behind the person's behavior, and realize that the person is trying to cope and express what he or she needs. There is much more in Chapter 9 regarding challenges in care.

CONCLUSION

Alice's attempts to continue to use her nursing skills were an expression of an aspect of her earlier life that continued to be very important to her in the present moment. Caregivers who are able to enter that moment and find ways to help persons with dementia express needs have discovered some of the joys of caregiving. In this chapter we have heard, through both the spoken voices and the actions of persons with dementia, something about what it is like to live in the moment.

Caregivers are invited to use these insights and guidelines to enter into the moment with persons with dementia, to capture the richness of that moment. The diagnostic and medical information in Chapter 3 will illuminate the reasons why persons with dementia primarily live in the moment.

3

Basic Information on Dementia

The following account describes how the relationships of and expectations for M. Wasserman, who was diagnosed with Alzheimer's disease at age 57, were shaped by symptoms he didn't yet have:

> His least and every move was watched intently by someone not in order to see what was right about it but only to wait for him to do something wrong. With the naming of his illness, his life had suddenly become a negative reversal in which only the shaded areas were observed, with all the positive images disregarded as exceptions to the darkness of his impending situation. (Buchanan, 1989, p. 43)

The following account shows another view:

> There are things I wish I could do, but on the other side, there are still things that I can do and I plan to hold on to them as long as I possibly can. Laughing is absolutely wonderful. A sense of humor is probably the most valuable

The information in this chapter is based on the following sources: Cummings (2000); Dodee (2000); Emery and Oxman (2003); Gauthier (1999); Gillick (1997); Huang, Svenson, and Lindsay (1994); Peterson, Mohs, Carli, and Galasko (2000); Snowdon (2001); St. George-Hyslop (2000); Swanberg and Cummings (2001); Weintraub (2003); and Wilcock, Bucks, and Rockwood (1999).

thing that you can have when you have Alzheimer's.
(Henderson & Andrews, 1998, p. 14)

OVERVIEW OF DEMENTIA

The symptoms of dementia are part of a global, progressive, cognitive impairment that is severe enough to interfere with social, occupational, and/or daily functioning. The cognitive deterioration associated with dementia is acquired later in life; it is not present since birth. Dementia itself is neither a disease nor a diagnosis but a syndrome, a descriptive term for a collection of symptoms that result from diseases of the brain. It may be helpful to think of *dementia* as a general category. Within the large category of soup, for example, there are many varieties—vegetable, mushroom, tomato and so forth. Similarly, within the general category of dementia, there are many different types, such as Alzheimer's disease, frontotemporal dementia, and multi-infarct dementia. Alzheimer's disease, sometimes called "AD," is the most common of more than 70 disorders that cause dementia. Alzheimer's is a disease of the brain that has primarily behavioral symptoms until its later stages.

Although there are important differences in symptoms and progression between Alzheimer's disease and the many other forms of dementia, the dementias are more alike than they are different. The differences between the various forms of dementia in terms of day-to-day functioning and coping strategies are more marked in the early stages. In the middle and later stages, the similarities between the types of dementia are the main consideration for guiding daily care. For this reason, this book uses the general term *dementia*. However, distinguishing between the different types of dementia can be critical in determining appropriate medical treatment and managing particular symptoms. A qualified medical practitioner determines the type of dementia as part of the assessment and diagnostic process. The most common types of atypical dementias are discussed at the end of this section. Distinguishing the dementias from each other is difficult. This task is further complicated by the fact that more than one type of dementia (e.g., Alzheimer's disease and frontotemporal dementia) may occur in the same person.

In many ways, our brain defines us; therefore, the effects of dementia are devastating and widespread. **However, caregivers must remember that a person is much more than a disease or diagnosis.** Each person is unique, and each person's experience of dementia is unique. Furthermore, many of the skills and habits acquired during a lifetime persist, despite the losses due to brain damage. The information in this chapter is intended to provide you with some basic information about the disease process; the ways in which this process is played out in the life of the person who you are caring for are highly individual.

David Snowdon, who studied the aging process in a community of almost 700 teaching nuns, summed up his research and personal experience in the following way:

> The Nun Study's real eye-opening findings, however, are the ones that add to the evidence that Alzheimer's is not a yes/no disease. Rather, it is a process—one that evolves over decades and interacts with many other factors. We have shown dramatically how pathology can mislead. Sister Bernadette had widespread damage and no symptoms, and our data now tell us that about of a third of the sisters in stages V and VI have shared her "escapee" fate. And then, there is Sister Maria, who had obvious symptoms and only modest damage. And finally, there is Sister Rose, the cen-

tenarian who taught us what may indeed be the Nun Study's most amazing lesson: Alzheimer's disease is not an inevitable consequence of aging. (2001, p. 100)

Bob Simpson, who has early Alzheimer's, said,

I am not invisible. I am not contagious. Or breakable. Or dangerous. I am the same person. Maybe I am a little different, but I am not just "Bob with Alzheimer's," I am Bob. And I am an adult. Don't treat me like a child. (cited in Simpson & Simpson, 1999, p. 137)

Definition of Dementia

Dementia describes a collection of symptoms. These symptoms are part of a large picture of numerous problems with memory and thinking. The problems worsen over time and are severe enough to cause difficulty with normal, daily activities. The formal definition of dementia has three parts:

1. A decline in cognitive ability
2. Widespread cognitive problems, which include memory problems and at least one of the following:
   - Problems with abstract thinking
   - Problems with judgment
   - Problems with speaking and understanding what others are saying
   - Problems with complicated activities (e.g., writing a check, driving a car)
   - Difficulty recognizing people or things
   - Difficulty drawing or building things
   - Personality changes
3. Being awake and alert as compared with exhibiting intermittent drowsiness

It is important to note that the person who "fades in and out" of confusion may be experiencing delirium. This can be caused by an acute physical illness (e.g., pneumonia), an imbalance in the body chemistry, or other factors and is reversible over time. However, it may take as long as 6 months after the cause is treated for the symptoms of delirium to fade. (If the person also has dementia, the brain is so fragile that the person may never return to the previous level of mental functioning.) It is essential that caregivers get immediate medical attention if they notice a sudden increase in confusion or decrease in function. Older people who have mental and/or physical frailties commonly experience reduced mental function, such as confusion, instead of the more usual symptoms of a physical illness, such as an infection. This occurs because of the loss of brain cells that happens with normal aging. When older persons who are frail become ill or undergo stress (e.g., surgery), they have less brain reserve to cope with the illness. The brain tends to sacrifice mental functioning to focus existing brain reserve on physical healing.

It is important to remember that dementia is NOT

- Part of normal aging
- Irreversible—approximately 3% of the causes of dementia (e.g., sensory deprivation; vitamin deficiency; alcoholism; a brain tumor; drug reactions; hypothermia; depression; a hormone, electrolyte, or thyroid imbalance) are treatable; furthermore, the treatment of other diseases (e.g., diabetes; high blood pressure; normal pressure hydrocephalus, or extra fluid around the brain and spinal cord, which is sometimes treatable) or an infection can sometimes improve cognitive functioning.

- Universal—not every person with dementia has every symptom
- Unilateral—for a particular individual, some symptoms may be severe and others barely noticeable
- Consistent—at one time of the day or week, the symptoms may be present; at another time, they may be absent

Also, although certain common characteristics describe the syndrome of dementia, there is no one description of a typical person with dementia. Each person is unique, with the severity and range of symptoms depending on many factors:

- The cause of the dementia
- The stage of the disease
- Preexisting lifestyle and personality factors
- Environmental supports
- Social supports
- The presence of other diseases (e.g., Parkinson's disease, heart disease) or an acute infection
- The area of the brain affected
- The level of fatigue or stress

Types of Dementia

Multi-infarct Dementia

For many years, researchers believed that 15%–20% of the cases of dementia were caused by multi-infarct dementia, which is sometimes called vascular dementia. This is a series of small, silent strokes (i.e., with no lasting physical symptoms) and used to be referred to as "senility due to hardening of the arteries." Persons with multi-infarct dementia have much the same symptoms as persons with Alzheimer's disease. However, the changes in skills and behavior usually happen in a more step-like fashion, compared with the gradual changes of Alzheimer's disease.

Research suggests that cases of pure multi-infarct dementia or vascular dementia are relatively rare (Snowdon, 2001). For example, participants in the Nun Study agreed to a brain autopsy at death; these autopsies showed that only 2.5 of the 118 persons with dementia had true vascular dementia. Furthermore, there is strong evidence that small strokes can trigger the symptoms of Alzheimer's disease. The long-held view that 20% of cases have a combination of Alzheimer's disease and multi-infarct dementia has been called into question. It is not a matter of having two separate causes; rather, it seems to be a matter of a complex interrelationship.

Atypical Dementia

The remaining 10%–15% of the cases of dementia are due to the potentially reversible causes previously described (accounting for approximately 3% or less of cases) and other diseases for which dementia is a primary or secondary feature of the disease. Diseases for which dementia is a primary feature are often referred to as the atypical dementias. Examples include dementia with Lewy bodies disease, frontotemporal dementia, Creutzfeldt-Jakob disease, or dementia as a secondary feature of a disease (e.g., Huntington's disease, Parkinson's disease, multiple sclerosis, AIDS).

Dementia with Lewy bodies, or DLB, is a form of dementia that is being increasingly recognized, although it is difficult to distinguish from Alzheimer's disease without an autopsy. However, it is important to make the distinction because of the extreme negative reaction of persons with Lewy body disease to neuroleptic drugs but the very positive response to anti-dementia drugs. The occurrence of visual hallucinations and agnosia (loss of the ability to interpret sensory stimuli) early on are two key clinical markers of dementia with Lewy bodies.

Frontotemporal dementia, or FTD, is sometimes referred to as *progressive comportmental dysfunction* and includes diseases such as Pick's disease. It is increasingly recognized by physicians and may account for as many as 10% of the cases of dementia. Persons with frontotemporal dementia typically experience problems with higher or executive functions (e.g., problem solving, planning, judgment, reasoning, social behavior) before memory loss. In some cases where the frontal lobe is affected, there may be a disinhibition of social control, which can lead to inappropriate communication or sexual behavior. Persons with frontotemporal dementia often appear apathetic and disinterested and have a great deal of difficulty organizing daily activities and paying attention.

Caregivers can support the person by providing organizational strategies that work for the person—perhaps a calendar, a list of things to do, or electronic reminders (e.g., watches or pill boxes that beep)—providing concrete directions for things to do to overcome problems with motivation, and planning ahead to avoid potentially embarrassing situations. One daughter caregiver said that her usually quiet mother became very outgoing and flamboyant when she developed frontotemporal dementia. She would talk to strangers in the mall, ask strangers personal questions, and be very talkative in restaurants. This caregiver decided to go with the flow unless there was a dangerous situation. She took a light-hearted approach, saying things such as "We are just out for fun today" and only redirecting her mother if others became upset. Another caregiver reported that she has learned not to take her husband's lack of emotion personally and not to get into arguments about small issues.

Some people have a form dementia that particularly affects language, resulting in primary progressive aphasia (the gradual loss of language abilities). People with this symptom can benefit in particular from Chapter 4's suggestions on communication. These strategies need to be used earlier with these individuals. Persons with another atypical dementia that affects primarily visual function (progressive visuospatial dysfunction) may particularly benefit from the environmental suggestions in Chapter 5.

Alzheimer's Disease

Alzheimer's disease was first described in 1906 by Dr. Alois Alzheimer. This first case involved Auguste D., a woman in her fifties who had the classical symptoms of dementia. For many years, Alzheimer's disease was thought to be a rare disease with onset before the age of 65 (presenile dementia). Dementia with onset after age 65 (senile dementia) was thought to be unrelated and due either to aging or arteriosclerotic disease (hardening of the arteries). For-tunately, this classification and the understanding of Alzheimer's disease have been greatly altered. Work begun in the 1960s has clearly established that

- Dementia of any type is not caused by "normal aging."
- Arteriosclerotic changes alone account for fewer than 20% of the cases of dementia.

Initially, it was thought that there was no difference—in either the pathological changes in the brain or the behavioral symptoms in Alzheimer's disease—with onset before and after age 65. However, more recent evidence suggests that there are significant differences; persons with early onset often experience a more rapid progression of symptoms and have increased language disturbances, among other differences (Emery & Oxman, 2003). Although Dr. Alzheimer identified the neurological changes of Alzheimer's disease in the early 1900s, Alzheimer's was not recognized as a major disease of aging until the late 1900s. The time that elapsed from the first identification of Alzheimer's disease until it became recognized as a major public health problem is most unfortunate. First, major research efforts regarding the cause, cure, and treatment of Alzheimer's disease were only undertaken when it became clear that it was a relatively common disease. Second, the system of classifying dementia into presenile and senile dementia contributed to a widespread and harmful misunderstanding that dementia, and particularly memory loss, is a normal part of aging.

The term *senility* has been widely and incorrectly used to describe dementia and/or confusion and memory loss among older people. In fact, *senile* simply means "old" or "aging." If an aging person becomes forgetful or shows other signs of dementia, it is NOT normal aging but a signal for a thorough investigation into the cause.

Alzheimer's disease is a disease of the brain. Because of the disease, over time, the basic brain cells (neurons) become less able to do their work. To understand what happens in the brain, it is important to understand what neurons are like. Figure 1 illustrates a healthy neuron.

Coming from the central part of the neuron are many fine root hairs, called *dendrites*. Dendrites make it possible for the brain to send messages from one part of the brain to another and to the rest of the body. The ends of these billions of dendrites in our brain communicate with each other because of chemical changes in the tiny spaces, or *synapses*, between the ends of dendrites.

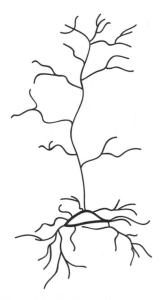

Figure 1. A healthy neuron.

It might be helpful to think of the whole brain as an electrical wiring system. Signals are carried over the lines and across the gaps in the lines because of chemical changes using chemicals found only in the brain, called *neurotransmitters*. This complex system works wonderfully when the brain is healthy. Although thousands of neurons die per day as we age (in fact, starting in our twenties), the brain still serves us very well. This is because we are so well supplied with neurons. There are as many as all of the stars in the Milky Way—more than 100 billion! Each of these neurons can have as many as 15,000 synapses or connections (Kolb & Whishaw, 1990). The brain does shrink, or *atrophy*, because of the loss of neurons during normal aging. However, it is very important to realize that because the brain has such a huge reserve of neurons and even more dendrites, this shrinkage by itself does not make a major difference in the way the brain works or in our daily functioning. In fact, it is now understood that with stimulation from involvement in mental and physical activities, dendrites continue to grow and form new connections well into old age (Diamond & Hopson, 1999).

Again, changes in mental ability or memory that cause significant problems in daily living are not part of normal aging. The brain changes that occur during Alzheimer's disease do cause major changes in mental ability and memory. There are three main changes in the brain that are caused by Alzheimer's disease:

1. There are deposits of discarded cell material outside of the neuron. These are called *senile plaques* and are the key pathological feature of Alzheimer's disease.

2. There are tangled growths within the neurons, which are much thicker and coarser than normal. These growths are called *neurofibrillary tangles*.

3. More neurons die and more dendrites are lost than in normal aging, which means that the shrinkage of the brain (atrophy) is much greater than in normal aging.

These changes in the brain happen gradually, but as the damage to the brain increases, the person has a harder time doing things in the usual way. This highlights a very important point about Alzheimer's disease: It is a disease of the brain, but most of the symptoms, especially in the early and middle stages, are changes in behavior. It is important to remember that these changes in behavior are a part of the disease and not a deliberate attempt on the person's part to be difficult. It is also important to appreciate that these changes only happen in certain parts of the brain and the amount of damage in certain areas of the brain can be quite different for different people. See Figure 2 for a quick reference on symptoms.

MAKING A DIAGNOSIS

It is essential to go to a qualified physician for a thorough assessment as soon as memory problems that interfere with normal daily living occur. Sometimes people fail to recognize that these symptoms indicate that something is wrong. They may mistakenly assume that such behavior is a normal part of aging—but, as noted previously, it isn't. It is also possible that symptoms may develop gradually and go unnoticed for a long time.

A diagnosis helps persons with dementia and their family members understand some of the changes and challenges that they are experiencing. Understanding leads to better relationships and an enhanced ability to make the most of each day. Caregivers can begin to acquire the skills that will be needed to help them and the person maintain an optimal quality of life. Available drug treatments also require a diagnosis. When a diagnosis has been made, the person may even be eligible (if he or she chooses) to participate in research studies and drug trials. Bob Simpson commented as follows:

> "Get a diagnosis," is the first thing I would say to those who suspect they have Alzheimer's. Then tell people. Don't try to hide it. When you feel anxious, share the feeling. Say you have Alzheimer's—people will be helpful. It takes the pressure off of you. I haven't had many bad experiences.
>
> Some people will be bothered, but most will be helpful; they may even warm toward you. Just say, for instance, "I have Alzheimer's, so I can't remember," or "I can't take too many directions," or "I'm tired now, and I have to rest."
>
> You get to know the people you can count on and those who stay away. They are embarrassed. People stay away from Alzheimer's patients if you are not open, because they don't know what to do with you. You get more isolated if you're not honest!

Alzheimer's Disease: 10 Warning Signs

1. Memory loss that affects day-to-day function

   It's normal to occasionally forget appointments, colleagues' names, or a friend's telephone number and then remember this information later. A person with Alzheimer's disease may forget things more often and not remember them later, especially things that have happened more recently.

2. Difficulty performing familiar tasks

   Busy people can be so distracted from time to time that they may leave the carrots on the stove and only remember to serve them at the end of a meal. A person with Alzheimer's disease may have trouble with tasks that have been familiar to them all of their lives, such as preparing a meal.

3. Problems with language

   Everyone has trouble finding the right word sometimes, but a person with Alzheimer's disease may forget simple words or substitute words, making his or her sentences difficult to understand.

4. Disorientation of time and place

   It's normal to forget the day of the week or your destination— for a moment. But a person with Alzheimer's disease can become lost on his or her own street, not knowing how he or she got there or how to get home.

5. Poor or decreased judgment

   People may sometimes put off going to a doctor if they have an infection, but they eventually seek medical attention. A person with Alzheimer's disease may have decreased judgment and may not recognize a medical problem that needs attention. Or he or she may dress inappropriately, wearing heavy clothing on a hot day.

6. Problems with abstract thinking

   From time to time, people may have difficulty with tasks that require abstract thinking, such as balancing a checkbook. Someone with Alzheimer's disease may have significant difficulties with such tasks—for example, not recognizing what the numbers in a checkbook mean.

7. Misplacing things

Anyone can temporarily misplace a wallet or keys. A person with Alzheimer's disease may put things in inappropriate places—for example, an iron in the freezer or a wristwatch in the sugar bowl.

8. Changes in mood or behavior

Everyone becomes sad or moody from time to time. Someone with Alzheimer's disease can exhibit rapid mood swings—from being calm, to shedding tears, to displaying anger—for no apparent reason.

9. Changes in personality

People's personalities can change somewhat with age. But a person with Alzheimer's disease can change dramatically, becoming extremely confused, suspicious, or withdrawn. Changes may also include apathy, fearfulness, or acting out of character.

10. Loss of initiative

It's normal to tire of housework, business activities, or social obligations, but most people regain their initiative. A person with Alzheimer's disease may become very passive and require cues and prompting to become involved.

Figure 2. Symptoms of Alzheimer's disease. (From Alzheimer Society of Canada. [2004]. *Alzheimer's disease: 10 warning signs.* Retrieved February 20, 2004, from http://www.alzheimer .ca/english/disease/warningsigns.htm; adapted by permission.)

Next, I must say this: some of the best days I have had have been the ones since I knew I had Alzheimer's. We have a good life! Bad days, yes, but now we know what we are dealing with. The worst times were before the diagnosis. I wish people would ask me . . . I might have time to tell them. It doesn't always go fast. (Simpson & Simpson, 1999, pp. 156–157)

Although information from the person with dementia, family members, and many other health professionals is essential, a diagnosis of dementia can only be made by a physician. Unfortunately, not all physicians have the expertise and experience to make this diagnosis. Persons with dementia and their care partners often report that in the early stages, their own observations and comments about difficulties with function were dismissed by doctors. They found that getting a diagnosis was a long, uphill battle, often taking 2–3 years of tests and appointments with specialists. Getting a diagnosis can be particularly challenging if the person is high functioning. Many of the standardized tests do not capture the problems experienced by high-functioning persons in the early stages and/or the day-to-day challenges experienced by persons with an atypical dementia. If a person has one of the atypical dementias, such as frontotemporal dementia, it may be even more difficult to find a clinician who recognizes the symptoms.

> Even standard neuropsychological tests may be insensitive to the comportmental changes associated with the so-called "Frontal Lobe Dementias" and it becomes important to review daily living activities and to speak to caregivers and other reliable informants to gather information about problems with judgment and customary ways of behaving. (Weintraub, 2003, p. 4)

If you believe that your concerns have not been addressed by a physician, I urge you to seek other opinions. Local or national Alzheimer's organizations can provide you with the names of physicians who are experts in Alzheimer's disease and other dementias. The United States has federally funded Alzheimer's disease centers (see Appendix B), which are excellent sources of diagnostic and other information. Most major

Canadian cities have geriatric assessment and treatment clinics associated with hospitals and/or university medical centers.

Under no circumstances should memory loss or other cognitive changes that significantly interfere with daily living be dismissed as part of normal aging. Seeking expert medical assessment and advice as early as possible is essential for everyone's well-being. It also avoids having to deal with a difficult diagnosis at the time of a crisis, such as an acute medical problem. The following account shows one person's feelings about the importance of getting a diagnosis and finding out the source of the problems that she was having.

> I'm sure almost every doctor I went to knew that Alzheimer's disease was a part of this, and they didn't want to deal with it. I'm very angry about that. I can understand that you could be cautious in some cases, but they need to give the person some idea of what they might have instead of protecting themselves. (Jean, cited in Snyder, 1999, p. 73)

Encouraging Loved Ones to Seek a Diagnosis

Like Jean in the preceding quote, some people realize that they are having problems and seek the advice of a doctor. In other cases, it can be challenging to encourage the person to go to the doctor for an assessment. The person either is not aware that he or she is having problems or realizes it privately but denies it publicly. Like many other aspects of dementia care, there is, unfortunately, no one way to handle this challenge. However, offering unconditional support and reassurance—letting the person know that you will stand by him or her whatever the circumstances—is invaluable. Caregiver support and encouragement throughout the diagnostic process are essential, especially if the diagnosis has been given in a less than compassionate way. Christine Boden spoke about the need for support:

It is very scary to be diagnosed with an incurable dementing disease. Try to imagine it—you are faced with the knowledge that you are going to lose all your normal mental functions over a period of years, and no-one can tell you exactly what will happen when, nor how long it will take. (1998, p. 54)

At the time of a memory loss episode, it may be possible to have a calm and sensitive conversation with the person that will let him or her know that you are concerned and would like to determine the source of the problem. Or other family members or friends whom the person respects may be able to play the same role. The key is to honor the person's feelings of fear and embarrassment and not be confrontational. Many caregivers report that although they were reluctant to approach the topic, the person was actually relieved to have a chance to talk about his or her concerns and to know that his or her family was supportive.

Remember that during routine office visits, it is unlikely a physician would notice the memory loss problems that friends and family see on a daily basis. However, it may be possible to sensitively and privately express your concerns to the physician in advance. There are, of course, issues of confidentiality in terms of the information that the physician may share with you. A similar approach could be used if the person has a trusting relationship with another health care professional, such as a visiting nurse or therapist.

For some people with dementia, especially those who have more advanced symptoms, it can be helpful to take a caring and positive but firm approach. A statement such as the following can be effective: "The doctor is going to see you today to see how you are getting along. I will help you get ready now and go to the appointment with you." More information on using this approach can be found in Chapters 4 and 6.

The Diagnostic Process

There is no single test or procedure that can diagnose dementia in a living person. The clinical diagnosis of Alzheimer's disease is based on a comprehensive history, the assessment of current symptoms, and the elimination of other possible causes of dementia. As noted, such a clinical diagnosis is 80%–90% accurate.

Determining the final diagnosis is the responsibility of the medical doctor, but the information necessary to make the diagnosis comes from many health professionals as well as from family members and significant others. The doctor (a family physician, a geriatrician, a neurologist, a psychiatrist, or another medical practitioner) is responsible for coordinating essential information from additional medical practitioners, lab technicians, and other health care professionals involved with social, functional, psychological, and physical assessment. Due to the progressive nature and variability of the disease and the hampered communication skills of persons with dementia, assessment must be ongoing. Working with a clinician who seeks and appreciates information from the person about daily living challenges is vital. Standardized and neuro-psychological testing often is not sensitive to these changes, especially with persons who are in the early stages. Many persons and their caregivers are understandably frustrated when they are experiencing enormous changes in daily life but are told that neuro-psychological tests do not show any changes.

Compiling a complete history is an essential part of the assessment and diagnostic process. This history must come not only from the person, who may not be a reliable source because of memory loss, but also from family members, friends, and other caregivers. Only through documenting changes in behavior over time can dementia be clinically diagnosed. Information about important life events, values and habits, previous personal coping styles, and personality factors (e.g., response to stress, style of sociability, temperament, self-image) is invaluable in explaining behavior and responses during the course of the disease as well as in indicating important areas of personal strengths and related treatments. For treatment planning purposes, an assessment must identify not only deficits but also persisting strengths and abilities. The assessment must include

- A complete history
- A neurological examination to identify possible neurological causes of the dementia
- A psychiatric screening for the presence of coexisting depression or depression presenting as pseudodementia
- A social and behavioral evaluation that includes the availability of family and social support systems
- An evaluation of functional performance in the activities of daily living and leisure pursuits, based on actual functional performance as observed by the evaluator or a reliable caregiver source
- An assessment of cognitive functioning, based on clinical observation and standardized assessment
- A comprehensive physical examination
- Laboratory investigations:
  Full blood count and differential
  Serum electrolytes
  Hepatic and renal functioning
  Serum calcium
  Thyroid functioning
  Syphilis serology
  HIV antibodies (depending on personal history)

Serum vitamin B_{12} and folate levels

Urinanalysis

Chest X-ray

Electrocardiogram

Electroencephalogram

Computerized axial tomography (CAT) scan of the brain

How Do You Know if It's Alzheimer's Disease?

The only way to be absolutely sure that someone had Alzheimer's disease is to have a brain autopsy after death. However, a clinical diagnosis can be made by a doctor who has a special understanding of aging and diseases such as Alzheimer's disease (e.g., a geriatrician, a neurologist, a geropsychiatrist). To make this diagnosis, the doctor will need to conduct numerous tests. In addition, the doctor will need to get information from family caregivers and other health professionals about how the person managed in the past and what he or she is able to do now. A diagnosis made by this process is 80%–90% accurate.

THE STAGES OF ALZHEIMER'S DISEASE AND OTHER DEMENTIAS

As noted, although Alzheimer's disease and the many other forms of dementia differ in symptoms and progression, the dementias are more alike than different. These similarities are especially significant for caregiving concerns. For this reason, the general symptoms of dementia, which includes Alzheimer's disease, follow. This same practice of using general symptoms has been followed throughout this book.

The average course is 7–8 years from the first symptoms until death. The person steadily loses skills and abilities during this progression. In some cases, however the course may be rapid (e.g., 2–3 years) or excessively long (e.g., 20 years).

There is much individual variation in the symptoms. It is impossible to precisely describe a "typical" presentation of dementia and to define in detail the symptoms at various stages of the disease. The course is one of progressive impairment in cognitive and functional abilities until death. The overwhelming consensus among clinicians and in the professional literature is that staging instruments are not very useful for education, care planning, and research because of the extreme variability among people regarding the onset, presentation, and severity of symptoms. In addition, staging can be destructive, undermining the person's abilities by setting expectations for decline. This can lead to a self-fulfilling prophecy. For example, many persons in the moderate stages have difficulty with dressing themselves. Yet, caregivers who expect this may dress the person from the first sign of difficulty instead of finding ways to adapt dressing so that the person can succeed. (See Chapters 6 and 7 for more information on helping the person succeed.) It is essential for caregivers to appreciate the variable nature of all dementias. Furthermore, persons with dementia have spent a whole lifetime acquiring skills and habits, and many of these persist despite the losses due to brain damage.

In addition to the variability in symptoms among different individuals with dementia, there is great variability from hour to hour and day to day for the same person. Kitwood (1997) suggested that staging is destructive because it emphasizes inevitable decline and doesn't account for the effects of interventions or treatments that emphasize continuing abilities. He suggested that with effective person-centered interventions (e.g., a supportive care environment), it is possible that the person can "re-ment"—that is, show improvements and fewer signs of dementia.

Assessment and care planning must be done individually, according to a person's particular strengths and weaknesses. Neuropsychologist Sandra Weintraub (2003), Clinical Core Director of Northwestern University's Cognitive Neurology and Alzheimer's Disease Center in Chicago, commented,

> One major challenge in working with this illness is the fact that, beyond amnesia, different patients may express entirely different symptoms. This is a fact that is very puzzling to health care providers and caregivers who may have the idea that there are "stages" of Alzheimer's that unfold in the same way in each patient.

With these important considerations in mind, caregivers do need a general framework of disease progression to plan for future care needs. A guiding principle is that losses occur in reverse order of the gains developed during infancy and childhood (Perrin & May, 2000; Thornbury, 1993). For example, the old axiom "You have to learn to sit before you learn to stand" is reversed. Individuals with dementia lose the ability to stand and walk before they lose the ability to sit independently. In addition, fine motor skills, such as using the fingers and hands to write, deteriorate or decline before gross motor skills, such as using the legs to walk. However, this rule of thumb is greatly tempered by the persistence of over-learned skills, such as feeding oneself.

It is also essential to appreciate that behavioral symptoms can be greatly reduced through the provision of supportive care, as described in Chapters 4–9 of this book. With this and the variability of progression and symptoms in mind, the general symptoms of each stage are described next. The format given by Volicer, Fabiszewski, Rheaume, and Lasch (1988), which divides the progression of dementia into four stages, follows.

Early Stage (Mildly Impaired)

In the early stages the changes are so subtle that neither the individual nor significant others may take particular notice. The person relies on long-term memory, lifelong routines, practiced skills, and overlearned behaviors. External structure and cues (e.g., calendars, reminder lists) enable function. With early diagnosis, many persons with Alzheimer's disease develop their own strategies that help them to continue with daily activities. In fact, a person may be so skilled at using these abilities in combination with social skills that others may not notice any difficulties. The person is able to carry out most routine activities (e.g., preparing a familiar meal) and may seek the assistance of others with more complex activities that involve abstract thoughts or cues or require higher cognitive skills, such as judgment and planning. If the person still has a job, difficulties may first appear at work. There may also be challenges with more complicated daily activities (e.g., managing finances) or hobbies such as planning a woodworking project or learning a new knitting pattern.

The hallmark symptom of dementia, memory loss, appears at this stage. This memory loss is periodic and inconsistent and occurs particularly in unfamiliar surroundings. The individual may forget how to get home, be unable to recall a particular word or name, be unable to locate personal items, or be unable to carry out a familiar but complex activity such as writing a check. Initially, these difficulties may be dismissed by the individual and others, perhaps as being due to fatigue or other stresses. The frequency of these incidents increases, and the individual begins having regular and noticeable difficulty with complex work or leisure activities requiring problem solving and high levels of judgment. Other problems during the early stages are more likely to occur in unfamiliar settings or when a novel situation arises. For example, the person may have difficulty making him- or herself a sandwich in a friend's kitchen or may easily get lost in an unfamiliar shopping mall.

Individuals react differently to these losses. Some may attempt to carry on as usual, making use of continuing abilities. Others may gradually withdraw from familiar activities with which they can no longer cope, appear apathetic, and be depressed. Depression is quite common in this early stage and may make the dementia symptoms appear worse than they actually are. It is essential to understand that there are effective treatments for depression, and the advice of a physician should be sought. Still others may express frustration at their incapacities and seek assistance from their physician or counseling from friends.

Middle Stage (Moderately Impaired)

The person continues to rely on overlearned skills and familiar routines and environments. However, this behavior in itself is no longer enough. The person uses physical and tactile cuing and requires a supportive, consistent care environment to call forth persisting skills. Nonverbal methods of communication take on particular significance, and the person increasingly relies on the caregiver to structure his or her day. Concrete activities (e.g., eating) that have one or two steps and don't require new learning are possible.

The difficulties with memory loss become much more pronounced in this stage, to the point that they interfere with daily living. The individual begins to need cuing and prompting for activities such as dressing and bathing. More complex activities, such as meal preparation, shopping, and financial management, require the direct assistance of others. Safe driving becomes impossible and should be discontinued. The individual becomes less able to cope in unfamiliar settings and experiences frequent disorientation to place and time, which may include day and night reversal. Difficulties with written and verbal communication become more apparent. For some, language difficulties become very marked during this stage. The physical ability to speak and use words persists, but the content may be hollow or involve problems such as perseveration (getting stuck on a particular word or phrase). Motor coordination problems appear and are more pronounced for some people than for others. Apraxia (the inability to carry out complex motor activities) may interfere with bathing, dressing, eating, and walking. Walking may be further impaired by perceptual problems (difficulty interpreting environmental information). Yet, motor restlessness, frequent pacing, and wandering also occur during this stage. For many people, these problems become much worse at the end of the day. This combination of restlessness and distress is known as *sundowning*. Although the exact cause of these symptoms is unclear, the symptoms are undoubtedly related to the individual's increasing inability to remember, and hence to locate, familiar places or people.

Frustration with progressive losses may lead to extreme emotional reactions, or *catastrophic reactions*, to seemingly minor events. Alternately, the individual may be apathetic and disoriented due to an overwhelming sense of his or her inability to cope. Some may express paranoia and blame others for misplaced items or misperformed activities. Much can be done to prevent the occurrence and associated distress of these behavioral symptoms. For more information, see Chapters 6, 7, 8, and 9.

Cognitive functioning is greatly impaired during the middle stage, and learning new material (especially verbal material) becomes very difficult. Concentration, attention, reasoning, and judgment are all noticeably deficient. The person recognizes but is frequently unable to name loved ones. Urinary incontinence may occur.

Advanced Stage (Severely Impaired)

By the advanced stage, the person relies on external sensory cues and is able to engage in repetitive one-step activities (e.g., brushing his or her hair) with the guidance of caregivers. Activities related to touch and movement provide pleasure. The person increasingly relies on the caregiver for emotional and physical support.

In this stage, verbal cues alone are usually not sufficient, and the individual requires constant supervision and physical assistance for personal activities such as toileting and personal hygiene. Both fecal and urinary incontinence are common. Language skills greatly deteriorate, and only simple phrases or familiar expressions persist. Language comprehension is limited. There is widespread loss of fine and gross motor skills, with assistance required for ambulation. Support is frequently required to maintain a normal sitting posture. Disorientation is constant. Some individuals may develop seizures. Some also may engage in hyperoralia—putting objects in their mouth. Primitive reflexes, particularly the grasp reflex, may return.

Terminal Stage

In the terminal stage, the person is totally dependent on others. The person may be unable to move, speak, or swallow. Particular attention must be given to maintaining caring human contact, giving comfort, and preventing complications such as bed sores, dehydration, aspiration pneumonia, and contractures. In this stage, family and professional caregivers must often make painful decisions about issues such as the initiation of tube feedings. In this stage, the complications of dementia, particularly those related to the control of the muscles used for breathing, lead to death.

THE CAUSES OF ALZHEIMER'S DISEASE

Although great advances have been made in understanding the brain pathology of Alzheimer's disease, the cause remains unknown. Numerous theories are currently undergoing further study. These theories attempt to explain the trigger that unleashes the formation of the senile plaques, which are the central pathological characteristic of Alzheimer's disease. Much current study of the biology of Alzheimer's disease focuses on the precursor protein for the formation of the amyloid beta-protein, which is at the core of these plaques. There is also study of tau proteins, which appear to be associated with the development of neurofibrillary tangles. Scientists do not agree on which of these two processes is most important, and this discussion is sometimes called the argument between the Baptists (those supporting amyloid beta-protein) and the Taoists (those supporting tau protein).

Scientists do agree on certain topics. It is now widely accepted that there are several types of Alzheimer's disease, each of which may have a different cause or combination of causes. A person may have more than one type of Alzheimer's disease. It is therefore highly unlikely that a single cause of Alzheimer's disease will be uncovered. Instead, it is similar to other chronic diseases, for which a variety of risk factors (triggers) interact in a complex way with each person's unique genetic makeup. As genetics and these various risk factors are better understood, it will be possible to determine individualized treatment and get a clearer understanding of preventive actions.

This understanding of Alzheimer's disease is rather like the model for the development of heart disease. For example, a person may be born with a genetic predisposition for the development of heart disease. However, other lifestyle or environmental risk factors (e.g., diet, exercise, smoking) play a major role in whether the person actually develops heart disease—that is, whether the genetic tendency is actually expressed. Conversely, someone may have a low genetic risk for heart disease, but if he or she smokes, is overweight, and does not exercise, the overall risk of serious heart disease is greatly increased.

David Snowdon described the role of these various factors in the development of Alzheimer's disease:

> You've heard about the nature-versus-nurture debate. We're now finding that it's more like nature *plus* nurture.
>
> Genes seem to be very important in early-onset Alzheimer's. But for late-onset Alzheimer's . . . we're finding other factors. I like to emphasize things people can do something about—always wear your seat belt!—or taking certain vitamins and antioxidants, or maintaining their cardiovascular health. There are good reasons for doing these things anyway—in addition, they may help to prevent Alzheimer's. (2001, p. 137)

There has been considerable investigation of the triggers for Alzheimer's disease. There is widespread agreement that age, genetic factors, having Down syndrome, and female gender are risk factors for the development of Alzheimer's disease. Other possible risk factors include a history of head trauma, low occupational/educational status, mild cognitive impairment, vascular disease, exposure to toxins, a high-fat/low-vitamin diet, smoking, lack of exercise, stress, and history of depression. Differences in study methods have led to different results regarding these risk factors. It is important to appreciate that these risk factors do not necessarily establish cause but represent links with the disease. An ongoing study of mild cognitive impairment and the factors that contribute to its stability or its developing into Alzheimer's disease (as it does in approximately 50% of cases) will add to the understanding of risk factors. Scientists throughout the world are studying specific risk factors, pooling the results of previous studies and developing predictive models for the risk of developing Alzheimer's disease.

It is important to appreciate that present findings do not show how to avoid developing Alzheimer's disease. Yet, the ever-expanding information in this area is exciting and offers much hope. The following subsections detail what is understood about the four known risk factors.

Age

The single greatest risk factor for Alzheimer's disease is age. The older we get the more likely we are to develop Alzheimer's disease. Although the percent of the population older than age 65 with Alzheimer's disease or another dementia varies somewhat from study to study (depending on study methodology), researchers agree that age is the most important risk factor. For instance, a review of 47 different studies found that the percentage of the population with dementia doubles every 5.1 years up to age 95 (Huang, Svenson, & Lindsay, 1994). However, it is not clear how the aging process is related to Alzheimer's disease. Because not every older person, even if advanced in age, develops Alzheimer's disease, there is clearly not a direct relationship between age and Alzheimer's disease. It is essential to remember that even when research that reports the highest numbers of persons with Alzheimer's disease is considered, more than half of persons older than 85 years do not have Alzheimer's disease. There is some evidence for a "hardy survivor" theory, supported by the number of persons older than 100 who do not have Alzheimer's disease (e.g., as in the Nun Study). Because the rate of occurrence of Alzheimer's disease stops increasing in the age 95 and older bracket, there is some suggestion that these individuals may be at reduced risk. That is, having reached age 95 and beyond, these individuals may be more hardy and less at risk of developing Alzheimer's disease than someone in his or her eighties.

Genetic Factors

Although there is a definite genetic link for Alzheimer's disease, the relationship is complex and far from clear. It is important to appreciate that there are two paths of genetic risks to consider. Furthermore, genetic factors operate with other risk factors to determine whether the gene is expressed. First, there are clearly established genetic links based on specific, inheritable chromosome abnormalities. To date, these abnormalities have been discovered on chromosomes 1, 14, 19, and 21, with 12 a possibility. Although these abnormalities have a strong genetic link, they account for a relatively small percentage (5%–10%) of Alzheimer's disease cases. This is called *familial Alzheimer's disease*, and in many cases, the disease develops well before age 65.

Late-onset, or sporadic, Alzheimer's disease is also influenced by genetic factors. A family history of Alzheimer's disease increases the risk of getting Alzheimer's disease, at any age, by approximately four times. The relationship with other risk factors is complex and not yet clearly understood. A component of proteins that is common in cerebrospinal fluid, apolipoprotein E (apoE), also plays a role in genetic susceptibility. Persons who carry the apoE4 form of this protein have increased risk of developing Alzheimer's disease. The gene for the production of this protein is found on chromosome 19. This the only clearly established genetic link with late-onset Alzheimer's disease. This relationship and the role of apoE4 in causing Alzheimer's disease are complex and still under investigation.

Because there is a blood test for apoE4, the discovery of this connection has furthered the complex discussion about genetic testing for Alzheimer's disease. Although it is possible to determine if apoE4 is present, it is not possible to say conclusively that carriers will develop Alzheimer's disease. Beyond this, there are complex ethical considerations about offering genetic testing for a disease that *may* develop in later life and for which there is, at present, no cure. This is particularly problematic in the absence of comprehensive counseling and support services. At present, genetic testing is only done at research centers.

Although the genetic links to Alzheimer's disease cause family members concern about their own risks, it is essential to remember that there are many well-accepted ways to prevent the development of Alzheimer's disease symptoms. These are the already well-known healthy lifestyle factors, such as keeping mentally and physically active and eating a healthy, low-fat diet that includes many servings of fruits and vegetables.

Down Syndrome

Down syndrome is a congenital disorder caused by an abnormality on chromosome 21. Virtually all persons with Down syndrome develop the brain pathology of Alzheimer's disease (i.e., senile plaques, neurofibrillary tangles, and brain atrophy) by age 40 or so. However, only about 50% of these individuals actually have the cognitive changes of Alzheimer's disease (i.e., a decline compared to earlier adult function). This observation is not clearly understood and is under investigation. Most individuals with Down syndrome are identified (i.e., have received a diagnosis), and many live in special care settings. Thus, study of the development of symptoms will not only help them and their caregivers to improve daily living, it will also provide some important clues about the development of Alzheimer's disease in general. For instance, it may help to determine the earliest symptoms of Alzheimer's disease, which occur before marked cognitive changes. In turn, this could lead to an early diagnosis and the possibility of early treatment.

Female Gender

Female gender as a risk factor was masked for some time by the fact that there are more older women than older men and, hence, more women with Alzheimer's disease. However, careful study has led to the conclusion that women are at greater risk for developing Alzheimer's disease than men. As with the other risk factors, the relationship is not yet understood. It may be related to postmenopausal hormone changes, genetic factors related to the X chromosome, or other unidentified environmental influences.

Possible Risk Factors

Head Trauma

Investigations suggest that head trauma with loss of consciousness is a fairly strong risk factor. Some have suggested that major head trauma, especially in early life, can speed up the development of Alzheimer's disease. However, not all studies have confirmed this risk, nor is the degree of risk understood.

Low Educational/Occupational Status

Numerous studies have found a relationship between a lower level of education and an increased risk of developing Alzheimer's disease. To express these findings in another way, education appears to be a preventive or protective factor in the development of Alzheimer's disease. The current understanding is that the stimulation of education, or indeed any challenging activity (e.g., one's occupation), increases the density of synapses (message connection points) in the brain and, hence, serves as an insulating effect against the onset of symptoms. That is, there is more reserve capacity in the brain. However, this is not a simple relationship. Persons with lower educational and occupational levels are also likely to have less healthy diets and to be more challenged by some of the written tests used to diagnose Alzheimer's disease.

Although evidence strongly suggests that stimulating and taxing the brain reduce the risk of developing Alzheimer's disease symptoms, it is erroneous to believe that these activities prevent Alzheimer's disease. Many highly intelligent and active persons do develop Alzheimer's disease, although the onset of symptoms may be delayed or never take place.

This is shown by the Nun Study, which has also provided excellent information on the role of activity in successful aging (Snowdon, 1997, 2001). The participants agreed to testing and study during their life and to a brain autopsy at death. They were all in their eighties and nineties and beyond, but for the most part also led very active lives. They continued to be involved with their families and community and to maintain physical and mental activities. Sister Mary, who lived to be 101, was mentioned as an excellent example of successful aging. She retired from active teaching at age 84; after this, she continued to teach family members and other sisters, maintained a keen interest in world events, and remained physically active. She also continued to have normal scores on cognitive tests. When she died, however, the autopsy results were surprising: Sister Mary's brain was riddled with plaques and tangles, the key markers of Alzheimer's disease! This case and others suggest that those who are involved in activities build up a rich network of pathways in the brain that serves as an insulating effect against the damage caused by Alzheimer's disease (Evans et al., 1997; Huang et al., 1994; Stern et al., 1994; White et al., 1994). It is also interesting to note that among the Nun Study participants, Sister Mary had one of the lowest levels of formal education of the sisters, and she didn't graduate from high school until she was in her forties.

In addition, the Kungsholmen project in Sweden found that being part of a rich social network decreased the risk of dementia by 31% (Winblad, Wang, Zenchao, & Fratiglioni, 2000). This finding is supported by the CSHA (Canadian Study on Health and Aging; see http://www.csha.ca) and the PAQUID (Personnes Agées Quid) study in France.

Mild Cognitive Impairment

Mild cognitive impairment (sometimes called "MCI") is a relatively new classification for the onset of mild memory problems in adulthood. The criteria and definition of mild cognitive impairment are still under development. As of this writing, the following criteria are suggested (Peterson, Mohs, Carli, & Galasko, 2000):

1. Memory complaint that is supported by a family member or significant other
2. Normal general cognitive functioning
3. Normal activities of daily living

4. Memory impairment greater than what would be expected for age and education
5. Diagnostic criteria for dementia are not met

The classification of mild cognitive impairment has come about because older individuals with memory loss are presenting themselves earlier and earlier to research centers and specialists. Individuals with mild cognitive impairment appear to be at an increased risk of developing Alzheimer's disease. Current data suggests that approximately half of those with mild cognitive impairment go on to develop Alzheimer's disease; however, it is important to note that approximately half do not progress. Some stay the same; for others, memory functioning improves. The factors that lead to the development of Alzheimer's disease from mild cognitive impairment are still under study but promise to aid in the understanding and prevention of Alzheimer's disease.

Vascular Disease

There is strong evidence that persons with vascular disease—that is, problems with blood circulation (e.g., heart attacks, artery disease)—have an increased risk of developing not only multi-infarct dementia but also Alzheimer's disease. Yet, treatment for high blood pressure has been shown to reduce the risk of developing Alzheimer's disease and to slow cognitive decline for persons with Alzheimer's disease. The lifestyle factors that reduce the risk of strokes and other vascular problems also reduce the risk of Alzheimer's disease.

Toxins

Aluminum was one of the earliest suggested risk factors regarding toxins. This is still under debate. Although there are elevated levels of insoluble aluminum in the brains of persons with Alzheimer's disease, there has been no demonstration of cause and effect or the source of the aluminum. Aluminum in drinking water is currently under investigation.

Lifestyle Factors

As noted previously, lifestyle factors may affect the development of Alzheimer's disease. The role of diet is just beginning to receive attention. A major retrospective study of almost 6,000 persons in Holland concluded that persons who ate a diet high in vegetables and vitamins E and C had a significantly lower risk of developing Alzheimer's disease (Englehart et al., 2000). Another controlled study of 376 people found that persons with the apoE4 allele and a high-fat diet had seven-fold higher risk of developing Alzheimer's disease (Petot et al., 2000). Investigations into the relationship between diet and Alzheimer's disease are ongoing.

Researchers from around the world strongly suggest that a healthy lifestyle, including a low-fat diet, regular exercise, stress management, and not smoking, helps to prevent and/or reduce the severity of Alzheimer's disease symptoms (Coleman, 2000). It is encouraging that this sensible approach to health and general well-being is being confirmed by research.

Depression

Information suggests that a lifelong history of depression is associated with an increased risk of developing Alzheimer's disease. Like other risk factors, the nature of this relationship is unclear and is under investigation. It is not clear whether this is a coincidental association or the result of neurochemical changes or whether depression is, in part, a very early expression of Alzheimer's disease symptoms. As pointed out in this chapter, however, it is clear that persons with Alzheimer's disease are at an increased risk of developing depression and that this depression does respond to treatment.

HOW COMMON ARE ALZHEIMER'S DISEASE AND OTHER DEMENTIAS?

Alzheimer's disease and related dementias form a major health issue for older adults. This issue, and the many others stemming from it, have been documented and detailed in the most comprehensive study of its kind to date, the CSHA. Information from this project is available in numerous publications (Clarfield, 1991; Clarfield & Foley, 1993; Eastwood, Nobbs, Lindsay, & McDowell, 1992; Gauthier, McDowell, & Hill, 1990; Lindsay, 1994a, 1994b; McDowell, 1994; Mohr, Feldman, & Gauthier, 1995; Tuokko, Kristjansson, & Miller, 1995).

Among any single disease, Alzheimer's disease and other types of dementia represent the highest cost of care and are the fourth leading cause of death (CSHA, 1994; Huang, Cartwright, & Hu, 1988). Approximately 5 million Americans and 300,000 Canadians have dementia, and these figures are expected to reach epidemic proportions as the number of aging persons continues to increase. CSHA (1994) reported an overall prevalence of dementia of 4.2% for persons older than 65. There is, however, considerable variation in occurrence rates among different studies. These differences are accounted for by differences in both diagnostic criteria and study methods.

CSHA found that the prevalence of Alzheimer's disease is 1% at age 65 and 26% at age 85 and older. Other studies with different criteria have found even higher rates. For example,

Evans et al. (1989) found a prevalence of 3%, for persons ages 65–74, and 47% for persons 85 and older. Persons older than age 85 compose the fastest growing population group in North America. To express this concept more graphically, by the year 2020, more 85-year-olds than 14-year-olds are expected to be living in North America. The prevalence of dementia may more than triple by 2050.

IS THERE A CURE FOR ALZHEIMER'S DISEASE AND OTHER TYPES OF DEMENTIA?

At present, there is no cure for Alzheimer's disease or many other types of dementia, although numerous promising drug trials are underway. At the same time, it is vital to remember that treatment is available to help the person with dementia live as healthy and active a life as possible. Caregivers can and do provide the most essential treatment available for dementia. The ways in which caregivers talk to, care for, and care about (or "treat") persons with dementia has an enormous impact on their quality of life and well-being. Bob Simpson shared how his wife Anne provides a treatment for him:

> You are really interested in what is happening now; you take me seriously; you want to understand, even if you don't always do what I want. If I say I am tired, you believe me. I go lie down, and then I get going again.
>
> What I appreciate is that you try to understand. Sometimes you interpret for me what I am feeling but can't put into words. That makes me feel really good! You're so helpful—you will play the game with me to help me remember someone's name. (Simpson & Simpson, 1999, p. 129)

Nonetheless, caregivers can find it very distressing that despite their best efforts, the person does not get "better." As suggested in Chapter 1, we need to rethink what we mean by *better.* Dementia is a brain disease for which there is presently no cure. From this point of view, the person cannot "get better." However, caregivers can and do help the person to be better—to have better moments, better days, better feelings, and a better quality of life.

> In Alzheimer's you come back to being very childlike, like an infant in your ability to function. But value lies not in what you can do, but in your being. People are valuable for what they are in the present, not just for their pasts or for their future potential. (Simpson & Simpson, 1999, p. 122)

The ways in which caregivers can provide treatment are described in the following chapters; however, one brief example is given here for illustrative purposes.

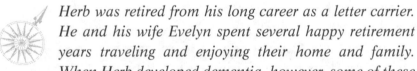

Herb was retired from his long career as a letter carrier. He and his wife Evelyn spent several happy retirement years traveling and enjoying their home and family. When Herb developed dementia, however, some of these activities had to be changed or stopped, and the couple spent more time at home. Although Herb had been retired for years, he began to get really restless in the mornings and kept telling Evelyn that he was going to be late for work. Evelyn tried to explain that he was long retired and suggested that they go for a walk instead. This wasn't enough for Herb, so Evelyn started saving all the junk mail and set up a "sorting station" for Herb. Each day after breakfast, Evelyn showed Herb his work and he spent several happy hours doing his job. When Herb had meaningful work and felt valued and worthwhile, the behavioral symptoms of dementia were less troublesome. When Herb moved to a long-term care facility, Evelyn helped the staff to set up a work station. This continued to play an important role in helping Herb to have meaningful days and the best possible quality of life.

Medical Drug Treatment

Four drugs are recommended for persons who are in the early and middle stages of Alzheimer's disease: tacrine (Cognex), donepezil (Aricept), galantamine (Reminyl), and rivastigmine (Exelon). At present, donepezil is the most widely used medication. Comprehensive study of donepezil's effects suggest that it has been modestly effective (i.e., for approximately 50% of people who tried it) in improving memory or delaying memory loss and other symptoms for 6 months to 1 year. It is important to note that donepezil's effect is to delay the progression of symptoms; it is not a cure. In addition, approximately half of those who tried it either couldn't tolerate the drug's side effects or had no observed benefit.

Presently, there is no way to tell in advance whether someone will respond to such a drug. In view of this, a trial period on the drug is sometimes recommended. However, there are other factors to be considered before this decision is made. Anti-dementia drugs are expensive, costing well over $100 (U.S.) per month. Some states and provinces have plans to assist with or cover this cost; others do not. In addition, not all private insurance policies cover the costs for these drugs. Some of the drug companies themselves have assistance programs. Furthermore, participants in clinical trials of these drugs typically receive the medication at no cost. However, one should not participate in a clinical trial solely for free medication. Information on clinical trials is available from national Alzheimer's organizations (see Appendix B).

In addition to cost issues, there are many personal and ethical considerations. Although these drugs offer promise, their use requires careful thought and consideration by the person and his or her caregivers. What does the person expect from this treatment? Will starting treatment create false hope for both the person and the caregiver? Is there a plan to support and encourage the person if he or she is unable to take the drug? Will the use of the drug divert caregivers from providing other essential treatment? It must also be remembered that a time will come when the drug is no longer effective; then, all must deal with the continued progression of symptoms. For further discussion of these issues, please see Bowlby Sifton (2001b) and Post (2001a).

Studies on the use of vitamin E and ginkgo biloba have shown some promising effects, and more studies are underway. Based on these early results, some physicians recommend the use of these nondrug treatments. To date, however, no conclusions have been reached.

The first trial for an Alzheimer's vaccine began in 1999 but was stopped in 2001 due to adverse reactions. Animal trials with this vaccine stopped further brain damage and, in some cases, even reversed existing damage. However, it remains to be seen whether further work will uncover a vaccine that is safe for people.

It is believed that scientists are very close to formulating a drug or combination of drugs that will prevent the later stages of the disease. For example, vitamin E, anti-inflammatories, donepezil, statin drugs, and ginkgo biloba are under study not only as ways to delay the symptoms but also as preventive measures for persons who have mild cognitive impairment but have not yet been diagnosed with dementia (see the subsection "Mild Cognitive Impairment" for more information on this condition). Trials with giving women supplemental estrogen as a preventive measure were inconclusive and have been halted because of serious side effects. The most current and valid information on these and other research projects and discoveries can be obtained from national Alzheimer's organizations or from other reliable resources found in Appendix B.

Caregivers are encouraged to keep up with new developments as well as to determine whether new reports, especially in the popular press, are accurate. Although there is much good news and much of it is accurate, inaccurate or misleading claims are possible.

TREATMENT FROM THE CAREGIVER

The way that caregivers care for (or "treat") persons with dementia has an enormous impact on quality of life and well-being. As the great humanist and neurologist Oliver Sacks (1990) said, "Persons with dementia have not really lost their personality or their memory, they have just lost access to it." This comment reminds us that everyone who comes in contact with persons with dementia has a vital role—enabling them to connect with the skills and resources that remain and to continue being involved in the web of life. Furthermore, it can lighten the caregiving day.

Other factors (e.g., the wrong medication, another illness, a confusing environment, caregivers who expect too little) can make it seem as though the person with dementia has a greater disability than he or she actually has. This is called *excess disability*. Caregivers can help provide treatment by remembering these tenets:

- The person with dementia still has many strengths and abilities.
- These strengths can be used to make up for some of his or her losses.
- There are eight general areas of strength. (See the following subsection.)

The Continuing Abilities of Persons with Dementia

The following subsections outline eight key continuing strengths of persons with dementia: 1) habitual skills and procedural memory, 2) humor, 3) emotional awareness and emo-

tional memory, 4) sociability and social skills, 5) sensory awareness and appreciation, 6) motor skills, 7) responsiveness to
music, and 8) long-term memory. Also included are suggestions for ways that caregivers can help the person gain access
to these skills. The book's remaining chapters provide more
details in all of these areas.

Habitual Skills and Procedural Memory

- Procedural memory is remembering how to do a familiar, often-repeated activity.
- Procedural memory is preserved in dementia.
- To encourage doing an activity based on procedural
  memory, make sure that the setting, the cues, and the
  way of participating are familiar, and use nonverbal cues
  instead of words.
- Persons with dementia are better at recognizing people
  than they are at recalling names.
- Always provide orientation information (e.g., your name,
  the date, the place) for the person with dementia.
- Memory for information that doesn't change (e.g., birth-
  days, holidays) is better preserved than new information.
- There is no evidence that quizzing the person or prodding him o her to recall things has any positive benefit.

Alice had always liked to sew. As long as anyone could
remember, she had made all of her clothes. In fact, she even
liked mending! In the very early stages of dementia, she continued to sew; however, cataracts on both eyes made it visual-
ly difficult for her to thread a needle. Finally, she had to stop
sewing altogether because of her poor sight.

About 4 years after the first symptoms of dementia
appeared, Alice had cataract surgery. Although just a few

hours afterward she couldn't remember having the operation, the surgery seemed to improve her sight in the long run.

About a year after her surgery, Alice attended a family barbecue. She disapproved of the cutoffs worn by one of her grandsons—which was absolutely in line with her lifelong take on such things. She asked for the "sewing thing" (a needle) so that she could fix the raggedy shorts. A needle and the shorts (off the grandson—this was the hardest part!) were produced. Alice, who hadn't sewn for more than 5 years, hemmed these shorts beautifully!

This is an example of what is called *procedural memory*. Procedural memory is remembering how to do something, such as the way Alice remembered how to thread a needle and make a hem. This can also be called an *habitual skill*—that is, remembering how to do something that the person has done repeatedly during his or her life. Activities based on procedural memory are simple, repetitive, familiar, and involve movement (i.e., motor activity). For this reason, procedural memory is sometimes also called *motor memory*. Some other examples of procedural memory include remembering how to sweep the floor, brush one's teeth, comb one's hair, eat, wash dishes, peel vegetables, or polish shoes.

Research indicates that persons with dementia remember how to do these familiar activities; however, often they are not able to do them completely on their own. There are three important tips for helping to get people started on these habitual activities:

1. Cues or hints that are connected with the activity should be used. Choose actual objects used in the activity. For example, with sewing, the cues were the needle and thread and the raggedy shorts. With sweeping, cues might be the broom and dustpan. Putting a fork or

spoon in the person's hand might cue eating. Feeding the cat might be cued by offering the person the can opener and the can of cat food. It is also important for the general surroundings (i.e., cues in the environment) to be familiar. For example, if the person always peeled vegetables sitting at the kitchen table, this should be continued.

2. The person should continue to do the activity the way he or she has always done it. Avoid changing the method; doing so causes confusion. For example, if the person has always cleaned the hall with a broom, do not suggest a vacuum or carpet sweeper. If the person has always listened to the news on the radio, don't suggest switching to the television news. If the person has always eaten supper on a tray in the living room, continuing this practice will help him or her to keep eating independently.

3. Action should be encouraged without using too many words. Use gestures, nonverbal communication, and actual activity objects. Procedural memory makes use of another less-damaged part of the brain, which does not rely on words as much as actions. Because understanding words is difficult for persons with dementia, keeping words to a minimum can help trigger procedural memory. In this way, a struggle to understand words does not distract the person from doing the activity. For example, to help the person get started watering the houseplants, hand him or her the filled watering can and point to a plant. To begin looking at photographs, open up the album and pat a place on the sofa with your hand. To get the person to put on a sweater, just hand him or her the sweater without saying anything.

Using these three methods draws on a continuing strength, helps the person to continue involvement in activities, supports self-esteem, and reduces behavioral symptoms.

Recognition Is Better than Recall

Although Melinda often visited her mother in the nursing home, she was never sure that her mother knew who she was. One day Melinda came to visit after getting her hair trimmed. She was amazed when her mother reached over, touched her hair, smiled, and said, "Nice." Even though her mother couldn't say Melinda's name, she knew Melinda so well that she recognized something as subtle as a slight change in hair length.

My experience with hundreds of persons with dementia has led me to have no doubt that the person recognizes others who are important in his or her life. The ability to name others (recall) may be lost, but persons with dementia know (recognize) their loved ones. Similarly, other caregivers, everyday objects, and events may be recognized or familiar, but the person may have difficulty recalling the appropriate names.

To understand this skill, think about a time when you were introduced to someone on a casual basis, such as at a party. Thinking that you will probably never see that person again, you put little effort into learning his or her name. Then, you see this person a few weeks later in the grocery store. The person greets you, and you smile back and make social conversation. The person looks familiar, but you can't think of why you recognize the person. If you are like me, you are flipping through the file cards in your brain, trying to place this person. Although we cannot see inside of the brains of persons with dementia, it is likely that they have such experiences dozens of times every day.

Caregivers should make use of the skill for recognition and compensate for difficulties with recall. Look for non-word signs of recognition—for example, a smile or gesture. It is essential that caregivers provide basic orientation information (e.g., their name, the date, the place) for the person during every conversation or interaction. This information is provided for reassurance—as we all need to know where we are and who we are talking to—not so the person will repeat or recall the information later. A conversation might begin like this: "Hi, Mom. This is your daughter Carol. I've brought you your breakfast on this beautiful Thursday in June." The conversation in this instance takes the pressure off by providing the recall information that Mother may be searching for and allowing her to make use of the skill of recognition to greet you. Thus reassured, she can relax and eat her breakfast.

By contrast, visits or conversations should never be turned into contests by asking questions such as "Do you know me?" "What's my name?" or "What day is it?" These questions put the person on the spot, cause embarrassment and frustration, and set a negative tone for the visit or the activity to follow. After all, how would you feel if the person in the grocery store whose name you couldn't recall interrupted your covering social conversation by asking, "What's my name, anyway?"

Caregivers can model this approach with other family members, friends, and visitors. When meeting an acquaintance or greeting someone at the door, caregivers can take the lead and take the pressure off the person with dementia by providing orientation information. They can say things such as, "Oh, look John, here comes Suzie. She used to live next door on Center Street and always had such a lovely garden."

Recall Is Better for Fixed Information

Recall of fixed information is another type of memory, sometimes called *fixed* or *crystallized memory*. Although persons with dementia have increasing difficulty with recalling specific events, especially recent ones, recall of fixed information is better. For example, the date of Christmas or various sorts of breakfast foods may be recalled, but the person may have difficulty recalling who he or she spent Christmas with or which foods he or she had for breakfast. Caregivers can make use of this skill by providing cues, such as decorations for holidays or photographs, that help the person to recall fixed information. These hints or cues help the person succeed, participate, and feel more secure and reassured. There is no evidence that quizzing the person or turning conversations into contests or prodding him or her to recall things has any positive benefit. In fact, this approach is likely to cause distress and embarrassment.

Humor

As noted previously, persons with dementia continue to be amused by the things that they always thought were funny. Although persons with dementia may not understand new jokes, favorite older jokes and stories will still lead to enjoyment. The lifelong tease will continue to find ways to exercise this skill. Most persons with dementia also enjoy and respond to mime and gestures.

A sense of humor is a wonderful skill with many benefits. A good laugh is therapeutic. Most of us know from experience that laughter brings good feelings and reduces stress, tension, and anxiety. Science has shown that a hearty laugh even has important physical benefits. It increases circulation, improves breathing, and increases the positive chemicals in the brain. These are important benefits for you as a caregiver, too. Perhaps you and the person can laugh together over familiar family stories, favorite comedy shorts (e.g., from Laurel and Hardy), or some new funny situation involving you both. Laughing together is an essential activity.

This brings up another important point about humor and the caregiver. So many funny things can happen when you are caring for someone with memory impairment. There isn't a thing wrong with laughing and enjoying these moments or sharing them with other caregivers, as long as you are laughing with, not at, the person. Finding this, and other ways, to bring humor into your caregiving is essential for your own health.

Many people with dementia are highly skilled at using humor to maintain dignity. Caregivers can share in the humor and use this same skill themselves to protect the person's dignity and avoid embarrassment when missteps happen.

As a caregiver, you can also use humor to make light of a situation and prevent distress. Say the person is becoming upset at bedtime because he or she does not want to go to bed. You can use gestures and amusing actions to indicate that you are tired and to suggest that the person tuck you into bed.

Pick up on personal jokes, encourage teasing, and encourage a light-hearted, playful tone during care and other times together. Both of you will feel better!

Emotional Awareness and Emotional Memory

Emotional awareness is the ability to experience the full range of human emotions: love, joy, anger, fear, sorrow, and so forth. Persons with dementia experience all of the normal human emotions. In my experience and in that of many others, persons with dementia are extra sensitive to emotional experiences and often highly skilled at reading others' emotions. However, as dementia progresses, they are likely to have difficulty with expressing their feelings, with letting others know what they are feeling.

Maybe Alzheimer's patients are like human barometers, sensitive like babies. When there is a change in the family their reaction is to cry. I don't cry because I am sad. It's because I am not clever or creative anymore. I don't know what I want or how I feel, but I sense how you feel. I know when you're busy and when you're anxious. (Simpson & Simpson, 1999, p. 116)

It is essential to let the person know that you are aware of his or her feelings. Examine the person's nonverbal cues (e.g., facial expressions) and the tone of his or her words to try to understand what the person is feeling. You might say, for example, "Katherine, it's good to see you so happy. Is it because you like the music?" or "John, you seem to be very upset. Is that true?" [Wait for a response.] "Are you upset because . . .?" Even if you can't determine what caused the person to be upset, letting the person know that you are paying attention to his or her feelings often helps to reduce distress. See Chapters 2 and 4 for more information.

It is important to provide activities that encourage the expression of emotions. Many activities can be nonverbal ways of expressing emotions. Some examples follow; the ensuing chapters contain many more suggestions.

- Caring for plants or pets (expresses feelings of caring, affection, and satisfaction and elicits responsiveness from living things)
- Listening to favorite music (recalls the happy or sad feelings associated with the music)
- Doing repetitive, physical activity such as walking, digging in the garden, or shredding papers for recycling (provides a release for feelings of frustration)
- Providing acceptable, adult expressions of caring and concern, such as hugging, holding hands, brushing hair, or applying hand cream (reassures the person; see Chapter 4 for other ideas on the use of touch)

- Doing simple household chores, such as drying the dishes or dusting (provides feelings of usefulness and self-worth)

It is to everyone's benefit to strive for a calm and positive care environment. When the environment and caregivers are calm, happy, and positive, persons with dementia are more likely to feel calm, happy, and positive. Conversely, when caregivers are distressed or angry or the care environment is chaotic and distressing, persons with dementia are very likely to become distressed. Chapter 1 provides suggestions to help caregivers cope with stress, express emotions, and achieve emotional balance. Chapters 2, 5, 6, 7, and 8 offer suggestions for creating positive environments and relationships.

In addition, highly tuned emotional and intuitive skills often enhance spirituality. Involvement in spiritual activities can be beneficial and of particular interest. Please see Chapter 8 for more details.

Emotional memory is recalling the feeling of an experience. Both research and practical experience show that persons with dementia have preserved emotional memory. For example, the person will probably remember having a good time with you even if he or she doesn't remember the context (e.g., a picnic). The person may not remember actually taking a bath but probably will remember if it was an unpleasant experience.

Creating positive emotional memories greatly enhances quality of life and well-being and encourages participation. For example, the person may not be able to remember the details of looking at a photo album or helping to make muffins, but he or she will remember the positive feelings of being with you and helping out. These positive emotional memories mean that the next time you suggest an activity, the person is more likely to respond enthusiastically.

Sensory items can help create positive emotional memories. For example, bath time can be a difficult experience. Yet, playing the person's favorite music and using soft, colorful robes and towels or scented powders and creams can create positive emotional memories of the activity (see Chapters 6, 7, and 8 for more details).

Alice was in the advanced stage of dementia and living in a nursing facility. Every Sunday, we would take her to church and then to our house for a family dinner. Alice always seemed happy on these occasions, singing along with the hymns in church, appreciating the greetings of friends after church, visiting with her grandchildren, and helping prepare the meal, for example, by tossing the salad.

One Sunday, she didn't seem to be having a good day. She sat with her head down during the whole church service, not even trying to sing the hymns, not looking up when friends came to chat. It was Easter Sunday, and we decided that the commotion of a special holiday meal would likely be too much for her. As we drove back to the nursing facility, Alice sat in the backseat beside me with her head down and her eyes closed. To my absolute amazement, Alice bolted upright when we drove up to the nursing facility entrance. In a clear voice she said, "What am I doing back here already?"

Alice couldn't have told anyone that every Sunday her son and his family took her to church and to their house for dinner—or even what their names were. However, she clearly had a strong memory in her heart of the feelings of Sunday—strong enough that she knew the day wasn't over yet.

This story, and others like it, carries a vital message for caregivers. First, it shows that even though persons with dementia may not remember an event itself, they remember the positive feelings associated with it. They remember in their heart. After all, this is the most important memory, and it tells you as a caregiver that despite memory loss, you do make a difference—a very important difference.

Sociability and Social Skills

 Before bringing her mother to an adult day program, Nina was invited to spend the morning getting to know the other participants and observing and joining in the activities. As she spent time singing, cooking, and reading the newspaper with the participants, she noticed one person who seemed especially skilled at getting everyone involved. Nina decided that she would join the lady at the coffee break to learn more about this energetic volunteer. Nina began by complimenting the lady on her ability to generate enthusiasm and participation. Then she said, "I'm sorry; I didn't catch your name." A look of panic overtook the "volunteer," who replied, "I forget." This person with exceptional social skills was herself a program participant who couldn't remember her own name.

As the preceding story illustrates, social skills that a person has practiced repeatedly tend to be preserved. These skills are a tremendous strength that can be called upon to bring pleasure, enable involvement and participation, and protect dignity. Caregivers who encourage and support the use of lifelong social skills are amazed at the resources and skills that the person is able to call on.

The handshake is an excellent example of a familiar social skill. I have worked with hundreds of people with dementia and have yet to meet someone who didn't respond to the offer of a handshake. A simple handshake has many possible positive effects—you can communicate warmth and caring by touch, the person usually smiles and makes eye contact, and usually when you say, "How are you?" you will get a, "Fine, thank you" in reply. Most important, by using the person's name and extending a hand in greeting, you are recognizing the person as an adult worthy of your attention. All of this from a 10-second activity! Another example is social conversation. Often repeated conversational phrases, such as "How are you?" "Nice weather, isn't it?" and "That's a pretty dress" are usually retained and make it possible for the person to be part of a conversation or a social get-together. If the person's day and the environment are set up to enhance sociability, there are virtually endless opportunities for social occasions, ranging from a friendly "hi" while passing by to hosting a friend for lunch.

Although persons with dementia usually don't take the initiative in social situations, these occasions are very important. Try to continue some form of the person's lifelong social activities. Examples include having coffee with a neighbor, a meal with family members, or a small party. Help the person to feel important and comfortable by giving him or her something to do and by providing information, such as names and dates. Tell others in advance that your relative has a memory problem, and suggest that they avoid asking questions but instead visit with the person by sharing news from their own life.

It is important to remember that social occasions require a great deal of energy, so they need to be balanced with rest and quiet times. Large crowds, noisy parties, or other gatherings where there is too much noise and confusion should be avoided. Persons with dementia can be become upset and overwhelmed in situations where there is more stimulation than they can manage. See Chapter 6 for more details.

Sensory Awareness and Appreciation

 Mr. D. only spoke every once in a while—sometimes saying "yes" or "thank you" or stuttering "I, I, I, I." Most of the time, he stared into space or sat with his head down and his eyes closed. He no longer fed him-

self. One day near Halloween, I placed a big pumpkin on the table in front of him. He still didn't lift his head or open his eyes. When I gently put his hands on the cool, ridged surface of the pumpkin, he hefted it with both hands and said, "My, that's a dandy. Wherever did you get it?" A few minutes later, after his hands were gently guided to his cup, Mr. D. stirred the milk and sugar into his tea and drank it down with enthusiasm. When Mr. D. had his attention drawn to the feel of the pumpkin, he was helped to speak a sentence. When he was stimulated by the movement of preparing his own tea, he was encouraged to hold the cup and drink independently.

This is just one example of the powerful effect that stimulating the senses can have on persons with dementia. Fortunately, the basic sensory areas of the brain are less damaged by the ravages of dementia than other areas. Caregivers can make use of this strength to bring pleasure and help the person respond to the world around him or her. A brief overview of sensory stimulation follows; see Chapter 6 for more details.

Sensory appreciation is the ability to get pleasure from the sights, sounds, smells, touches, movements, and tastes of everyday life. This is an essential part of life for all of us; we understand and respond to the world around us through our senses. For example, the wonderful aroma of stew reminds us that it is suppertime; the green grass and singing birds remind us that it is spring. We all need sensory stimulation until we die.

Sensory stimulation is essential for brain functioning; it helps us to pay attention to the world around us and to respond (e.g., by talking or eating). As dementia progresses, however, the person will have increasing difficulty paying attention to sensory information and responding to sensory messages. In addition, persons with dementia are at risk of not getting enough sensory stimulation because

- Their difficulty in paying attention leads to difficulty in interpreting the sensory stimulation of everyday life
- The effects of aging may mean that their senses (e.g., vision, hearing) aren't as sharp as they used to be
- Persons with dementia are less likely to respond independently, which may mean that others make less effort to provide the necessary stimulation

Nevertheless, research has shown that providing a level of sensory stimulation that the person can understand improves alertness and responsiveness. It can even improve the person's ability to do everyday activities, as occurred with Mr. D. Thus, using the continuing ability of the brain to receive sensory information is a way to overcome some of the losses of dementia. To make use of the senses for stimulation, it is important to follow these steps:

1. Use familiar, everyday objects and materials (e.g., a cup of tea).
2. Focus on only one sense at a time (e.g., the warmth of the tea in the cup).
3. Draw the person's attention to the object (e.g., gently place his or her hand on the cup).
4. Encourage the person to respond (e.g., by drinking the tea).

Everyday activities provide thousands of opportunities for sensory stimulation. Using Steps 2, 3, and 4, caregivers can provide pleasurable sensory experiences and help the person to be more responsive and involved in life. Please see Chapter 6 for more details.

Motor Skills

Generally, the motor areas of the brain and basic motor skills, such as those used for walking, are preserved until the later stages of dementia. (In a few cases and with particular types of dementia, motor skills may be affected in the earlier stages.) In the later stages, when independent movement become difficult, it is essential to continue helping the person to move for as long as possible. Movement helps to prevent complications such as bed sores, problems with breathing, and painful contractures of muscles.

Furthermore, the human body is not meant to be still for long periods. Whenever you have to sit for several hours, such as at a meeting, you really appreciate the need to move. You may find, as many people do, that you are more tired after sitting all day than if you had been doing physical work. Conclusive research has shown that movement and exercise help people to be physically healthier and mentally sharper. This is true even for people in their nineties who are frail and for persons with dementia (Bowlby Sifton, 2000f; Cress et al., 1999). It is never too late to begin to exercise. Even 5 minutes of mild exercise can make a huge difference. (A doctor should always be consulted before beginning a more strenuous exercise program.)

As noted, the ability to move continues until the later stages of dementia. Yet, difficulty getting started on things or loss of initiative is a symptom of dementia, so persons with dementia often need help to get moving. It is as if the person has a broken starter. Caregivers can act as the starter for movement activities, using the suggestions in Chapters 6, 7, and 8. For example, a walk might be started by saying, "It's a gorgeous day. I would like you to walk with me to the park."

Familiar activities that involve movement are excellent motivators. Household activities such as sweeping the floor, raking leaves, folding laundry, hanging clothes, or digging in the garden provide good exercise and involve familiar movements. Try to continue familiar sports activities, such as swimming, at least in part. Encourage use of the automatic reflex to catch something, which persists for some time. Use soft items, such as beanbags or Nerf balls, and introduce the activity in an adult way—as exercise to keep the hands moving. As dementia progresses, the person will need increasing help to move, including hands-on physical assistance. Movement is, however, even more vital at this stage. Caregivers should consult a qualified therapist for help with adaptive equipment and the best ways to help the person move. (See the information on occupational and physical therapy associations in Appendix B.)

Music is one of the best stimulants for movement. Dancing, clapping hands, tapping feet, and swaying are movements that can be triggered by music. The next subsection offers more on using music.

Responsiveness to Music

The areas of the brain that respond to and appreciate music (generally in the right hemisphere) are frequently preserved. The continuing ability to respond to and appreciate music opens the door to many possibilities. Music has an amazing capacity to speak, to enliven and enrich, to bypass the many communication deficits of dementia. In doing so, music brings pleasure not only by sound but also by taking the person back to the rich emotional associations with favorite and familiar music.

Music is a whole different language, another way of communicating. Matching the music to the person's mood helps the person to express feelings. Listening to favorite music takes the person back to the positive feelings and experiences that are connected with songs. Favorite, calming music can help the person to relax and get to sleep at night.

Music is sometimes called a universal language. However, this is not exactly true. Not all types of music appeal to every person. Everyone has his or her own musical tastes—country, pop, classical, and so forth. To get the most benefit from music, pick the types of music that the person has always preferred. Music from the early years of life—mid-teens to mid-twenties—is usually best remembered and the most favored. It is important to share these musical tastes and favorite songs with other caregivers; using the All About Me form in Appendix A is a good method for sharing such information.

Because of the problems that persons with dementia have getting started or involved in activity, just putting on music isn't enough. It is essential to help the person connect with the music. Some ways to do this are humming and singing along, clapping your hands or tapping your toes in time with the music, or sitting beside the person and taking his or her hand and gently swaying to the music. Dancing is also an excellent way to help the person get involved with and respond to music.

Long-Term Memory

 Eric had been "existing" on the special care dementia unit for approximately 2 months. The staff members were caring and conscientious and the setting was cheerful, but Eric was heartbroken. He spent most of his time sitting slumped in a chair. On occasion, he would shuffle around the living room, glance sadly out the window or pick up a book, and return to his chair. No one could remember seeing him smile. He responded to questions or attempts at conversation with a simple "yes" or "no"—if he responded at all. The staff members

tried their best, but it seemed that nothing alleviated Eric's great sorrow at having to leave his ailing wife of 52 years and their home.

I too had tried everything I could think of to bring Eric some joy and to get him involved in daily life. He would come to reminiscence groups, but all attempts at getting him involved fell flat. Then, one day I hit pay dirt. I had brought some copies of old car ads. When I first showed these to Eric, he responded as usual with a sad nod. However, after a few others had contributed their memories about these cars, Eric stunned us all by commenting that one particular model pictured there had never caught on. Pointing to this picture he explained that the doors had opened from a back hinge (instead of from the front). Although it was a good car, nobody liked the way the door opened, so it went out of production. Building on this surprise response, I went on to involve Eric and the others in a lively conversation about getting a driving license, first cars, car trips, favorite cars, the cost of cars, current cars compared with cars from years ago, the participants' current dream cars, and so forth.

Eric loved to share his stories; it was a gift to see a smile on his face and to hear his lively voice. Through calling on past memories, Eric was enabled to feel pleasure and joy in these present moments. Subsequently, I (and other staff members) called on the connection made during this reminiscence session to bring pleasure in many other interactions with Eric.

Long-term memory recalls events that happened in previous years. Like Eric, people with dementia have better preserved memories of their childhood and young adult years than of more recent memories. Things that happened 5 minutes ago or 5 years ago may not be recalled, but significant events from 50 years ago likely will be remembered. There are gaps in these memories, and these gaps increase as dementia progresses; however, by using what you know about the person as a hint or a cue, you can help to recall his or her past.

Reminiscence is a very important activity that can become part of daily routine. The value of reminiscence is not just that it gets people talking; it also takes them back to the feelings associated with these memories. By recalling important life accomplishments with the person, you help to take him or her back to a time when he or she was in charge, productive, and successful. It helps the person to feel worthwhile and improves mood and self-esteem. Reminiscing—that is, sorting out past life experiences and putting them in perspective—is an essential activity at all life stages. Yet as people age and look back over the past, summing up their life is a vital developmental activity. The memory loss caused by dementia means that assistance from others to reminisce is needed and appreciated.

Of course, not all memories are happy. It is important to also provide an opportunity to recall unhappy memories and to express sadness. This helps people to release the feelings and to get on with the present.

When you know about the important events of a person's life—winning the championship game, the first day of school, building a home—these can be used as verbal reminders to help him or her to recall these experiences. Actual objects from long ago are very important triggers for memory: photographs, kitchen utensils, tools, clothes, hats, books, magazines, catalogs, jewelry, watches, and so forth. Allowing the person to handle and use the objects provides sensory stimulation and further enriches the experience.

When helping to trigger memories, it is important not to ask questions that might have right and wrong answers. Questions such as "What is this called?" are difficult for persons with dementia, so they might become upset and withdrawn. However, everyone can offer an opinion. Questions such as "Does this look familiar to you?" "What do you like best about this?" and "What is you favorite . . .?" give the person a chance to participate and be successful. See Chapter 6 for more information on reminiscence.

Ways the Caregiver Can Address the Symptoms of Dementia

No two people are alike. It always amazes me to think that we humans are more alike when are born then we ever will be again. More general statements can be made about a 6-month-old than about a 65-year-old. The vast range of life experiences in those years has a powerful effect on how a person thinks and acts. Then, when we add in the effects of dementia, the picture gets even more complicated. Recalling that wise adage "It is not what disease the person has, but what person the disease has" can help caregivers to stay focused. Family caregivers know the person better than anyone else ever will. This knowledge can help you and other caregivers to support the person in maintaining a familiar lifestyle, to make use of the person's continuing abilities, and to understand the sometimes puzzling changes in behavior. Dementia care is person-centered care.

No one person necessarily experiences all of the symptoms. There is not a fixed pattern to the way in which the brain is damaged by dementia. For instance, some will have difficulty recognizing objects early on; others will not have this problem until later in the disease.

Like all of us, persons with dementia have some days that are better than others. The person's ability to do things may vary on different days and at different times on the same day. It depends on many things, such as how rested the person is, how familiar the surroundings are, and whether the person is physically healthy.

With these important considerations in mind, ways for caregivers to address the general symptoms of dementia are outlined under the following main categories: cognitive, behavioral, and physical skills. (These skills are all interrelated, so separate categories are somewhat artificial.) A brief description of each symptom is followed by comments on how the person may feel, what the person can do, the ways in which caregivers can help compensate for these symptoms, and references to other chapters for more details.

Cognitive Skills

Even if I try my hardest, events and phrases just disappear from my consciousness . . . my sieve brain leaks too much! There are simply huge gaps, where I don't register an event—the memory is not laid down anywhere in my brain. So it is not that I have forgotten and you can remind me. It is as if it never happened. Even if you tell me what happened, it means nothing to me. I'll just smile politely and try to pretend I remember all about it. (Boden, 1998, p. 65)

The key symptom of dementia is memory loss. In the preceding quote, Christine Boden described what this feels like. At first, the memory loss is for more recent events (e.g., yesterday's visit from a friend). The person may also occasionally misplace things, forget people's names, forget appointments or directions, repeat the same questions or stories, or get lost in familiar places. As the disease progresses, the memory loss increases and includes longer-term memory. When this happens, the person may feel embarrassed. The person is still able to recognize people that are important to him or her and shows this, for example, by greeting these people with a smile. You can help by always using his or her own name and others' names in conversation and by not putting the person on the spot. (See Chapter 4.)

Another cognitive symptom is **difficulty understanding things that are not concrete.** This includes abstract ideas, such as making plans about money. When this happens, the person may feel frustrated that he or she can no longer manage things such as personal finances. The person may still be able to do part of the activity with help from others. You can help by quietly taking over activities while giving the person a chance to participate—for example, by paying the bills yourself but asking the person to sign the checks. (See Chapter 7.)

Difficulty with judgment is also apparent in dementia. For example, the person may go outside on a cold day without a coat. When this happens, the person may believe that he or she is being treated like a child if the caregiver just tells him or her what to do—for instance, to put on his or her coat. The person is still able to understand nonverbal suggestions. You can help by using a positive way to suggest wearing a coat, such as holding out the person's coat and saying "I got out both of our coats so that we will be all ready for our walk on this cold day." (See Chapters 6 and 7.)

Difficulty paying attention is another cognitive symptom. For example, the person may be unable to attend to a conversation or a television show and may be easily distracted. When this happens, the person may feel overwhelmed by normal daily commotion and have difficulty doing a task. He or she may also become upset and agitated or withdrawn. The person is still able to get pleasure from and respond to quiet daily stimulation. You can help by limiting noise and stimulation, especially during important conversations and mealtimes. (See Chapters 4, 5, and 6.)

Difficulty starting activities is a symptom of dementia. It may appear that the person has lost interest in doing things. When this happens, the person may feel sad and depressed because he or she doesn't have anything to do. The person may also be afraid to start something because he or she does not want to make mistakes or be embarrassed. The person is still able to do many familiar activities if the methods for doing them can be changed. You can help by gently taking the initiative in starting an activity and assuring the person that he or she will not be alone. For example, take the person's arm and say, "I would like you to come for a walk with me." (See Chapters 6, 7, and 8.)

The person with dementia will have **difficulty solving problems.** For example, he or she may not be able to determine that a lamp won't work because the bulb has burned out. When this happens, the person may feel frustrated and angry that he or she can't figure out things that used to be easy. The person may still be able to do many things that solve a problem in the same way every time (e.g., turning on the light to illuminate a dark room). You can help by trying to make sure the person doesn't encounter problems that he or she can't fix. In addition, the caregiver can provide chances for the person to be helpful (e.g., asking the person to help put in a new light bulb). (See Chapters 6, 7, and 8.)

Difficulty planning and organizing tasks or activities is another symptom of dementia. At first, the person may have problems organizing a complex task, such as preparing a meal. The person may lose the thread between the many steps of this task and forget what to do next. Over time, other less complex activities, such as brushing one's teeth, also become challenging. When this happens, the person may feel so frustrated and embarrassed that he or she gives up. The person is still able to do many familiar activities with guidance. You can help by adapting the activity so the person can succeed (e.g., break the activity into steps and give hints or cues for each step). (See Chapters 6, 7, and 8.)

Dementia leads to **difficulty describing or explaining things to others.** When this happens, the person may feel frustrated, embarrassed, and angry. The person is still able to use other ways of communicating. You can help by trying to understand the person's emotional message. This can be done by reading facial expressions and other nonverbal ways of communicating. (See Chapter 4.)

Dementia also causes **difficulty understanding what others are saying.** When this happens, the person may feel embarrassed and frustrated. The person is still able to understand the speaker's emotional message and make standard social responses. You can help by using other ways of communicating and making use of the person's social skills to preserve dignity. (See Chapter 4.)

The person will have **difficulty organizing familiar coordinated activities,** such as getting dressed, sitting in a chair, and walking. The person has the physical ability to do these activities, but he or she is unable to carry out the coordinated movements and steps required. This is called *apraxia.* When this happens, the person may feel frightened about falling and be embarrassed at seeming so clumsy. The person is still able to engage in simple movement activities and, with help, can get dressed. You can help by providing guidance (e.g., taking the person's arm and saying, "The chair is right behind you") and making the living space as safe as possible. (See Chapters 5, 6, 7, and 8.)

Another symptom of dementia is **difficulty recognizing things or people, especially when they are not in their usual settings.** This is due to perceptual problems—that is, problems the brain has in understanding messages from the senses. The senses may take in the information and send them to the brain, but the person's damaged brain just cannot sort out what the sensory messages mean. The person may have difficulty with one or all of these types of perception: vision, touch, spatial orientation, and body awareness. For example, the person may not be able to recognize a spoon when it is jumbled up with other silverware but can recognize it by feel when the spoon is in her or his hand. A person who has problems with proprioception (awareness of the body's location in space) may, for instance, have difficulty sitting in a chair because he or she doesn't know where his or her body is in relation to the chair. When this happens, the person may feel frightened, frustrated, and distressed. The person is still able to recognize and appreciate offers of help and concern. You can help by maintaining a living space that looks as familiar as possible and always naming any persons present. (See Chapters 4, 5, 6, and 7).

Persons with dementia will have **increasing difficulty with recalling orientation information.** The person may have problems with stating the date, the place, the time of day, or his or her name. When this happens, the person may feel embarrassed, frightened, and frustrated. The person is still able to appreciate being reassured. You can help by always providing orientation information for reassurance. (See Chapter 4.)

The person will have **difficulty making decisions,** even about simple things such as what to wear. When this happens, the person may feel sad and discouraged as well as frustrated by the feeling of not being in control, of not being able to make choices. The person is still able to make choices between two things (e.g., if asked "Would you like to wear this white shirt or this green shirt?"). You can help by finding ways to offer choices that the person can make. (See Chapters 6, 7, and 8.)

There may be **changes in personality** due to all of the changes in the brain. Some persons may have marked changes—for example, the normally cheerful and easygoing person may become tense and anxious. When this happens, the person may be aware that something's changed and feel distressed about it, or he or she may be unaware of the changes. The person is still able to respond to a supportive care situation. You can help by understanding that the changes are the result of brain damage. (This topic is covered in all of the book's chapters.)

Behavioral Skills

Changes in behavior result from damage to the brain and/or to the person's problems coping with lost abilities. Behavioral changes are a symptom of dementia. Please remember that the person is not trying to be difficult or annoying on purpose. Often, what may seem to be unusual behavior is the only way the person can let others know his or her needs. Chapter 9 provides more on how to understand, prevent, and/or respond to behavioral symptoms.

Difficulty sleeping occurs because of damage to the sleep–wake area of the brain and problems with time and place orientation. When this happens, the person may feel restless and upset at night. The person is still able to get rest at other times of the day or in another location at night. You can help by determining ways to improve the person's sleep, such as keeping a familiar bedtime routine. (See Chapter 7.)

The person may experience **pent-up energy,** which can lead to restlessness, fidgeting with clothing, pacing, and so forth. This restlessness can increase at the end of the day (sundowning). When this happens, the person may feel anxious or frightened and be unable to sit still. The person is still able to enjoy using his or her hands for simple, familiar activities such as sweeping the floor or folding clothing. You can help by providing familiar activities and a calming, welcoming environment, especially at the end of the day. (See Chapters 5, 6, 7, 8, and 9.)

The person will have **difficulty keeping track of things or explaining puzzling situations.** Because the person still tries his or her best to explain things, this can sometimes lead to blaming others for hiding things or for not sharing information. When this happens, the person may feel upset that he or she can't find things. The person is still able to realize that something he or she values is missing. You can help by being nonconfrontational, providing reassurance, and having extras of things such as glasses or keys. One caregiver said, "My mother is always losing her purse, so now I have a whole closet full of purses!" (See Chapters 5, 6, 7, 8, and 9.)

The person with dementia may experience **hallucinations (sights or sounds that seem real to the person but are not really there) or delusions (fixed but untrue ideas)** (e.g., a man insists that his wife is having an affair). Although symptoms are rare, they are extremely upsetting to everyone if they occur. These misperceptions can be extremely fixed, despite memory loss. Hallucinations and delusions are a direct result of damage to the brain. When this happens, the person may feel absolutely sure that these experiences are real and become frightened and/or angry. The person may still be able to respond to pleasant distractions. In some cases, medication may help. You can help by seeking the advice of a doctor, understanding the person's distress, offering reassurance and favorite activities (e.g., eating a favorite snack, listening to a favorite song), and avoiding arguing (See Chapters 2 and 9.)

Perseveration can be a symptom of dementia. This involves getting "stuck"—repeating the same phrase or movement. In this case, the brain is acting like a broken record that can't move out of a groove. When this happens, the person may feel content that he or she has something to do or frustrated by not being able to get "unstuck" from a particular activity. The person is still able to be involved in interesting, repetitive activities. You can help by using perseveration as an aid to do things or by offering another repetitive activity if necessary. For example, if the person claps continually, the caregiver can offer a familiar, quiet movement activity, such as sanding a board or drying dishes with a cloth. (See Chapters 6, 7, and 8.)

The person may have **difficulty feeling "at home."** This can lead the person to search for home and risk becoming lost. When this happens, the person may feel frightened and lost. The person is still able to appreciate being reassured that someone is going to look after him or her. You can help by providing reassurance (e.g., giving hugs, providing a homey environment). (See Chapters 2 and 5.)

The person may feel extremely discouraged, and/or he or she may have clinical **depression.** Anywhere from 30% to 50% of persons in the early and middle stages of Alzheimer's disease are depressed. When this happens, a person may feel overwhelmed by all that is happening to him or her. The person is still able to respond to the reassurance and support of caregivers and to medical treatment (i.e., counseling and/or medication), if necessary. You can help by seeking medical treatment for the person if the symptoms of depression (e.g., change in appetite or sleep patterns, extreme tearfulness or feelings of hopelessness, apathy) exceed 3–4 weeks and by helping the person to feel supported and be successful. (See Chapters 2, 6, 7, and 8.)

A **catastrophic reaction** is an unexpected bout of distress—such as tearfulness, shouting, or striking out—that seems out of proportion to the circumstances (e.g., the person yells when he or she has difficulty putting on shoes). When this happens, the person may feel overwhelmed by tasks or circumstances that he or she can't manage. The person is still able to benefit from reassurance. You can help by trying to avoid circumstances that overwhelm the person and providing reassurance and distraction if the person does become overwhelmed. (See Chapters 2, 6, 7, 8, and 9.)

Physical Skills

Changes in cognitive and communicative abilities—and, later, in physical ability—make it increasingly difficult for persons with dementia to remain independent in work, leisure, and self-care activities. Initially, the person will be challenged by more complicated activities that require planning, problem solving, and decision making, such as developing a new project at work, managing finances, or following a complicated knitting pattern. As the disease progresses, the person will begin to have increasing difficulty with routine physical activities, such as bathing, getting dressed, and, eventually, eating. At the same time, continuing to be involved and as independent as possible in daily activities is vital to the person's well-being. Fortunately, there are many ways to help the person to do so. (See Chapters 6, 7, and 8 for details and suggestions for supporting involvement in daily activities.)

As dementia progresses to the later stages, brain damage begins to affect basic physical abilities such as walking, going to the bathroom, and even swallowing. As noted, the person usually loses these abilities in reverse order from the way that they are acquired in childhood. For example, persons with dementia will have difficulty doing fine motor activities, such as fastening buttons, before they will have difficulty doing gross motor activities, such as holding a spoon to eat. Or, they will have problems walking before they have problems sitting up. However, the continuation of lifelong skills and supportive interventions from caregivers help preserve day-to-day abilities and, most important, a sense of self-worth. All of the chapters of this book offer suggestions in this regard.

Difficulty with walking and balance becomes evident in the middle to late stages. When this happens, the person may feel frustrated with the loss of independence but may be unable to appreciate the risk of falling. The person is still able to benefit from regular physical activity and supportive interventions such as walking aids, wheelchairs, or bathroom safety equipment. You can help by ensuring that the person gets plenty of physical activity and that a qualified therapist conducts an assessment for the use of adaptive equipment. (See Chapters 5, 6, 7, and 8.)

The person will experience **difficulty with coordinated hand movements.** When this happens, the person may feel embarrassed and frustrated, which may lead him or her to stop trying to do things with his or her hands. The person is still able to use his or her hands when activities are adapted. You can help by setting up activities for success. (See Chapters 6, 7, and 8.)

Difficulty controlling bladder and bowels is a physical symptom of dementia in the later stages. When this happens, the person may be extremely embarrassed and angry at the loss of independence. The person is still able to appreciate respectful treatment as a dignified adult and may benefit from a toileting routine and/or incontinence products. You can help by always treating the person with respect and dignity and never causing shame or embarrassment or mentioning the problem in public. (See Chapter 7.)

In the end stages of dementia, some individuals (about 10%) may have seizures. Caregivers should consult a physician for the management of seizures. Some may also have a **return of primitive reflexes** (Altman, 1987; Burns, Jacoby, & Levy, 1991; Volicer et al., 1987). These reflexes are referred to as "primitive" because in infancy they are basic movements that are automatic or preprogrammed. Infants rely on these automatic movements, such as the sucking and rooting reflexes in search of food, for survival. As an infant's movements become more skilled and planned, these reflexes disappear. In the later stages of dementia, when more skilled movements have been lost, these primitive reflexes may reappear. Skilled caregivers can use these reflex movements to assist in care and for the person's survival. Above all else, it is essential that you appreciate that these movements (e.g., grasping tightly onto one's arm or hair) are not deliberate; they are automatic in the same way an infant might grasp onto whatever touches his or her palm. The most common of primitive reflexes are discussed next.

Grasp Reflex

This familiar reflex is stimulated by light touch in the middle of the palm. It is what causes infants to hold onto a rattle, toy, or a parent's hair or glasses. When the grasp reflex is present, the person's fingers will automatically flex or close around whatever object has lightly touched the person's palm, often the caregiver's hand or wrist.

If the grasp reflex has been triggered, do not struggle to release the person's grasp; this just increases the stimulus to hold on tighter. The best approach is to offer something interesting to the person (e.g., a snack, a favorite interesting object) that will encourage him or her to reach out and take it. If this doesn't work, gently rub or tap on the muscle bulk on the outside of the forearm, just below the crease of the elbow joint. These are the muscle bodies that extend the fingers. You can locate this area on your own body by bending your fingers, laying your forearm on a table, and feeling the change as you straighten your fingers.

As with all primitive reflexes, it is best to avoid creating the stimulus. However, some ways the grasp reflex can be useful are as follows:

- Holding on firmly during transfers or while rising from lying to sitting or standing
- Grasping a spoon for eating
- Grasping safe, interesting objects for self-directed activity

Suck Reflex

The reflex to close the lips around an object is stimulated by a light stroking of the lips. This is what stimulates a newborn to nurse or drink from a bottle. If present, this reflex can be used by a skilled professional to assist with feeding during the late stages of dementia. However, caregivers generally should avoid triggering this reflex. If present, it can interfere with eating and may cause persons with advanced dementia to put dangerous or inedible objects in their mouths.

People who have a positive suck reflex should only be fed by a skilled professional or by someone who has been properly trained. The suck reflex can be used to assist drinking fluids through a straw or a special cup. Some professionals recommend providing adult soothers to satisfy the reflexive need to suck, but this approach is not yet widely accepted.

Rooting Reflex

This reflex causes the movement of the corner of the mouth toward a light touch on the corner of the mouth or the cheek. Like the suck reflex, it can interfere with eating. All but professionals or trained caregivers should avoid stimulating it.

Gegenhalten Response

The Gegenhalten Response is quite common. Persons with late-stage dementia often hold their arms close to the body and in a flexed (bent) position. Naturally, caregivers who want to assist with dressing will attempt to straighten the person's arms. This movement of the forearm from a flexed position to an extended (straight) position is the stimulus for a reflexive movement to resist straightening the arm. Clearly, this reflex can interfere with offering hand-over-hand guidance during dressing and exercise activities, such as throwing a ball or a beanbag. Avoid stimulating this reflex during care and other activities. Offer the object and encourage the person to extend his or her own arms. Putting on blouses, shirts, and sweaters will be easier when the person is standing and his or her arms are already extended.

Positive Supporting Reaction

When the positive supporting reaction is present, the person's legs extend in response to firm pressure on the bottom of the feet (e.g., from the footplates on a wheelchair). Obviously, this is helpful when moving the person from sitting to standing, but it can be problematic when changing from standing to sitting—for instance, while seating the person for a meal or an activity. The person may remain standing and rigid as a board. The best way to break up this reflex is to provide a stimulus that encourages an automatic response to bend the knees and sit down. Having the table prepared and others seated around it helps in overcoming this reflex. Gently guide the person into a chair by placing your hands on his or her hips and his or her hands on the chair arms or table. Use gentle downward pressure on the hips. It is essential not to use force; above all, do not push down on the person's head and shoulders.

Startle Reflex

When the startle reflex is present, a sudden noise or movement will cause the person to fling his or her arms and legs into extension and throw the head back while extending the neck and back. Most everyone jumps at the unexpected slamming of a door. However, the startle reflex is an extreme exaggeration of this response and can be stimulated by what seems to be only a slight, sudden sound (e.g., a sneeze). It is very distressing to the person and may lead to agitation and/or a catastrophic reaction. As Chapter 5 details, extra care must be taken to provide a calm and quiet environment for all persons with dementia. It is particularly important to never move a person's chair without first telling him or her and to ensure that the person is aware that you are in the room.

CONCLUSION

Because there has been an explosion of information about Alzheimer's disease and other dementias since the 1980s, this chapter has provided an overview of some of the basic information that may be of assistance to caregivers. When considering this information, as well as information from other sources, it is essential to remember two things above all else: 1) Each person with dementia has many continuing abilities that can be used to overcome some of the deficits caused by dementia, and 2) the most important focus is on the *person* with dementia and not on dementia, as each person's experience of dementia is unique. Chapter 4 provides suggestions for ways to continue to be connected with the person through communication.

4

Communicating with Someone Who Has Dementia

On her birthday, Micheline was rushing around the house doing a treasure hunt Ianthe had prepared, and a clue was hidden under the smoke detector. I said, 'Get the tissue!' (to stand on, instead of the stool).

And now, imagine this is happening to you nearly *every* time you speak—and you know it's only going to get worse. Often you wonder whether it's worth trying to speak, because it always comes out wrong and everyone laughs at you.

That's what its like to have Alzheimer's. (Boden, 1998, p. 75)

LESSONS ON LISTENING: THE ART OF COMMUNICATION[2]

In the modern world, we are constantly bombarded with a cacophony of messages—from 24-hour news on 24-inch (or 48- or 64-inch) screens, piped-in music and infomercials at malls, junk mail that consumes acres of trees, e-mail spam,

---

[2]Portions of this section previously appeared in Bowlby Sifton, C. (2002). Lessons on listening: The *art* of communication. *Alzheimer's Care Quarterly, 3*(2), iv–vi; adapted by permission.

voice mail, and so many others. In the midst of this bombardment, I wonder, "Does anybody really *listen* anymore?" Has the effort required to get our own message across or to evade unsolicited messages from so many sources obscured our ability to listen? Have we forgotten that true communication requires both listening and speaking/writing skills to arrive at a shared meaning?

Reflecting on and responding to these questions is important to all aspects of our daily lives and to every vocation. However, when our daily lives involve spending time with persons with dementia, the preceding questions take on critical significance.

Persons with dementia have decreasing ability to speak our language; caregivers must learn to speak theirs. Above all, we are called upon to listen with our ears, our eyes, our heads, and especially our hearts. An example of this type of listening follows.

Mary:	"This time it is not the place to . . . you know . . . It is always, well . . . very nice."
Helen:	"Mary, I'm glad that it was nice. You look very nice yourself in that beautiful dress."
Mary:	"Yes, it is the one that wasn't hard, you know it came from the one."
Helen:	"Well, just the same, you always look so smart. That blue looks great on you. Is blue your favorite color?"
Mary:	"Blue, red . . . red . . . ah red, white and ah, yes that was always it, you—well, the way when that happens it goes like—hmm."
Helen:	"Oh, what a good idea, Mary—the red, white, and blue. Shall we sing the national anthem?"
Mary:	"Well, that's just the thing—it's too, ah far the hmmmm, and then it's, well you know all that."

Anyone who has spent time with a person with dementia has probably had a conversation similar to this exchange between Mary and her caregiver, Helen. At first blush, most probably would not consider it a conversation. After all, can you really say that there was any kind of meaningful exchange of information, that Mary understood or responded to what Helen was saying? In usual terms, this was not a conversation. However, taking into consideration all of the nonword pieces, it is clear that significant communication has taken place.

Mary: "This time it is not the place to . . . you know . . . It is always, well . . . very nice." (*Mary is pacing in the living room; she looks puzzled and anxious as she mutters these words—seemingly to no one in particular.*)

Helen: "Mary, I'm glad that it was nice. You look very nice yourself in that beautiful dress." (*As Helen speaks to Mary in a warm and reassuring voice, she gently touches Mary's arm and moves so that she is in Mary's line of vision. Mary stops pacing, looks at Helen, and smiles hesitantly.*)

Mary: "Yes, it is the one that wasn't hard, you know it came from the one." (*Mary meets Helen's gaze. Mary's face and body look less tense. She gestures with her hands and shrugs as if to say, "Well, there was nothing to it."*)

Helen: "Well, just the same, you always look so smart. That blue looks great on you. Is blue your favorite color?" (*Helen touches Mary's dress admiringly and gently takes Mary's arm as she starts walking to the kitchen. Mary responds warmly, smiling widely at Helen, and starts to walk with her.*)

Mary: "Blue, red . . . red. . . . ah red, white and ah, yes that was always it, you—well, the way when that happens it goes like—hmm." (*Mary looks a little puzzled and ends with a hesitant humming.*)

Helen: "Oh, what a good idea, Mary—the red, white, and blue. Shall we sing the national anthem?" (*Helen hugs Mary with enthusiasm, and Mary responds with pleasure, still trying to hum something.*)

Mary: "Well, that's just the thing—it's too, ah far the hmmmm, and then it's, well you know all that." (*Mary is struggling to answer and to get started on a tune. She looks to Helen as if asking for help. Helen smiles warmly and starts singing the national anthem. Mary beams and joins in with great enthusiasm as they happily march toward the kitchen.*)

When "stage directions" are added, it is obvious that meaningful communication occurred in this moment. Even more important, for Mary, the moment moved from anxious concern to happiness at sharing a well-known and loved song. Mary and Helen had a moment of significant connection, and each was able to recognize the other as an important person in her life.

Helen was highly skilled at active listening, at looking beyond Mary's words—using facial expressions, body language, gestures, and the feel of what Mary was saying to fill in the blanks and communicate with Mary in a meaningful way. Helen demonstrated that she is a great master at what some call the *language of Alzheimer's*.

Communicating—sharing thoughts, ideas, and feelings—is the foundation of human relationships. It is the core of living in the community, of being with and relating to another person. Over time, persons with dementia lose the ability to speak in words and to understand our words. As these conventional communication skills diminish, other ways of communicating, of maintaining connections with people, become strengthened. Persons with dementia become skilled at intuitive language; they understand and speak the eloquent voices of the heart. By listening to gestures, touch, actions, created words, facial expressions, body language, and emotional expression, persons with dementia learn to read others like an open book. The following is one example from the experience of my colleague, Anna Ortigara, R.N.

Anna was having a happy conversation with Louise. Both were enjoying being connected and sharing thoughts and feelings, although an inexperienced listener would think that nothing meaningful was being exchanged. This conversation was taking place at one end of the corridor of a busy nursing facility. This corridor was full of activity, with residents and staff talking and going about their daily rounds. At the far end of the corridor, a male employee from the laundry department was talking enthusiastically "at" a female care aide, who didn't seem interested. Anna noted that the young man was trying his best to get a date with the staff member but was not having any success. With all that was going on in this corridor, Anna was amazed that Louise could pay attention to what Anna was saying. Then, Louise made a comment that absolutely floored Anna. Shaking her head and smiling ironically, Louise said, "Mmm, mmm, mmm. He's sellin', but she ain't buyin'."

Against all odds, Louise had used intuitive listening skills to understand the events at the far end of a busy corridor. Even after all of the time that I have spent with persons with dementia, I continue to be amazed by their creative and skilled ways to communicate beyond words.

We are invited into this rich world of understanding and sharing that goes beyond words, that requires active listening. There is much to be shared and celebrated if we can open ourselves to other ways of communicating; there is much to be heard and understood if we can still ourselves and the urgency of our personal agenda and open our hearts to listen. We need to learn about the art of listening from the grand masters—persons with dementia.

Active listening is an essential skill that enhances all of our relationships, particularly those with persons who have dementia. It is vital for affirming and acknowledging the ongoing worth of persons with dementia who steadily lose their ability to speak and understand words. This need to continue to be connected, to communicate with others, was noted in Chapter 2 when Marie, who had dementia, tapped on her heart and told her husband, "Michael, don't you forget that I'm still in here." We are reminded that persons with dementia are still very much present and in need of recognition and connection with others.

Although language losses can make it seem that the person with dementia is lost to us, that we cannot reach him or her, nothing is further from the truth. Never has the need to maintain communication and connection been greater. Caregivers are invited to learn about and share the nonverbal ways that persons with dementia use so richly and skillfully. Keeping connected—communicating through words and in these other ways—is vital, as is pointed out by Bob and Anne Simpson:

> We decided to jot down what had been helpful in our experience, because when someone has a loss, of any kind, we all wonder what to say. And many times we are not at all sure that we will say the "right" thing, so we say nothing at all.
>
> Our suggestion, first of all, is say *something*. Say, "I'm sorry"; say, "I'm thinking of you"; say, "You are in our prayers"; or say, "How are you doing?" If it is said with love and concern, the words don't matter. If you feel that you

might blubber, don't worry. When you express your emotions about our loss, we know that you are trying to understand our feelings and that you are willing to share them.

Talk to us in person. Come to visit, go out of your way to start a conversation in the grocery store, on the sidewalk in town, at church, at a friend's house—wherever we may run into one another. If you say nothing when we meet, we will think you do not care. (Simpson & Simpson, 1999, p. 64)

NONVERBAL COMMUNICATION

In Western society, spoken and written language tend to mean the same thing as communication. We celebrate as children struggle to form their first words and, later, first sentences. As we move through the stages of life, spoken and written words celebrate life's happy and sad occasions: a toast to the bride and groom, a eulogy, and so forth. Years of schooling, community events, and book stores and libraries have elevated the spoken and written forms of communication to a high art. Much of what we want to know, understand, wonder, and feel is shared in the spoken and written word.

With this emphasis on speaking and writing, the powerful, unwritten, nonverbal language of tone of voice, facial expression, body posture, touch, and gesture often goes unnoticed. Yet, before they can ever utter a word, infants are able to tell us when they are happy, hungry, or distressed and need comfort. They are also able to make us happy. Nonverbal language was our first way of communicating, and it continues to be an essential part of all communication. Many experts suggest that nonverbal communication makes up as much as 55%–97% of all communication (Gross, 1990).

If you think about our own experiences, you can probably appreciate that this is true. Have you ever had the experience of doubting someone's apology or excuse because the look on his or her face or in his or her eyes said something quite different? Who can forget the powerful nonverbal messages from parents—a beaming face in the audience at a Christmas concert or stern looks for bad manners at the dinner table? In addition, think about how reluctant we are to deliver sad news, such as a death, over the telephone; without the nonverbal element, it is very difficult to convey feelings of caring, support, and concern. Sometimes, we even hide behind a telephone or e-mail message or perhaps even the inaccessible language of the law to deliver difficult messages while keeping our feelings in check. I invite you to make your own list regarding the power of nonverbal communication; thinking about this can help you to appreciate the value and use of nonverbal messages, an avenue that is still open to persons with dementia.

For persons with dementia, nonverbal communication—first language, the unspoken language of the body—again becomes the most important language. This is similar to sight, touch, and smell becoming a lifeline for someone with a hearing impairment. With the progression of dementia and increasing difficulty in using spoken words, caregivers who make nonverbal language the first language enable the person to continue the sharing and understanding of thoughts, needs, and feelings. When caregivers use and attend to nonverbal communication, persons with dementia have a channel of self-expression, understand what is expected of them, and have their self-worth supported. Listening to and using nonverbal communication relieves anxiety and frustration, and it can often trigger the use of words. By using these eloquent voices of the heart, persons with dementia and others are able to communicate person to person.

The return to first language is difficult because of our life-long, adult focus on verbal communication. If your personal communication style has always included much touch and gesture, it may be easier. Others may require more practice and conscious thought, but it is possible. Furthermore, it is essential.

When using the first language modalities of touch, facial expressions, voice tone, body posture, and gestures, the following must be appreciated:

1. Return to first language is NOT a return to childhood and childish ways. I have no doubt that persons with dementia retain their adult sense of themselves. Any caregiver use of first language that suggests that the person is childish (e.g., patting the person on the head) is an offense to dignity.

2. Personal, generational, and cultural traditions need to be respected. Although sharing hugs and touches now tends to be an accepted practice among family, friends, and acquaintances, this is not the experience of many older people. Hugs and other forms of touch may be viewed as an invasion of personal space or something that is shared only with the most intimate family members and friends. When the person requires assistance with personal care or is in a communal living situation, such as a nursing facility, respecting privacy and personal space becomes even more important.

3. Caregivers need to observe the types and combinations of first language and verbal language to which the person responds. For example, some people find the use of gestures and pantomime easy to follow; others may be able to follow written directions.

Touch

The power of touch is astonishing and begins very early; a fetus first responds to touch at 8 weeks (Huss, 1976). Infants begin to experience, explore, and understand the world through touch—the security of Mother's womb, the comfort of cuddling in Daddy's arms, the feel of the warm blankets or a wet diaper on the skin. Touch remains a powerful medium of communication throughout life even though we develop other ways of communicating. Although greeting others with a hug has become common, touch is mostly reserved for intimate personal relationships—parents and children, lovers, spouses, and dear friends. In most cases we use a handshake to touch from arms' length. Even still, this handshake speaks volumes: the warmth and caring of a lingering firm grasp; dominance or anger from the too-firm grip; anxiety and fear in the weak, hesitant offering of a limp hand.

As Mary Judd said so eloquently, "TOUCH is a language seen by the blind, heard by the deaf and felt by everyone" (1983, p. 13). If we think about it, the word *touch* comes up everywhere in conversation: "Let's keep in TOUCH," "Your comments TOUCHED me," "We need to "TOUCH base," or "That's a TOUCHY subject."

The need to be touched and to touch others continues throughout life. This need is especially powerful when we are ill or distressed. Think about the tremendous comfort that is provided by the touch of a loving hand when we are sick or distressed. Perhaps you can remember a parent's healing touch. As we age and experience losses and sickness, we especially need this touch, with its wordless reassurance and nurturing. Yet, as time goes by, spouses, children, lovers, friends, and other people with whom we have shared touch may not be with us. In addition, when a spouse takes on the caregiver role, it can be difficult to continue in physical or sexual relationships. This can become more difficult still if the spouse with dementia misinterprets a caring touch as an invitation to intercourse. Spouse caregivers should be reassured that these feelings and responses, both their own and those of the person with dementia, are natural. Chapter 7 has more on this topic.

A touch on the hand, a hug, a gentle arm around the shoulder, or an extra snuggling in the blankets often calms a frightened and distressed person; offering a caring touch reassures and can be understood without words. Yet, friends and family members, disturbed by the changes caused by dementia, often have less personal contact with the person. Except for practical caregiving tasks, paid caregivers are often reluctant to touch older people, recoiling at their wrinkled, sagging skin. Touch is further discouraged by the physical fences erected by frailty, geri-chairs, wheelchairs, and bed rails. As a result, the people who are most in need of a caring touch— persons with dementia (especially those in long-term care facilities)—are least likely to receive it. Expressions of this need for touch can be seen in persons with advanced dementia—in the hands that reach out to passersby, in behaviors such as rubbing a chair tray, clothing, pieces of fabric, or stuffed animals. In professional care, efforts are being made to overcome this lack of touch. For example, nurses are being trained in the use of Therapeutic Touch, as developed by Doris Krieger (1979). The results of a few research studies in this and other approaches have been very positive (Griffin & Vitro, 1998; Woods & Diamond, 2002).

Guidelines for the Use of Touch

Because it is so powerful, caregivers must take care not to use touch in ways that may have negative effects. The following guidelines are offered for the use of touch.

*Respect the Person's Dignity
and Cultural and Social Background*

Touch can be negative if it is not offered in a way that respects the dignity, adulthood, and privacy of the person. For example, many of us have been offended by the touch of an overly familiar salesperson. The possibility for offense becomes even greater when the person has dementia, especially when assistance is needed for personal care. Caregivers must always ask permission before invading personal space to provide care.

This can be especially difficult and sensitive when spouses or family members become caregivers and help with personal activities such as bathing. Stand in the other person's shoes for a minute. Whatever our previous relationship, it seldom would have involved assisting with bathing or other personal activities. These activities are our most private. In the case of some older persons, even their spouses may have never seen them naked. When the caregiving role calls for assistance with these activities, it can cross a threshold that both the person and the caregiver find challenging. For instance, one caregiver's mother agreed to help with her bath but came to the tub wearing her bathing suit! In another much more challenging situation, a husband caregiver reluctantly resorted to holding his wife's arms still so that a paid caregiver could do her personal care. In this case, touch was far from therapeutic; instead it communicated power, control, and humiliation. Fortunately, with the advice of a third party, the husband was able to reassume a therapeutic role by, among other things, gently holding his wife's hand and singing her favorite song while the paid caregiver used warm cloths and gentle touches to wash her. For more information on touch and communication during personal care activities, see Chapters 6 and 7.

It is vital to share with paid caregivers information about touch, personal habits, and values. This should include not only personal information but also cultural and social information. For example, in some European cultures, hugs and kissing on the cheek are an accepted form of greeting between adults; in others, a handshake is the only acceptable form of touch.

Begin the Use of Touch Gradually, Constantly Assessing the Person's Reaction

In Western cultures, a handshake is an acceptable and familiar greeting, and it should be used frequently with persons with dementia. I have yet to encounter a person, even in the most advanced stages of dementia, who does not respond in some way to this familiar use of touch. First and most important, this touch recognizes the person as a valued adult, especially if the person is also addressed by name. If the person responds well to this contact, further caring can be communicated by adding the other hand on top, a double handshake.

The usual acceptable distance for social conversation is approximately 3 or 4 feet. If the person feels comfortable with this distance, you can gradually move closer. Other hints about how the person responds to touch include facial expression, muscular response in areas touched (relaxed muscles mean the person is comfortable, tight muscles mean that the person is not comfortable), and body posture (leaning back means withdrawal, leaning forward means acceptance).

Be Aware of the Emotional Component of Touch

Although we may not be consciously aware of it, we often learn a great deal about how the other person is feeling during a handshake. As with verbal communication, how you say it is as important—or more important—than what you say. Touch needs to be caring and compassionate, gentle but not hesitant.

Be Aware of Where You
Touch the Person with Dementia

A touch on the hand or a handshake is the most familiar and least threatening touch, especially from strangers. Although it is distressing, family caregivers need to remember that a person with advanced dementia may not recognize them by sight alone and that they should touch from a distance at first. Read the person's response (e.g., facial expression) to a touch on the hand as a guide to the appropriateness of a more intimate form of touch (e.g., a touch on the arm, shoulder, or back). A touch on the head or face is much more personal, and many older persons find this invasive, especially if they believe they do not know the person well. The sense of touch in the fingertips and the palms is likely to decrease with aging and/or the progress of dementia.

Use Conventional Approaches
and Activities that Involve Touch

Touching and hugs had never been part of one caregiver's family culture when she was growing up 65 years ago. It had, however, become very important in her own family with her sons and her husband. One time when she visited her 96-year-old mother with advanced dementia, the caregiver initially was unsure of how to relate to her mother. Words neither communicated the care and the love that she felt nor relieved her mother's distress. She also noticed the terrible state of her mother's nails. Because it caused such distress, the nurses no longer tried to cut them. This caregiver pondered how to connect with her mother as she set about repairing the state of her mother's nails—soaking, clipping, polishing—all the while speaking gently and reassuringly and lovingly caressing her mother's hands.

This caregiver had unconsciously discovered a way to connect, to communicate love and concern. Not only did her mother allow her daughter to give her a manicure but also the activity relieved her mother's distress and helped her relax. Some other familiar activities that include touch are

- Taking the person's arm while walking
- Helping with grooming activities (e.g., washing, setting, and brushing the person's hair)
- Rubbing in hand cream or after-shave
- Gently massaging the person's feet, hands, arms, or shoulders
- Dusting the person with talc or powder
- Dancing

Suggest or model activities that encourage acceptable touch to other family members and visitors. Encourage them to communicate through touch as well.

Use Light Touch for Stimulation and Firm Touch for Reassurance

Gently touching the person with your fingertips or brushing him or her with soft fabric gets the person's attention and increases stimulation. This might be used to help the person to respond or to participate in activities such as eating or getting dressed. Conversely, firm touch is reassuring and calming (e.g., giving a firm handshake, placing your arms around the person's shoulder, snugly tucking the person under the blankets). This type of touch can be used to help calm the person when he or she is distressed. In instances of extreme distress, however, it is often best to give the person sufficient personal space and to avoid touching him or her in case this touch is misinterpreted as the use of force or restraint.

Ensure that the Person Is Aware
of Your Presence Before You Touch Him or Her

Because of perceptual changes and possible hearing and visual loss, persons with dementia often are not aware of someone
approaching beside or behind them. As a result, they may be
startled if you touch them—this touch may seem to come out
of nowhere.

Be Careful: The Fragile Skin
of Older People May Tear Easily

Helping the person to transfer from one surface to another or
to move around in bed is an opportunity to provide caring
personal touch. However, it is essential to be very careful with
an older person's fragile skin, which can tear easily.

Be Sensitive and Open
to Appropriate Touch from the Person

It is especially important for caregivers who are not family
members (e.g., paid caregivers, neighbors, acquaintances) to
be open to appropriate touch from the person with dementia.
Paid caregivers usually accept the right and need to touch the
person with dementia. Conversely, there is an assumption
that it is inappropriate for patients to touch service providers
such as personal care aides, nurses, doctors, or therapists. The
seemingly unpredictable behavior of persons with dementia
may add to this assumption. Please see Chapter 9 for further
information about caregivers' essential role in understanding
and preventing these behaviors, which serve to communicate
a need.

Persons with dementia also need to express their thanks, to
nurture and to care for others. Touch is a way for them to
meet this need. Paid caregivers may find that it takes some

time and good rapport to become comfortable with this expression, but it is well worth the effort. Some of my most precious moments involve the gentle caress of a frail hand on my cheek.

Be Extremely Careful so that Caring
Touch Does Not Take on a Sexual Meaning

Due to difficulties with interpreting the environment, persons with dementia may misinterpret touch. Caregivers should avoid touching hips with the person if sitting beside him or her on a bed. A hand on the shoulder or arm is more neutral and less likely to arouse sexual feelings then an arm around the waist.

Be Aware that Touching in Certain
Areas May Stimulate Primitive Reflexes

Primitive reflexes sometimes return in the later stages of dementia. Please see Chapter 3 for more information on these reflexes.

Gestures

Most of us unconsciously talk with our hands or use gestures to illustrate our point. Many family members and friends suggest that I, for one, would not be able to talk on the telephone if they were to tie my hands behind my back! They are probably right.

When persons with dementia begin to have difficulty with spoken language, you can deliberately add gestures to help understanding. For instance, when suggesting a walk, you can get the person's coat and walk toward the door. By modeling the use of gestures, you can encourage persons with dementia to do the same.

Some common gestures that are useful include

- Waving hello or goodbye
- Beckoning
- Indicating a chair or place at the table with an out-stretched hand
- Mimicking and exaggerating movements that indicate activities such as washing one's hands and face, eating, brushing one's teeth, combing one's hair, and using the telephone (to avoid confusion, use these movements only in the appropriate context)
- Identifying yourself and others by name while pointing or gesturing your whole hand toward the appropriate person
- Sliding your arm gently under the person's elbow to indicate that you want the person to come with you

Many of the guidelines for verbal communication apply to using gestures. Be sure to alert the person that you are there and don't move too fast; use slow, exaggerated movements. Speak your message at the same time and use appropriate facial expressions.

Remember the Physical Environment

Touch from the physical environment can also communicate caring and reassurance. Familiar and favorite furnishings and carefully selected new pieces and decorative items can offer a variety of pleasing touch experiences. Upholstery on furniture should be warm, soft, and comfortable. There are new breathable, washable or water- and stain-resistant fabrics that are much more pleasant than plastic and vinyl. If necessary, a favorite chair can be protected with a washable fabric cover that has plastic underneath. Please see Chapter 5 for more information on the environment and Chapters 6 and 7 for more information on using things such as plants, pets, and fabrics for touch stimulation.

GUIDELINES FOR ENHANCING SPOKEN COMMUNICATION WITH PERSONS WITH DEMENTIA

Interpersonal Approaches

The following subsections detail interpersonal approaches for enhancing communication with someone who has dementia.

Always Speak to the Person as an Adult

Persons with dementia remain acutely aware that they are adults. Given their vulnerability and fragile self-esteem, they particularly need to be treated as dignified adults and to have their personhood honored. Recognize them as worthwhile adults by making eye contact; addressing them properly; and offering genuine compliments on their clothing, hairstyle, smile, or other personal attributes. Behavior remains a powerful way of communicating, so speaking to persons with dementia without expressing the dignity and respect that they deserve leads to understandable distress and/or withdrawal. *Never* use unfamiliar nicknames (e.g., "Pops," "Babes," "Gramps," "Grannie"), which can sound condescending, or baby talk (e.g., "Are we ready to go wee-wee now?"). The following example shows the negative impact that such terms can have.

Reverend Donald Jamison had advanced dementia and was unable to dress himself or find the bathroom. Nonetheless, Reverend Jamison retained the personal dignity and decorum of his profession. It was hard to

imagine what could suddenly cause this calm, genteel, polite gen-
tleman to curse and wave his arms. However, further investiga-
tion revealed that some staff members had developed the habit of
referring to Reverend Jamison as "Donnie Boy." When they told
"Donnie Boy" to go to the bathroom, shave, or go to lunch, he
rebelled against this insult to his dignity with the only means
available to him.

Although this example is a very dramatic and obvious violation of respect for the person's dignity and adulthood, other
more subtle offenses can unconsciously taint communication.
For instance, caregivers need to think about the language of
caregiving and how this may affect the person. Words have a
powerful impact, not only for the person but also for caregivers. For instance, we can talk about aprons and briefs or we
can talk about bibs and diapers. We can say that the person is
distressed, upset, or angry or we can say that the person is agitated, aggressive, or out of control. These differences also
affect attitude. For example, when someone is distressed, he
or she needs to be comforted. Conversely, when someone is
agitated, he or she is doing something "bad"—perhaps on
purpose—that has to be stopped.

Address the Person Properly

Family members can play an important role by telling other
caregivers what name and/or title the person prefers. Many
older adults are not accustomed to being addressed by their
first name, except by close friends. Using a nickname is fine if
an individual was willingly known by it all of his or her adult
life. For example, one person may have been called "Pops" his
entire adult life, and this is the best way to address him. For
someone else, this name would be very insulting. It is also
essential for all staff to know the proper pronunciation of

people's names. This signifies respect. Also, it helps avoid the incorrect assumption that the person doesn't respond to his or her own name, as shown in the following example.

Mrs. Watson was in the advanced stages of Alzheimer's disease and also had significant hearing loss. Friends and family members were able to communicate with her by using familiar expressions and long-practiced techniques. Nursing facility staff members were frustrated, however, because they couldn't even get her to respond when they tried to tell her that it was mealtime. They had to resort to feeding her the few bites of food that she would take. A dear friend who visited one day at lunchtime was astounded to hear the staff saying, "Lois, eat your lunch," and becoming frustrated when they got no response. The friend gently suggested that Mrs. Watson wouldn't answer because "Lois" wasn't the proper pronunciation of her first name. She had always been called "Loise" (pronounced like "noise"). When addressed by her friend in this way, Mrs. Watson lifted her head and smiled. Unfortunately, despite this discovery, which both the friend and—later—family members shared with the charge nurse, staff members continued to call Mrs. Watson "Lois" and to get no response.

Acknowledge and Affirm the Emotional Message

We do have feelings and we do have some kind of knowledge. It may not be very profound, but nevertheless I think we do have experiences which might be worthwhile, especially to anybody who had any reason at all in this world to want to know a little bit about Alzheimer's. I do suspect that we do know more than we seem to know because it gets so hard to express what we know. (Henderson & Andrews, 1998, p. 56)

As Cary Henderson pointed out, even if the words aren't making any sense to us, it is essential to listen to the feeling message of what the person is saying. The person is sending an emotional message, making a very powerful "I" statement about what he or she is feeling and experiencing. By attending carefully to nonverbal communication (e.g., voice tone, facial expression, body posture, gestures) and combining it with any understandable words, caregivers can uncover the feeling that the person is trying to express.

Check your interpretation with the person by saying something such as "Jack, you seem to be sad." If you get agreement, acknowledge the feeling by a caring touch and an applicable reply, such as "I'm sorry you are sad. Is it because you are missing your friend Joe?" Continue to reassure and explore the reasons for the feeling. In some cases, the source will never be uncovered, but just acknowledging that you are aware of the person's feelings is often calming and reassuring. It is particularly important to discover whether the person is in pain or feels ill because as dementia progresses, even these expressions become impaired.

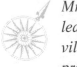

Mr. Cormier's native language was French, but he had learned to speak English quite well in the small fishing village where he had lived all his life. As his dementia progressed, Mr. Cormier could no longer live on his own and was placed in the only available nursing facility. Unfortunately, this was in a city that was 100 miles from his life-long home and where only English was spoken. Mr. Cormier did not do well in this unfamiliar setting. The bathroom didn't look like the outhouse he was used to, so he urinated in corners and doorways and on potted plants. He missed the fresh air and his active life in the village, so he constantly paced the unit, moving furniture and rummaging in drawers. The once-familiar English words of his caregivers lost their meaning.

Because the laundry cart was late one morning, Mr. Cormier was still wearing his pajamas while pacing the corridor. He came to me in great distress and pointed to his pajamas, saying, "Ce, ce non, non terrible, this, this jacket."

Taken at face value, these words didn't make any sense. However, by paying attention to the nonverbal cues, I was able to understand what he meant. I replied, "Yes, I agree it is terrible that there are no pants for you to wear yet. I'm sure it's very upsetting for you to be still in your pajamas long after breakfast. I will help you to change as soon as your clean pants come from the laundry."

When he realized that I was listening to his concerns, Mr. Cormier calmed down.

At times, persons with dementia are searching for someone or something that is not part of the present reality. For example, a woman may desperately search for her long-dead husband and her now-grown children, a long-retired man may believe that he needs to get to the office, or a person who has spent years in a long-term care facility is desperate to go home. The most natural response to these "mistaken" searches is to set the record straight, to tell the woman her husband is dead and her children grown or tell the man that he retired long ago. For years, this reality orientation approach was considered the best way to respond to such statements. However, experience and research have shown that this approach only causes further distress (Bowlby, 1993). These responses do not match the person's reality; even more to the point, they do not meet the person's needs, do not answer the longing that is tormenting him or her.

Caregivers are called on to look at the emotional message behind these seemingly confused statements, to try to understand the need that underlies them and respond to this need. Responding to the need behind these searches brings the person reassurance and calm. Although the need may reappear later, the person is more content for the moment (see Chapter 2). For example, the woman who is looking for her spouse undoubtedly misses him and the caring and support that this relationship provided. She needs to talk about her husband, to remember him, and to be reassured that you are there to care for her now. Searching for children or the office are often powerful statements of the need to be needed, to have something meaningful to do. In this case, you can discuss and affirm the valuable work that the person has done and provide opportunities to do meaningful things now (see Chapters 6, 7, and 8). Searching for home is often a statement that the person needs the comfort and reassurance associated with home (see Chapter 5).

Respond Warmly and Appreciatively to Communication from the Person

As Christine Boden noted, "Often you wonder whether it's worth trying to speak, because it always comes out wrong and everyone laughs at you. . . . That's what its like to have Alzheimer's" (1998, p. 75). Responding with a smile, a touch, or positive words is vital to help overcome the embarrassment and frustration that people with dementia experience. Even if you are not able to understand what the person is saying, recognizing the effort is essential for maintaining a connection. By responding, you acknowledge the person's worth and value. You offer reassurance that you are interested in what the person has to say and that you can be trusted not to humiliate him or her. This encouragement and assurance can often, in turn, lead to additional and clearer responses. Yet, if the person is ignored or dismissed because you can't understand what he or she is saying, the feelings of failure—of being ignored and devalued—will discourage further attempts. This situation may also lead to anger and distress.

Be Aware of Every Aspect of Presentation

It's not so much what you say; it's how you say it.

This piece of folk wisdom stresses that the nonverbal parts of communication are very powerful and can either enhance or overwhelm the spoken message. The words "I'm so glad to see you" can be entirely overwhelmed if spoken in an angry or indifferent tone of voice, with a disinterested facial expression, and without eye contact. Conversely, this same phrase—accompanied by a warm smile, a happy tone of voice, and eye contact—carries an entirely different message and will receive an entirely different response. Because persons with dementia are highly sensitive to feelings and emotional messages, the nonverbal aspects of communication—such as voice tone, posture, and facial expression—take on extra importance.

Include the Person in Conversations

People have to understand about Alzheimer's patients. We're still here. We still have ideas and can express them. Just be patient and listen to us. We are real people! There is a difference between the people and the disease. The disease is what makes us different. (Simpson & Simpson, 1999, p. 52)

Excluding a person with dementia sends a powerful message that he or she is a nonperson and is not worthy of respect. In many cases, the person with dementia understands our words much more than we imagine. If you have been in such a situation yourself—in which people have talked around you—you can appreciate how humiliating and degrading this experience is.

When there is a need to discuss care concerns or other matters privately, arrange for a meeting or telephone call. On all other occasions, make every effort to include the person in conversations by using nonverbal cues such as turning to the person, seeking his or her opinion, and sharing meaningful things that have happened. Such actions enhance self-esteem and reduce distress.

Content

Begin with Orientation Information for Reassurance

I don't seem to have space in my brain any more for that sense of 'Thursday-ness' (or whatever day it might happen to be), or 'April-ness', or '1998-ness'. . . . I'm finding this limits my ability to chat. I struggle to find the words in response to questions like 'how has your day been?' I usually have to think frantically to remember what day it is?—is it morning or afternoon?—what have I done today?! (Boden, 1998, p. 62)

Communication is about information sharing and relationship building. Caregivers must set the stage and provide the information that the person with dementia needs to feel reassured and ready to participate. When the person begins to have difficulty remembering names and dates, caregivers need to provide this information at the start of every conversation to help put the person at ease. This can be done in a sensitive, conversational manner by saying something such as, "Hi, Mom. It's me—your daughter Carol. I brought you a cup of coffee on this cold December afternoon." In this way, the person isn't troubled by trying to recall who you are or other information and is freed to respond to the conversation and the visit.

Remember that this information is given for reassurance, not for later testing of facts (e.g., names, dates). Avoid taking away the pleasure of the conversation by turning it into a memory contest. This serves little point and causes the person to become distressed, embarrassed, and confronted by his or her losses and disabilities. It is important to stimulate the person and help him or her remain mentally active; however, there is no evidence that quizzing leads to beneficial outcomes.

Emphasize Recognition, not Recall

It is natural for caregivers to want recognition by name from persons with dementia. It is also natural for persons with dementia to have difficulty recalling their caregivers' names, even early in the course of dementia. For example, Alice began to call me "that other woman" (You know, the one who took her son away!) in the very early stages, even before she was diagnosed. Caregivers need to call on the person's strength for recognition, to look for other comments and nonverbal responses such as a smile or a warm embrace. As discussed in Chapter 3, persons with dementia recognize those who are important to them, right to the very end. Here is an example from my family experience.

We made a very difficult family decision to spend 13 months in California for study and research when Alice was in the later stages of Alzheimer's disease. Alice remained in Nova Scotia in the nursing facility where she had lived for more than a year. During our time away, Alice lost a lot of abilities: She no longer walked independently, was incontinent, and was restrained in a chair most of the day. Although staff reported that Alice spoke very little, she brightened at the mention of her son. During calls from California, Alice amazed staff with her ability to carry on a telephone conversation, using favorite phrases such as "It's so wonderful to hear from you" and "How are the kids?" Eight months into the California trip, her son returned for a short visit. When he took Alice's hand and said, "Hi, Mom," her entire body came alive in recognition. Six months later, when the whole family returned, this scene was repeated with every family member—even our teenage son and daughter, who had grown considerably during this time.

Although we all wept tears at the frail figure that Alice had become, we had no doubt that she *knew* who we were without naming us. She also knew that our visits were happy and reassuring occasions for her.

These simple but eloquent expressions of recognition are the ways in which persons with dementia express that we are recognized, as are our efforts. Confronting persons with dementia with recall questions (e.g., "What's my name?" "Do you know me?") sets a negative tone by confronting them with their disabilities. Try to imagine the person's embarrassment at not being able to name a son, daughter, spouse, or dear friend. Perhaps you have experienced this by temporarily forgetting the name of a colleague or an acquaintance in a social situation.

This same principle applies to all aspects of conversation with the persons with dementia. When caregivers provide the orienting cues and prompts and establish a positive tone for the conversation, the stage is set for the person to use his or her strength of recognition (see Chapter 3). This example shows the difference that enacting this principle can make.

Due to the effects of advanced Alzheimer's disease, Henry could no longer walk independently and frequently had great difficulty settling to sleep at night. Although Henry spent much of the day dozing in his chair, sometimes he called out in a booming voice, often for his sister Emily. Emily and her husband had lived near Henry; for

years before his illness, Emily had provided meals for her bache-
lor brother. Given that Henry was so frequently calling for Emily,
it was curious that when she did visit, he didn't recognize her. Or
did he?

One winter's day, Emily and her family, still wearing their
coats and hats, crowded around Henry, who was seated in the
busy day room. Eager to be recognized, Emily stood above Henry
and said, "Do you know me?" Henry boomed, "No, who are
ye?"

When I saw Emily's distress at not being recognized, I suggest-
ed that the family move to a quieter room and remove their hats
and coats. Emily took off her coat and hat, bent down to Henry's
level, took him by the hand, and said his name. In response,
Henry boomed, "Why, Emily, how are ye?"

Speak Positively, Avoiding "Don'ts" and Commands

You can catch more flies with honey than with vinegar.

It can be easy to forget this folk wisdom when we are challenged with caring for someone with memory loss—someone
who needs direction and assistance to move through the day.
The natural tendency is to be directive when the person
seems unable to do something or is doing something that we
wish he or she wouldn't do. However, you need to remember
that despite the help that may be needed, the person with
dementia retains his or her sense of being an adult and values
independence. No one likes to be ordered around. By phras-
ing suggestions or directions in a positive and respectful
way—one that implies that the person will follow us and that
we are there to support them—you are more likely to get a
positive response. You can say, for example, "Your favorite
lunch—tuna salad—is ready; I'll help you to the table" rather
than "Sit here and eat your lunch." Offer an arm and say,

"John, I'd like to show you the pictures of your boat that just came back from the shop" rather than, "John, get out of that cupboard—you are making a terrible mess." See Chapter 6 for more information about invitations to activity.

Don't Argue with, Contradict, or Belittle the Person

The caregiver who said, "I won my last argument with Sam before he got Alzheimer's disease," expressed the futility of arguing over an issue or idea that is incorrect. For persons with memory loss, the world must seem to be constantly changing—confusing, frightening, and totally unpredictable. Because we all need to feel anchored and secure about some things, persons with memory loss often use their own unique logic to fasten onto a few constants. As noted previously, it may not be our logic, but it is still logic. Although every fiber of reason within us cries out to persist, to set the situation straight, arguing is almost guaranteed to cause nothing but distress to both parties. Caregivers need to perfect the art of mild statements of interest, such as "Mmhm," "That's interesting," or "Imagine that" while counting to 10 and changing the subject. As discussed previously, it is also important to respond to the feeling need, the "I" statement in what is being said.

It is particularly important not to argue if the ideas are expressions of paranoia. As inaccurate as the information may be, the person has arrived at it through his or her own reasoning and perception processes. Direct attempts to correct the faulty information will be threatening and will probably cause distress and agitation. Instead, try to identify with the feelings associated with these statements and to make positive connections with the people or things mentioned. The following story from my caregiving experience is an example of what *not* to do.

Early in my career as both a professional and family caregiver, Alice stayed with us following cataract surgery.[3] This coincided with Christmas vacation and many social and family activities. After one such happy occasion, during which Alice was an accomplished cohostess, she wearily headed to bed. I told her that she hadn't taken her pills yet. She insisted that she had. I disagreed with her, at which point she became very angry, insisting that she had taken her own pills for years and couldn't possibly have made such a mistake. At this point, her agitation was so great that she threw the pills across the room, an act that was completely out of character. The situation was resolved by her son, who sat with her for some time and reassured her. Then, he gently gave her the pills while saying that he was very concerned about her health.

The longer-term solution was discussing dosages with Alice's doctor so that she could take medication only once per day. After that, we gave Alice a week's supply of daily doses. This way, it was easy to determine whether that day's dose had been taken.

My mistakes in this situation were many. I should have begun by thanking Alice for all of her help during the party. Next, I should have calmly said that I had her evening pills while handing her the pills. In all likelihood, this would have prevented the altercation. If Alice still insisted that she'd taken the pills, I should have diverted the topic by talking about what a busy and happy day we had. Then, I should have gradually changed the conversation to how easy it is to forget things, like pills, when life gets busy. Following is an example of how another caregiver learned not to argue.

---

[3]A previous version of this story appeared in Bowlby Sifton, C. (2000e). Meeting needs. *Alzheimer's Care Quarterly, 1*(4), iv; adapted by permission.

Frieda had a lifelong love of stylish and fancy shoes. She had an amazing collection—shoes for all occasions. When Frieda developed dementia and could no longer live on her own, she happily agreed to live with her daughter Kathleen. Before the move, Frieda and Kathleen sorted the lifetime collection of shoes and gave away many pairs—those that no longer fit or that Frieda didn't wear anymore. Frieda and her still-substantial shoe collection settled in happily with Kathleen and her family.

However, as Frieda's brain deteriorated further, she began to have trouble keeping track of her shoe collection and remembering which pairs she still had. Sometimes Frieda would come storming into the kitchen shouting that Kathleen had been taking her shoes again, that her favorite black patent ones with the bows were missing. After a few disastrous attempts to remind her mother that she had given those shoes away 2 years before, Kathleen changed her approach. Instead, she calmly and empathetically said, "I know, Mom. That is a very special pair, and you never can have too many pairs of shoes. Let's go have a look and see what we can find." Kathleen would put an arm around her mother and head to the shoe rack. As Frieda began sorting shoes and commenting on each pair (e.g., how lovely this pair was, what a good buy that pair had been), she forgot her distress and became involved in admiring her collection.

Another example follows, this time from a conversation that occurred in a nursing facility elevator.

It was Sunday afternoon, and the nursing facility was full of visitors. An older lady, who was frail and accompanied by a nurse, got on the crowded elevator. Both were wearing their coats, and it seemed that they were returning from a visit to the hospital emergency room. One visi-

tor politely asked the lady which floor she wanted. She replied, "Six, please." After this her nurse said abruptly, "No, we're going to three." The lady looked puzzled and asked the nurse, "How come?" The nurse could have said something like "I know it's hard to keep track of things after all the rushing around this afternoon, and especially because you aren't feeling well, but your room is on the third floor." Instead, the nurse patted the lady on the head and said, "Because you're 90 years old and you're all confused." The lady was needlessly humiliated and embarrassed in front of strangers, and she still hadn't been provided with reassuring orientation information.

Use Lead-In Information and Opinion-Seeking Questions

Everyone can offer an opinion. Persons with dementia can successfully reply to questions that call for opinions, such as "What do you like best about or least about _____?" "What does this object make you think of?" or "Does this color remind you of anything?" They have more difficulty with questions that have right and wrong answers, such as "What is this called?" and "What color is this?" So, for example, a caregiver could say, "Marjorie, that's a lovely dress—is blue your favorite color?" as opposed to "Marjorie, that's a lovely dress—where did you get it?"

Questions that narrow down the options and help to focus responses should be used instead of open questions. For example, a caregiver could say, "Mom, the house looks wonderful, but you look tired—have you been busy cleaning today?" instead of "Mom, what have you been doing today?" The second question may be overwhelming to the person with dementia, whereas the first one narrows down the choices and gives directions for responses.

Use Short, Simple Adult Sentences

As dementia progresses it becomes increasingly difficult for the person to focus on more than one or two ideas at a time. As a result, it becomes important for caregivers to keep sentences short and simple so that the person is able to focus on the content. Descriptive and complex words as well as long phrases should be eliminated. For example, "John, see the beautiful sunrise," would replace, "Good morning, John, dear, it is going to be a glorious day; as I look out the west window in the living room, there is just the most magnificent sunrise taking place."

At the same time, it is vital to ensure that the tone and structure of the sentences—and all communication—are adult. Simple does not mean childlike.

Use the Name or Term
that Is Most Familiar to the Person

It is important to appreciate the subtle meanings of language as it has been understood and used by the person. Phrases, figures of speech, expressions, dialects, and the language spoken during childhood (i.e., the person's native language) may become the best remembered and most preferred language. Languages and ways of speaking learned later in life may fade, even if the person has used this language for years. You can enhance communication by learning and using these better retained language skills. It is essential to share this information with paid caregivers, using something like the All About Me form in Appendix A. Paid caregivers should take care to avoid technical or professional jargon.

Regional expressions, unique local names, and pronunciations—within just one language—offer a wide variety of names, even for everyday items. This can be confusing enough for those who do not have cognitive difficulties. For example, I recall the frustration of a friend from South Africa who had recently arrived in Nova Scotia. She went shopping for "cotton wool" and was presented with cotton batten, yarn, and yard goods before she finally got what she was looking for—thread! The following example illustrates how language misunderstandings can occur between care providers and persons with dementia.

> *A Russian-born and trained psychiatrist was having great difficulty understanding the source of her patient's agitation at bedtime. The man with dementia kept insisting that he had to be "tucked in." Several minutes of team meeting time, with team members adding their own personal accounts, were required to explain the many nuances of security and comfort which were associated with these two simple words.*

For persons with dementia, such situations are even more complex, as shown in the following story.

> *At 3:00 P.M., a Canadian lady with advanced dementia asked a fellow resident's out-of-province visitor, "Have we had our dinner yet?" In the visitor's province, dinner is the evening meal, so he said "No, not yet. Dinner will be in 2 hours, at 5:00." The lady was very distressed and muttered that she had never heard of waiting until 5:00 for her dinner.*
>
> *Another visitor, who was a local, attempted to calm the lady's agitation by reinterpreting her question about dinner. According to local use, dinner was the noontime meal. The visitor told the lady, "Yes, you had your dinner at 12:00. You will have supper in 2 hours." Unfortunately, it was too late to relieve the lady's agitation entirely. She continued muttering, "One person says 'yes'; one says something else." When she passed another person in the hall, she asked, "Have we had our dinner yet?"*

Caregivers can help alleviate such situations by taking note of lifelong terms and local expressions that may not be understood by others.

Use Phrases or Mannerisms
that the Person Once Used or Still Uses

Family members and significant others will be familiar with a person's favorite expressions and phrases, and it is important to share these with paid caregivers. In addition, observant caregivers will be able to pick up these expressions from overheard conversations or fragments and will reinforce their use by repetition. The following vignette is one example of how this practice can enhance communication.

Alice was in the advanced stage of Alzheimer's disease. Verbal communication was reduced to some single words and occasional short phrases. A few weeks before her death, we talked with her about her upcoming birthday. She barely opened her eyes when the arrangements were being discussed. It had been a long-standing family joke that Alice had remained age 39 for the past 43 years, so, suddenly inspired, I asked, "How old are you going to be on your birthday, Mom—39 again?" Alice instantly became alert. With her eyes open and a mischievous grin on her face, she joined in the full spirit of the joke by replying, "Well, yes, of course."

Use Nouns and Descriptors, not Pronouns

It is important to use descriptive terms. Instead of saying, "We are going out to eat," the caregiver should say something such as "You, Tom, and I are going to eat at the Red Star restaurant—the place where you always liked the clam chowder."

Use Concrete, Clear Language

Doris had remarkably well-preserved social skills that charmed everyone. These skills often made her language skills appear to be more intact than they actually were. One day, I offered to help Doris get up from a chair by saying, "Can I give you a hand?" Confused, she replied, "Well, now, wouldn't I look silly with three hands?" Despite her high level of social skills, Doris couldn't understand figures of speech or abstract language.

Expressions such as "Hold onto your hat" or "Jump into bed" may be taken literally. It is best to avoid sayings and figures of speech that may be misunderstood.

Physical Aspects

Eliminate Distractions

Confusion reigns. And I would guess it's pretty common that somebody with Alzheimer's really can't cope with more than one thing at a time. And that one thing at a time has to be reasonably easy to understand. (Henderson & Andrews, 1998, p. 74)

We live in a noisy world. Many older persons with dementia probably find the sounds that now fill modern households overwhelming. In addition, dementia damages the brain in a way that makes paying attention difficult when there are too many noises or other distractions. As dementia progresses, even the sound of traffic coming through an open window, the refrigerator's hum, or another quiet conversation at the dinner table may make it difficult to pay attention. Too much visual stimulation, such as the television on with the volume muted, can also distract the person.

To have a conversation or help the person to be involved in an activity (e.g., eating), every effort must be made to reduce all unnecessary distractions.

Face the Person When You Speak

Persons with dementia need every possible nonverbal cue (e.g., facial expression, body posture, lip movement) to help them to interpret the message. Something that is said while passing in the hall or called from another room will likely be lost or misinterpreted. If the person is seated, squat down or bend over so you are on his or her level. Yet, don't get too close, as this is not socially acceptable. It may also be interpreted as threatening or as a sexual gesture.

Alert the Person to Your Presence

Over the course of dementia, people have more difficulty understanding things that happen around them. It becomes increasingly important to use hints to let the person know that you are there, such as a touch on the hand and saying the person's name, before beginning a conversation.

Speak Slowly and Clearly

It takes longer for persons with dementia to process information, so it is important to speak slowly. They also need every possible cue, and some may have unconsciously come to rely on lip reading.

Speak in a Rhythmical Manner

As words fail, persons with dementia become more skilled at other channels of communication. As discussed in Chapter 3, music and rhythm compose one of these channels. When the natural rhythm of music is used in speech, some persons with advanced dementia can understand messages from others. As with all other adaptations, this should be used with sensitivity and in an age-appropriate way. Several caregivers have shared that when the person doesn't respond to a spoken message, they sing it, and the person can follow and respond. In one case, the caregiver used this approach for doing exercises and then continued it in other situations. The person with dementia responded positively and often began to sing as soon as the caregiver appeared.

Lower Voice Tone and Speak a Bit Louder, But Don't Shout

This suggestion about voice tone also applies to communicating with persons who have hearing impairments. With increasing age, higher voice tones commonly become difficult to hear. There is a natural tendency to shout when someone doesn't seem to hear or understand. However, shouting should be avoided, especially with persons with dementia. The person still may not understand the verbal message, but shouting may send a nonverbal message of anger and irritation. This can cause further distress and a communication breakdown. In addition, shouting distorts sounds and words, making it even harder to understand what is being said.

Maintain a Normal Conversational Style with Turn Taking

Although persons with dementia sometimes have difficulty understanding content, they continue to follow standard patterns of conversation, such as turn taking and most other social conventions; changes in tone of voice to indicate the end of a sentence or ask a question; the rhythmic quality of language; and lifelong patterns of pronunciation, syntax, and grammar. Following the lead of persons with dementia—fitting into their conversational style—helps to maintain communication.

Techniques

Use Ample Nonverbal Communication and Seek it from the Individual

As discussed at the beginning of this chapter, persons with dementia remain highly skilled in interpreting elements of nonverbal language, such as facial expressions, reassuring touches, gestures, voice tone, symbols, and familiar music. Caregivers who encourage, attend to, and use these ways of expression can open many avenues of communication. For instance, one paid caregiver of persons with advanced dementia who have very limited spoken language has found that she can get a window on thoughts, feelings, and recollections by using paper and pencils. At times, a person with dementia draws something and as the "conversation" continues and the caregiver teases out the drawing's meaning, the caregiver draws something in response. She has found that, despite the fact that these people have advanced dementia, most have very definite ideas about the meaning of particular symbols in the drawings. These visual representations of thoughts and ideas encourage further expression in symbol and in word.

Repeat Messages by Using the Same Words

It is automatic to rephrase something when the person we are talking to doesn't understand our message. For instance, we may say, "Lunch is ready," and if this isn't understood, we may then say, "It's time to eat lunch." This approach works well with persons who have a hearing impairment. However, it is not a good practice for persons with dementia, who are likely still trying to figure out the first comment. Repeating can be helpful, but only if the same words are used the second time.

Reassure the Person and Move on if He or She Becomes Frustrated

It is easy to become like a dog with a bone—completely unwilling to let go—when there's a communication misfire. However, to avoid frustration for everyone, it is best to drop the subject after a few tries. A break may give insight into what the person was trying to express or how you can share your message.

Encourage the Use of Gestures and Demonstration

Gestures and demonstration can be very helpful, especially for encouraging the person to do activities. With practice, a common language of basic gestures can be developed. Because of their physical nature, gestures tend to be more easily recalled and understood than words.

Supplying the Word that the Person Is Trying to Recall Is Sometimes Appreciated

Persons with dementia may substitute a similar-sounding word (e.g., saying *pin* for *pen*) or describe an item for which they cannot name the word (e.g., calling a pen "the writing thing"). Or they may stall or get stuck on a certain word. When the person is stuck, it may be helpful to supply the missing word. However, the use of this technique needs to be decided on an individual basis. Some people appreciate such help; others find it embarrassing. In almost all cases, there is little point in turning the word search into a contest by quizzing the person.

Repeat the Last Words that the Person Has Said

Repeating the last words that the person has said helps maintain his or her train of thought. This technique also needs to be used individually, however, as some find it helpful and others find it frustrating.

ENHANCING COMMUNICATION DURING VISITS

Christine Boden (1998) shared her challenges with day-to-day conversation, a skill that was second nature before she developed Alzheimer's disease. Christine was a senior administrator in the Australian government and was therefore accustomed to chairing meetings, speaking to the press, presenting papers, and having highly focused social conversations. After developing Alzheimer's disease, she found social conversations taxing. However, she and others with dementia share that it is essential to have social times, such as visits and conversations with family and friends. Visitors are asked to step into the person's world and enable a time of sharing that meets the need for connection without overtaxing or humiliating the person. Ann Davidson shared some lovely thoughts about the value of visiting for both her and her husband, who has advanced dementia:

> Recent visits drift through my mind: Julian sitting in the little music room, asleep in an armchair, listening to Mozart. Kneeling before him, I wiggle his knees, say "Julian, hello darling, hello Julian."
> Slowly his blue eyes open but stare off to one side. "Julian . . . hello . . . it's me . . . I'm happy to see you."

Finally his eyes focus on mine. Pausing, he inhales. "Oh... good!" he sometimes manages. His hands, clenched in his lap, won't open to receive the Hershey's Kiss I've brought. So I pop one in his mouth, and he chews, silent again, closing his eyes, savouring the chocolate.

Perched on the arm of his chair, I comb my fingers through his hair, massage his shoulder. Just sitting close and touching him fills me with familiar warmth. Impaired as he is, the way he relaxes and sighs suggests my touch and presence comfort him too.

Pressed together, we listen to both sides of the Mozart tape, quartets in D minor and D major. Violins and cellos chase each other. From time to time, Julian unfolds his hands and in time to the cello gives several loud claps. (2001, p. 3)

In addition to the previously discussed communication guidelines, the following suggestions are offered for visiting. Family caregivers are reminded to share and model these ideas with other visitors who may not be as familiar with the person's needs and abilities. These suggestions should also be shared on the All About Me form (see Appendix A) or a similar form. This becomes especially important if the person is in a residential care facility and family members are not there to guide visitors.

Preplan the Visit

Most of us appreciate the courtesy of visits organized in advance. This gives us a chance to suggest a time that is convenient—a time when we will be best able to appreciate the visit. This factor becomes even more important when someone has dementia. A surprise visitor may arrive when the person or the caregiver is especially tired or overtaxed or busy with someone else. Although persons with dementia tend to have well-preserved social skills, making use of these skills requires a lot of energy and focus. Visits at an inconvenient time may overwhelm the person, either during the visit or later, thus destroying the possible benefits of enjoying another's company.

At some point, home caregivers need to take the lead in letting friends, relatives, and neighbors know that visits are much appreciated but must be prearranged. Visits should be planned for a time of day when the person is most rested and there is little else happening. Similarly, when visiting the person in a care facility, family caregivers should ask staff when the person is likely to be rested and when care activities are not too demanding.

As dementia progresses, caregivers need to decide how far in advance to share news of a visit with the person. Sometimes giving this information too far in advance causes the person to worry and become distressed about how he or she will cope. Caregivers who are concerned that visitors may overstay their welcome can organize visits at times when there will be obvious deadlines (e.g., a little while before a meal or an appointment).

Keep the Visit Short

As you probably have discovered, after a long visit or social occasion, the person with dementia is extremely tired and more likely to become upset and distressed. One effect of dementia is that the person tires easily, especially from expending the effort that goes into visiting. Some visitors may be sensitive to this; others may need to be informed and even reminded of it. You can watch for familiar signs of fatigue and sensitively intervene to bring the visit to a close. In some cases, the person with dementia may seek an end to a visit. I have seen persons with dementia suggest that it is time for their walk or for a certain television program or that they would like a cup of tea. In other situations, they simply withdraw from the conversation or become distressed and ask to go home or leave. You should strive to intervene before the person reaches this stage.

As the person becomes more frail, energy levels and the ability to concentrate further decrease. In turn, the length of visits should decrease. Brief visits also become more important if the person lives in a long-term care facility, as coping with the stimulation of the extra people and activity in this setting requires even more energy.

Establish a Calm and Quiet Atmosphere

In the early stages we tend to avoid what are for us difficult situations. Conversations, chats, children playing, background music—all these are very hard for us to deal with because our brains work so much harder to sort out the competing sounds and sights in our surroundings so as to make sense of them. (Boden, 1998, p. 52)

Visitors are called on to remember the needs of persons with dementia. Visits are appreciated but need to be conducted in ways that are comfortable for the person as he or she is now. Too much commotion is difficult and causes distress. Visits should be quiet and calm, conversations should be one to one, and the number of visitors should be small. If there is a large gathering, such as a family get-together, find a quiet place where the person can visit one to one or just rest.

Be Comfortable with Silences

I know you're busy now. You have so much to do. And I can't even help you! Do you remember when we first met—

how we could just *be* together? We'd talk and laugh and not really do anything. (Simpson & Simpson, 1999, p. 99)

The most valued part of a visit is spending time with another person. When words and conversation become difficult, just sitting quietly with the person, gently holding his or her hand, and perhaps listening to music is very meaningful. Visitors must try to be comfortable with silences. There is no need to fill every minute with conversation, except perhaps for visitors to overcome their discomfort until they become accustomed to another way of being with the person who has dementia.

Take the Lead in the Conversation

Although there is no need to fill every minute with conversation, visitors will probably need to take the lead in sharing news or views of mutual interest. Following the communication guidelines in this chapter can provide guidance to help this time be as positive as possible.

Share an Activity

When words become difficult, both visitors and persons with dementia can enjoy special times together by doing simple activities that are prepared by the visitor. You can model the activities with visitors. Such activities can be especially important for visiting people in long-term care facilities. Some long-term care facilities now provide visitors with activity or memory boxes that are suited to each resident's abilities and interests. Working together to develop these boxes can be a meaningful project for the person with dementia, family members, family caregivers, and paid caregivers. Nonetheless, many meaningful activities can be spontaneous, making use of little or no materials. A few suggested activities follow; for many more, see Chapters 6, 7, and 8.

- Look at a photo album or memory book.
- Sing a favorite song.
- Rub on hand cream.
- Give a manicure.
- Brush the person's hair.
- Polish the person's shoes.
- Look at an interesting picture in a magazine or on the wall (use communication suggestions).
- Prepare and share a drink and/or a simple snack.
- Look at or write greeting cards. Persons with dementia who are not able to write their own greetings often would like others to write for them. Some even may be able to write a greeting better than they can speak it.
- Take care of and/or admire a plant or flowers.

As with conversation, however, bear in mind that there isn't a need to fill every second with activity. Doing so would likely be too stressful for the person.

Keep a Guest Book

Encourage visitors to write in a guest book that has columns for the date, the visitor's name, and a brief description of what was shared during the visit. Looking at the book becomes a meaningful activity and may reassure the person that others care. Such a book becomes especially important if the person is in a long-term care facility.

TELEPHONE USE

The phone. That's the most frustrating thing on earth. I get nervous trying to use the phone. I get tongue-tied. I can't figure out what the heck I'm doing. If I am the only one at home, it's trouble. Even if people eventually hang up—even if they're important people we'd like to talk to, I still can't do it. When they hear that I'm fumbling for words for a long time, they usually give up. (Henderson & Andrews, 1998, p. 79)

Things that I could do almost by instinct now take a lot of effort. For instance, it's the hardest work to make a phone call. All those numbers . . . remembering who I am going to talk to . . . what to say . . . It didn't used to be so hard! But I want to keep doing it. (Simpson & Simpson, 1999, p. 79)

Cary Henderson and Bob Simpson expressed the difficulty that most persons with dementia eventually experience in using the telephone. This is likely so difficult because it involves the spoken word only; the person with dementia does not have access to vital nonverbal cues. As a result, telephones should be reserved for emergency contact or for keeping in touch with distant friends and family. There is a wide variety of telephones—some with large number buttons, emergency contact systems, or automatic dialing features—that can be helpful if the person learns to use them during the early stages of dementia. Caregivers should concentrate on finding a telephone that is simple. Then, they should work with the person to practice using the system several times. If there's an automatic dialing system, instructions and any necessary codes should be posted next to the phone.

Caregivers should find ways to save the person embarrassment related to using the telephone. Taking messages can be difficult for the person, so caregivers might encourage the use of an answering machine while they are out. Brief telephone calls to out-of-town friends and family can be a good way of keeping in touch; however, caregivers may need to stand by to support and encourage the conversation.

Guidelines for Enhancing Spoken Communication with Someone who has Dementia

A Adult: Remember that the person is one!
Avoid arguing, confrontation, questions with right or wrong answers, negatives, direct commands

L Lower your tone of voice and speak loudly (but do not shout)

Z Zero-in the person's attention; help the person to focus

H Holistic: Take a positive approach; respect personal values
Humor: Use It!

E Emotional message of "confused" speech: Needs to be identified
Emotional memory: Is a strength

I Identify missing or misplaced words
Introduce yourself every time

M Maximize the use of touch and nonverbal communication
Maintain normal conversational structure

E Eliminate distractions

R Reality reassurance information (e.g., who, what, why, when, where): Must be provided
Repeated comments should use the same words

S Slow and Simple: Keep your speech that way

Figure 3. Mnemonic reminder of guidelines for enhancing spoken communication with someone who has dementia. (Copyright © 2004 by Health Professions Press, Inc.)

CONCLUSION

The many ways to continue to maintain connection and communication, both verbal and nonverbal, have been reviewed in this chapter. By using these and other techniques that may be unique to their situations, caregivers can continue to connect with persons with dementia who may otherwise become distanced from people. The mnemonic in Figure 3 highlights key points for enabling communication; you may wish to put a copy on your refrigerator as a reminder. Communication is not the only area for maintaining a connection, however. Chapter 5 focuses on establishing an environment that enables continuing connection with the people and the places they live in.

5

Creating a Supportive Environment

Sometimes I just get overloaded with things I think ought to be thought. I feel so much—I guess you might say in the way. I feel sometimes very much in the way. Someone with Alzheimer's I don't believe can participate fully—sometimes I think I'm doing a pretty good job of it and other days I'm totally at a loss. Confusion reigns. And I would guess it's pretty common that somebody with Alzheimer's really can't cope with more than one thing at a time. And that one thing at a time has to be reasonably easy to understand. (Henderson & Andrews, 1998, p. 74)

SEARCHING FOR HOME[4]

"Home is the place, where, when you have to go there,
They have to take you in." (Robert Frost)

 Every day after supper, Bill tipped back his chair, looked at Eva, his wife of 45 years, and said, "Thanks for the lovely meal, but I'd better be getting home now."

[4]Portions of this section previously appeared in Bowlby Sifton, C. (2000b). Caregiving challenges: Searching for home. *Alzheimer's Care Quarterly*, *1*(1), 81–85; adapted by permission; and in Bowlby Sifton, C. (2000d). It is in the shelter of each other that people live. *Alzheimer's Care Quarterly*, *1*(1), iv; adapted by permission.

Bill was in the same home that he and Eva had shared for 45 years, the same home that Bill had built with his own hands. As a result, this was the saddest part of Eva's caregiving day because she was devastated all over again by the terrible losses that Alzheimer's disease had created for her and Bill. Nonetheless, every day she patiently explained that she would take care of Bill and that she needed him to stay here with her now. Although this moment was always full of sorrow, Bill would respond to Eva's gentle reassurance. The worry would leave his face, and they both would enjoy cuddling on the couch while listening to some of their favorite music. The sorrow would give way to a moment of contentment.

Persons with dementia often search for home, whether they live at home, like Bill, or in a long-term care facility. Phrases such as "I have to go home now," "I can't stay here—I have to go home," and "Can you tell me how to get home?" may be repeated. The person may become restless and search for home, sometimes by attempting to leave or actually leaving the care setting. This is very distressing for family and professional caregivers and can be a serious safety risk for the person.

The first step in any caregiving challenge is try to understand the meaning behind the behavior. For persons with dementia, whose ability to communicate in conventional ways may be compromised, behaving in certain ways can be their only means of communication. Searching for home is especially distressing and puzzling in cases like Bill's, when the person is in fact at home. We may need to think about the meaning of *home* in these circumstances. What words come to mind when you think of the word *home*? Some ideas that might come to mind are warm, friendly, caring, comfortable, relaxed, welcoming, and nurturing. Descriptions of home tend to relate to feelings rather than to tangible things; people seldom say that home is blue walls, an oak bureau, or 220 Elm Street. If the description is concrete, it usually has a strong emotional association, such as "my favorite chair." Home is more of a feeling, more of an emotional place than a physical place.

What persons with dementia may be searching for is emotional shelter from the fearful storms of living with dementia. Persons with dementia describe it as *Home Is Where I Remember Things* (the title of Gwyther's 1997 book) or "Home is where I can be myself" (Fazio, Seman, & Stansall, 1999, p. 81).

When you have had a long, stressful day and are absolutely exhausted, would you rather go home or to a party with people you don't know very well? Most people would say home, hands down. When we are feeling overwhelmed, tired, sick, fragile, or stressed, there is nothing like the predictable reassurance of our own home and the people in it. For most of us, home is a place where we can feel free to be ourselves and still be accepted, warts and all.

This helps to explain why persons with dementia often want to go home. With all of the stresses and strains of coping with the symptoms of dementia, they must have a terrible longing for a place of total comfort and acceptance. For a person with memory loss who has difficulty in recognizing the people and things around him or her, the world must be a very confusing and frightening place.

For the most part, home is also where we can do what we want when we want. Home is where we are in control and make decisions—from small ones, such as having supper on a tray in the living room instead of at the table, to large ones, such as redoing the kitchen. The changes due to the brain damage caused by dementia are beyond a person's control.

Undoubtedly, the feeling of having your life controlled by a condition over which you have no power adds to the need to find a place—usually home—where you are in control.

Caregivers notice that searching for home can be especially strong at the end of the day. Where do we like to be heading at the end of the day? Home. The person with dementia has the same need but has more difficulty in getting there. As noted, this end-of-the-day searching, often called *sundowning*, is complex. There are many interconnected explanations and responses, which are detailed in Chapter 9.

Thinking about home in these ways, it is understandable that persons with dementia might be eager to find a place where life is comfortable, sure, and predictable. They may be looking for a place where life can get back to normal. Sadly, because they have a progressive condition of the brain, this can never happen on a permanent basis. Fortunately, much can be done to help the person feel normal, at ease, and at home in the present moment (see Chapter 2). The next section explores some immediate ways that caregivers can respond to the challenge of a person who is searching for home. Later sections offer suggestions for setting up the environment so that the person will feel at home.

Helping the Person with Dementia Find Home

The suggestions in this and other chapters help to reduce the amount of time that the person spends searching for home. However, because of damage to the brain, there will still be times when the person feels a need to find home.

Family and frontline caregivers can become so overwhelmed by the demands of everyday caregiving that it can be difficult to step back from a situation, such as the person attempting to leave the care environment, to carry out systematic problem solving. The following discussion outlines some problem-solving steps that have been adapted for dementia care challenges and applied to the situation of a person attempting to leave his or her current residence. This approach is based on the foundation that the sources of the challenge need to be understood before action is taken. See Chapter 9 for extensive problem-solving details and examples.

Step 1: Identify one challenge.

Providing care for someone with dementia is rewarding, but it also holds many challenges. When caregivers feel overwhelmed, it can be difficult to focus on one challenge, difficult to see the one tree in the forest. However, you are only human and can only do one thing at a time, so it is important to step back from the situation and focus on just one challenge or difficulty at a time. In this case, the most serious challenge is that in continuing to look for home, the person may wander off and get lost.

Step 2: Identify the owner of the problem. Is it a problem for the caregiver or the person with dementia? If it's a problem for the caregiver, can it be ignored (i.e., is it really a problem)?

The caregiver needs to think carefully about the particular person and the situation. For example, a person with dementia who walks about is actually getting exercise and exploring the environment. Research has shown that persons with dementia who walk about are healthier than those who don't (Cohen-Mansfield, Werner, Marx, & Freedman, 1991).

However, you may find the person's walking and pacing challenging. It's possible that the person with dementia may be so emotionally distressed by the need to find home or to leave that the caregiver needs to intervene. If the person is at physical risk (e.g., for exhaustion, falling, or getting lost), caregivers need to take further steps to understand and respond to this problem. The caregiver must ensure that the person has a safe place to walk and explore and that he or she is eating enough to make up for the extra calories burned.

Step 3: Identify what is going on with the person that may explain the problem.

There are several common themes that may give the caregiver direction in determining why the person is searching for home:

- The person may not be in his or her *own* home (i.e., he or she is in a care setting), or the person may have recently moved.
- The person may not have things to do that bring meaning to his or her days and support a feeling of contentment.
- The person may not have enough opportunity for making choices, being in control, and making decisions that support dignity and a sense of self.
- Daily routines may differ from the ones that the person is used to and would prefer.
- The person may not feel valued and respected.
- There may be a lack of free access to the outdoors.
- There may be a history of traumatic experiences, causing the person to feel especially vulnerable and insecure.
- The person may be uncomfortable—for instance, he or she may need to go to the bathroom or may be too hot, too cold, hungry, thirsty, dressed uncomfortably, or seated uncomfortably.
- The person may be getting sick.
- The person may be experiencing a reaction to medication.

Step 4: Identify aspects of dementia's progress that may explain the problem.

Again, although the reasons need to be determined on an individual basis, there are several possibilities why the person may be searching for home:

- The person may be frightened and traumatized by the losses that he or she is experiencing and is searching for emotional shelter.

- Brain damage may have caused perceptual losses so that the person no longer recognizes the people and the things around him or her.

- The person may not recall moving or may have shifted back in time to an earlier or childhood home.

- Sounds, sights, or people in the environment (e.g., the sound of a siren outside) may be misinterpreted and cause alarm, and the person may feel the need to get to a safe haven.

- Trying to cope with daily activities with a damaged brain takes a tremendous amount of energy. Persons with dementia become easily overtired and, hence, are more in need of "home."

- Judgment and reasoning may be clouded by brain damage. The person may not be able to appreciate that he or she cannot travel, say, the 100 miles to his or her family home.

- Memory loss and difficulty interpreting the environment may make it seem that past traumatic experiences are happening now (e.g., sounds from a war movie on television may trigger in a former soldier the need to leave for combat).

Step 5: Ask yourself how you would *feel* if this were you.

It is essential to take a moment and put yourself in the shoes of the person who you are caring for and try to imagine how you would feel if you were in similar circumstances. This demonstrates not only more empathy and compassion for the person but also often provides solutions to the challenges. For instance, how stressful would it be if you *knew* that you had to be at work or at home caring for your children but you could not get there because you are in a place that you do not recognize and nobody will let you leave?

When we appreciate how stressful and real these feelings are, we can find ways to reassure the person that his or her work was valued in the past (i.e., by talking to him or her about the work) and now (i.e., by finding ways that he or she can help you).

Step 6: Decide whether a change is needed or the behavior can be accepted.

The decision depends on the situation. It is really pointless to expect that persons with memory loss will learn not to ask to go home if they don't feel at home. However, putting in place the ideas found in this and other chapters does reduce how often and how urgently the person searches for home. Of course, if the need to find home causes emotional distress for them or others or if they are at risk of physical harm, the caregiver needs to think about ways to reduce the distress and the risk.

Step 7: Determine what happens just before and just after the challenging behavior.

Thinking about the people and places that surround a challenging behavior can help with understanding it and often provides some solutions. Does the difficulty occur at a certain time of day, with a particular caregiver, or when the person is tired? Keeping a record is helpful.

Some events and activities that may cause the person to want to go home are

- The coming and going of caregivers
- Being told of an event or an appointment that is not immediate, leading to worry about getting there on time
- An environment that is too stimulating (e.g., a noisy family gathering, a large institutional dining room at mealtime), leading to distress
- An understimulating environment, causing the person to go in search of stimulation
- Expectations that are too much for the person (e.g., trying to find the bathroom when it is beyond the person's ability to do so)
- Time of day (e.g., the start of the day, which is associated with going to work; the end of the day, which is associated with going home) or other environmental triggers (e.g., a coat hanging by the door)

It is important to remember that some caregiver responses may reinforce the person's need for and attempts to find home. If the person feels that his or her needs are being ignored, he or she will continue trying to find home, where needs are met. In addition, the person may keep trying to leave the care setting if he or she gets attention (even if negative) only when attempting to do so and not at other times (e.g., when sitting quietly).

Step 8: Generate a list of possible solutions that use persisting strengths.

This step relates to on-the-spot responses to the person who wants to find home. (Chapter 9 presents other suggestions for preventing and responding to this challenge.) A starting point for generating a list of solutions is asking, "How can we caregivers help the person with dementia to find home?" When I try to answer this question, I go back to the notion of home being a feeling and to thinking about the emotional need behind wanting to go home.

Dementia symptoms constantly assault the person's abilities to remember, understand, and do. Thus, the person needs to feel accepted and loved for who he or she is, to be reassured that someone will take care of him or her, to be reassured that his or her feelings have been heard, to feel needed, and to find comfort. The person does not need to be hit yet again with losses by having others say, "You are at home." The person cannot recover his or her memory and understanding and obviously doesn't feel at home, so constantly hearing that he or she is home is not helpful.

The words and ways to best reassure the person are individual. For example, an earlier story in this chapter illustrated how Eva had learned not to argue with Bill. Instead, she reassured him with words and touches and, later, with the comfort of familiar music and sitting together. The content of verbal reassurances should be specific to the particular person and to his or her history and needs. It is always helpful to start by letting the person know that you have heard his or her expression of feelings and needs by saying something such as, "You sound really sad, Joan. I am sure you must miss your lovely home."

Deciding what follows requires an intimate understanding of the person and a careful assessment of the reason and the urgency of his or her need to find home. Think about which aspects of home the person is longing for at this time (Fazio et al., 1999). A person who is looking for particular people, such as children or a spouse, may be missing the shared aspect of home. In this case, reminiscing about home and the people in it—by looking at photos or personal mementos—is reassuring. For others, reminiscing just causes further distress. A person may miss the experience of creating a home and may respond well to being needed. In this case, it helps to involve the person in some aspect of creating a home, either in his or her room or elsewhere. This can be done by saying something such as, "Joan, you have such a flair for decorating. I would really appreciate it if you could stay and help me arrange the sitting room pictures."

Sometimes persons with dementia seem unsure of where home is and are upset about what they are going to do. They may need reassurance that they have been given a home and that someone is there to take care of them. They may also need to be reassured that they will always have a place to go and someone to look out for them.

At times, persons with dementia may need to share their home by offering hospitality to others. Whether they are in a community home or long-term care facility, they must be able to share their home with others by being a host or hostess in ways such as showing someone their pictures. Visitors and family members can support this need by respecting personal space, especially by knocking before entering the room.

In some instances, a favorite activity, such as a walk or eating a snack, can be used as a distraction and the person can be gently redirected from the urgency of the need to find home. Yet, sometimes the need is so strong that distraction won't work. Some suggest that as a last resort, a therapeutic fib or a white lie may help quell this urgency for people living in long-term care facilities. This approach is illustrated in the following vignette.

Mona often expressed an urgent need to leave so she could pick up her children. When it was impossible to distract Mona from this need, staff could reassure and calm her by saying that the babysitter had called to say that she had taken the children to her house for supper. The staff then involved Mona in helping to prepare for supper by asking her to set the table, and they talked about and looked at photos of Mona's now-grown children. Mona always enjoyed these activities and left her distress behind.

It is essential to remember that this technique requires a great deal of skill and intimate knowledge of the person. With some individuals, this approach may totally backfire: They may not remember what you said, but they may well remember feeling deceived. This situation can lead to distrust. This approach also requires the person using the technique to be comfortable with it. Persons with dementia have heightened emotional awareness and can quickly sense discomfort and fraudulence in others. Because I personally never feel comfortable lying to someone, even for a therapeutic purpose, I don't use this approach and tend not to recommend it. However, as noted in the vignette about Mona, it can work when used skillfully.

Step 9: Evaluate the possible solutions and pick the best one.

Because you know the person best and know what you have tried in the past, you are the best judge of what might work. The word *might* is really important here. You will never know if something works until you try it.

Step 10: Implement the selected solution.

Unless a possible solution was a total disaster, you may need to give it several tries to see if it is going to help.

Step 11: Evaluate the effectiveness of the solution; if it was unsuccessful, try another.

As pointed out previously, problem solving is a way to come up with a range of possible solutions. If one thing does not work, backtrack and try again. Sometimes it is a combination of several solutions that may finally work.

Chapter 9 provides additional details on the problem-solving process.

ENVIRONMENTAL GUIDELINES FOR PERSONS WITH DEMENTIA

We are all profoundly affected by our environment—we can feel very happy and content in the warmth of a friend's home or threatened and miserable in a corporate office for a job interview. Physical or cognitive disabilities tend to make us even more dependent on our surroundings. Anyone who has spent time in a wheelchair or on crutches and has confronted stairs, uncut curbs, and heavy doors probably has a personal understanding of this. The losses caused by dementia also make a person more dependent on a supportive environment. For example, good lighting and use of contrast become even more important to overcome perceptual problems. Clear pathways and signs help to overcome problems with orientation. A calm, welcoming environment overcomes distress.

On a positive note, a supportive environment can be an ongoing source of care and treatment, 24 hours per day. Unfortunately, as with most other areas of treatment, there is no set of absolute rules for designing a safe and supportive environment. Research and clinical experience (Brawley, 1997; Calkins & Marsden, 2000; Lawton & Maddox, 1985; Warner, 2000), however, provide guidelines. These guidelines can be divided into three areas: setting up surroundings for success, balancing needs, and compensating for losses. The guidelines are not intended as a comprehensive approach to setting up the environment, but it is hoped that they will help to get you started. See Appendix B for additional resources on this topic.

Setting up Surroundings for Success

These guidelines are intended to make use of the person's continuing abilities and enable the person to be as successful as possible. Surroundings that are set up for success focus on familiar faces and places.

Familiar Faces and Places

Alice had increasing problems coping in her own home, so we had to make the difficult decision to sell her home and move her several hundred miles to be near us, her only immediate family. We were very concerned about how this move would affect Alice, and there is no doubt that leaving her home of 45 years was difficult and stressful. I made some huge mistakes, such as telling Alice that it was too expensive to move her hoarded supply of bargain canned goods. Alice was a survivor of the Depression, so this was like stealing from her bank account and upset her greatly. In fact, there was no need for me to even mention this to Alice because I was doing most of the packing and unpacking. By the time her belongings were unpacked, she would have forgotten all about her special supply of cans and been delighted with the bargains I put on her shelves.

One thing we did manage pretty well, however, was finding an apartment near us that was laid out like Alice's previous home. I then arranged her favorite furniture and precious collections from over the years in a similar pattern. This was a tremendous comfort and seemed to help Alice adjust to this big change. The first day in her new home, with all of her things around her, Alice sat with me at the kitchen table and thanked me for all of my work. To my surprise, she said that she had never been so happy and that she didn't miss "that other house" at all. The following suggestions may help you set up the environment so that the person you are caring for doesn't miss "that other house."

Keep the Environment as Familiar as Possible

Although the person may often be looking for home, care-givers shouldn't think that the surroundings don't matter. It is essential to try to keep the care environment looking as famil-iar as possible. This includes the placement of furniture and decorations, the organization of cupboards and drawers, and the location of often used objects (e.g., grooming supplies). Although the person may not verbally recognize where he or she is, having a physical setting that is familiar helps to trig-ger nonverbal recall. Unfamiliar settings can be disorienting, as illustrated next.

With the support of his family and other caregivers, a prominent businessman with dementia was able to con-tinue functioning very well with his daily activities at home. Because he was well versed in public presentation and social skills, his activities often included entertaining and going to public functions and dinners. At one service club dinner in a large hotel, he excused himself to go the bathroom, something he managed to do at home with no problem. His wife was dis-mayed, however, when she heard her husband and others shout-ing in the men's bathroom. When she ran to investigate, a fellow dinner guest told her that he had tried to stop her husband from urinating in the men's room trash can. Apparently, the unfamiliar bathroom—with its many mirrors, lights, stalls, and urinals—had totally confused her husband, rendering him unable to function.

This is definitely not the time to redecorate or renovate in ways that involve drastic changes in furniture arrangements, color scheme, or design. Practical objects within the home should continue to look and work just as they always have. For example, although lever sink taps may be physically easier to operate, the person with dementia may not recognize that they are taps.

If the environment needs to be changed—for example, for safety reasons or to move the person's bedroom nearer to the bathroom—this should be done as gradually and discretely as possible. Try to avoid rearranging the basic furniture layout in main living areas (i.e., kitchen, bathroom, living room, bedroom), particularly the person's favorite places to sit. Keep favorite pictures and special treasures in easy view.

We are all creatures of habit. I hadn't realized myself how deep this need for consistency goes until I made a trip to my childhood home. When I sat down at the kitchen table, I instinctively ducked to make way for the old crank telephone above the chair. Yet, that telephone had not been there for 30 years and had been gone for at least 10 years before I had moved! For persons with dementia who are losing the ability to take in things around them, these old patterns and habits become even more important.

Introduce Changes Gradually and Subtly

If a move is necessary, try to arrange furniture and other objects in familiar ways. Involve the person in decorating his or her new room, in ways that he or she can manage (e.g., by asking, "Would you like your mother's picture hung here by the door or over by the dresser?"). However, some things are related to safety and are not open for discussion—for example, removing a pile of old magazines scattered on the floor by the sofa or installing grab bars by the bathtub and toilet. If these changes are made subtly and without much fuss, the person may scarcely notice. However, if making the changes becomes a point of discussion and argument, resentment can result.

The move from a community home to a long-term care facility can be especially traumatic for everyone. Caregivers can do a great deal to smooth the way by arranging the environment. Some basic suggestions follow; see Chapter 10 for more information.

- Bring as many of the person's own furnishings and possessions (e.g., dresser, chair, comforter, photos, mementos) as possible.

- Make every effort to arrange the new bedroom like the person's previous bedroom. For example, use the same organization for his or her dresser drawers. An easy way to do this is to move the drawers as is so their contents aren't rearranged.

- Involve the person in arranging and decorating his or her new room.

- Ensure that favorite photos and other precious objects are easy to see.

- Share a pleasant time in the new environment. Have a snack and visit with the person, looking at photos or participating in other favorite activities. If the person is able, he or she could host a small open house.

- Explore other surroundings (e.g., the dining room, the patio) and then "go back home."

Encourage Independent Activity

Regardless of what time it was or whether Gerry had just eaten, dozens of times per day he would ask his caregiver if it was time for supper yet. No answer ever really satisfied Gerry; he always seemed anxious that he wasn't getting his meals. A new caregiver decided to get Gerry to help set the table on a daily basis. A few days later, Gerry started to ask if it was time for supper, then stopped and answered his own question by saying, "Oh, wait now. I helped set the table, so I guess we must have eaten." Sometimes Gerry was able to answer his own question and sometimes he needed hints from his caregiver, but he was always reassured that he ate because he remembered setting the table.

In this and countless other ways, a home environment that encourages the person to be involved in meaningful daily activities helps to overcome some of the losses caused by dementia, thereby improving the quality of life for the person and his or her caregiver.

Have you ever asked the person with dementia, "What would you like to do today?" What answer did you get? Probably something such as, "Nothing," "Whatever you would like to do," or "You decide." As noted previously, such replies can lead caregivers to think that the person has lost the desire to do things. This is not true; what the person has lost is the ability to determine what to do and how to get started. He or she has lost the ability to independently plan and organize "doing." However, if the person's environment is set up to encourage participation in familiar, meaningful activities, some of these problems with initiative can be overcome. Having meaningful things to do in the home connects the person with his or her past, reassures the person about who he or she is, and supports self-worth.

Providing these opportunities becomes especially important if the person moves to a long-term care facility. In addition to providing opportunities for doing, family caregivers can play an important role in helping paid caregivers to learn more about the person and his or her interests. This information should be included in the All About Me form in Appendix A.

The focus in this section is on ways to structure the environment to promote self-directed activity. Chapters 6, 7, and 8 provide many more suggestions that can help keep the person "doing." Caregivers in long-term care facilities are directed to *Therapeutic Activities with Persons Disabled by Alzheimer's Disease and Related Disorders* (Bowlby, 1993).

Focus on Previously Enjoyed Activities

Think about what brought the person comfort and pleasure in the past. How did the person relax and unwind before developing dementia? Gardening, listening to music, reading the newspaper, listening to the ball game, resting on the couch, cooking, swimming, walking—the possibilities are endless. Previously enjoyed activities come naturally to the person, bring the most pleasure, and are easy to help continue.

Make Activity Opportunities Easy to See

Once you have determined which activities are most important for the person you are caring for, try to set up opportunities for the person to still do these activities independently. As a rule, if persons with dementia can see something, they are likely to be interested in exploring it. Having simple activities set up and ready to go serves as a "kick start."

For example, suppose the person used to find gardening relaxing but can no longer manage it independently. In addition to using the suggestions for doing gardening together (see Chapter 8), consider these or other garden-related activities that could be ready for the person to do on his or her own:

- Fill a mister bottle and set it near potted plants.
- Place an opened gardening magazine or seed catalog near the person's chair.
- Fill a small photo album with favorite pictures of the person's garden.
- Help the person to start picking the dead leaves off a plant.
- Set out a tub of potting soil to be mixed.
- Set out sprigs of dried herbs to be crushed and put in bottles.

In this same way, other favorite activities can be set up in the person's surroundings and adapted so that he or she can still have meaningful things to do independently. This can offer a great deal of reassurance and comfort and can help the person to feel at home, both with him- or herself and with the surroundings. The businessman needs papers and files to organize and a desk to sit at; the teacher needs papers to mark and books to read; the homemaker needs dishes to wash, laundry to hang, and things to dust. See Chapters 6, 7, and 8 for additional suggestions.

Set Up a Work Station

For reasons of safety or orderliness, it may be better to have a separate work area that is specifically set up for the person's interests and abilities. It's best to choose an area that will be near you but also is open and obvious to the person, inviting him or her to get involved. Again there are endless ideas; here are a few suggestions:

- Provide a desk with papers, files, books, envelopes, pens.
- Fill a bureau with socks to sort and handkerchiefs to fold.
- Stock a work bench with safe things to take apart and put together and tools to sort.
- Arrange a sewing table with buttons, yarn, and fabric.

Provide Opportunities to Reminisce

When Edna moved from her home to a long-term care facility, her daughter Rosemary traveled thousands of miles to do everything she could to help make this move as comfortable as possible for her mother. This move occurred many years ago, long before long-term care facilities allowed people to bring personal furniture. However, Rosemary insisted that Edna needed to have family photos with her, and she hung these on the wall of her mother's room. Several months later, Edna needed a higher level of care and was moved to another unit in the same facility. Unfortunately, Rosemary was unable to help with this move, but she was confident that the devoted care staff would help smooth the way. They did indeed do a wonderful job of comforting and reassuring Edna as the move took place.

After the move, everyone was very surprised when the normally sweet and pleasant Edna became agitated and resistive to care. She started wandering the halls day and night and constantly searched others' rooms. At first, care staff believed that this behavior was caused by Edna's difficulty adjusting to her new room. After 3 weeks, however, they became concerned and called Rosemary, who made an emergency trip. As soon as she entered Edna's new room, she realized the source of the problem. Her mother's cherished photos had not yet been hung on the walls of her new room.

Without these treasured photos to help her connect with her past, Edna was distressed and disconnected from an important part of herself. Staff verbally reassured Edna that all was well and that maintenance staff would soon hang up her photos, but Edna forgot this reassurance almost immediately. When she couldn't actually see her photos, she began a frantic search for them.

As detailed in Chapter 6, recalling the past is important to everyone, but the opportunity to reminisce is especially important for older people. For older persons with dementia, concrete reminders of the past take on special significance.

The surroundings play an important role in helping the person to "remember when." Having an environment that stirs memories can offer reassurance. This provides an opportunity to look back and recall people and experiences from the past, to relive a time before dementia made life so difficult. Remembering is enhanced with the caregiver's help, but having family photos on the walls and in albums and favorite possessions set out in easy view encourages the person to get in touch with his or her past. If photos and personal treasures are labeled, the person can often go on his or her own sentimental journey. This also invites visitors to share in the memories with the person. Creating and looking at a labeled, handheld, photo album or memory book is an excellent family project and shared activity.

Fragile items can be displayed on plate racks, on high decorator shelves, or in a china cabinet with locking doors. Caregivers can provide opportunities for the person to touch and look at breakable items such as dishes.

In addition to personal items, interior design and decorating play an important role in supporting reminiscence. Furnishings, fabrics, wall coverings, and decorator items can help to trigger memories. I worked in a unit that had an old crank telephone that had been donated by a family member. Residents spent happy hours cranking their old ring or that of a friend and recalling the party-line days.

Balancing Needs

Certain areas—manageable choices, "welcome to my place," and sensory stimulation without stress—involve a need to establish an individualized balance (between two opposing needs) that is suitable for the person.

Manageable Choices

Home is where we decide how things should be arranged. At home, we feel free to decide when to eat, where to hang a new picture, and whether we will make our bed now or later—or not at all! The expression "A person's home is his or her castle" suggests that whatever home is like, the person should feel like the master of a great castle, the person in charge of the kingdom.

To feel at home, to feel like the ruler of the castle, persons with dementia also need to make decisions. Although making decisions out of a wide range of choices eventually becomes too difficult, offering manageable choices (usually between two options) supports the person's sense of feeling at home. The following story from my experience illustrates some other pitfalls regarding choices. See Chapter 6 for more on providing manageable choices.

Everything connected with her son's life was important to Alice. So, well in advance of his birthday, I took Alice shopping for a gift for him. Because I knew that he wanted a portable telephone, I helped Alice select one, giving her frequent reminders about who it was for and so forth. Going shopping was a major excursion—traveling through February snow and slush and arranging to get Alice into the crowded mall on a Saturday when I was off. It would have taken about a quarter of the time and a tenth of the energy for me to go shopping by myself and buy the telephone on Alice's behalf. However, I knew how important this was and felt that Alice should be involved. Because I was concerned about her safety, and that of the telephone, we wrapped the gift and kept it at my house until the big day.

After all of this effort, you can imagine how exasperated I was when Alice called later that day to say that she didn't have a present for her son's birthday. These calls took place daily and then more frequently as the day approached. I always gave Alice the same reassuring reply, "Yes, we have a gift; it is safe at my house," and recounted our adventures in shopping for it. None of this had much effect; on the big day, Alice arrived at the family party proudly carrying a wrapped gift. In a panic that morning, she had persuaded her housekeeper to help her get a gift. Alice was pleased as punch with her efforts—a shaving kit for her son with a beard!

It is only now, years later, that I understand a little bit of what went wrong. I had involved Alice and offered choices. However, the gift choice was so far removed from anything that she would ever buy for her son that the choice had no meaning to her. In addition, she didn't have a wrapped gift as a concrete reminder that her shopping was done. She also may have been so overwhelmed by the whole shopping expedition that it was a negative rather than a positive memory. The short trip to the local drug store with her housekeeper made a lot more sense.

Suggestions follow for involving the person in making choices around the house.

- Ask the person about the placement of photos or pictures. Say, "Do you think we should put it here or here?"
- Ask the person to choose between two different sets of sheets when changing the bed linens.
- Offer a choice between two different decorator items (e.g., wallpaper, paint colors, fabric). If it becomes too

overwhelming for the person to go shopping to make these choices, bring home samples.

- Offer a choice between two places to sit.
- Ask the person to choose between two sets of napkins or placemats for the table.

Access to the Outdoors

Everyone needs the opportunity to make a choice to go outside. This is such an important choice it warrants a separate discussion.

Exposure to natural light is essential for maintaining many bodily functions. In particular, sunlight is needed to manufacture vitamin D. Vitamin D is now added to many foods, but there is evidence that these supplements are not as effective as natural light (Brawley, 1997). Only 10 minutes of protected hand and face exposure are required to produce a day's requirement of vitamin D.

Exposure to natural light is also essential in helping the body to break down and use calcium and to enable and support the immune system. The setting of one's internal clock, also known as the sleep–wake cycle or the circadian rhythm, depends on several minutes of exposure to natural light per day. Seasonal affective disorder is a form of depression that is triggered by the shorter days—hence, the decreased hours of sunlight—in winter.

There is compelling evidence that many older people who are frail are in fact suffering from sunlight starvation (Brawley, 1997; Gill, Williams, & Tinetti, 2000). This leads to decreased levels of vitamin D and calcium as well as to disturbances of the sleep–wake cycle and depression or seasonal affective disorder. Natural light deprivation can be particularly negative for persons with dementia, who already have disrupted sleep–wake cycles and problems with orientation. Several controlled experiments have found that exposure to bright light is effective in reducing agitation in persons with dementia and that increased lighting is effective in reducing sundowning behavior (Volicer & Bloom-Charette, 1999). It is heartening to know that the design or renovation plans for long-term care facilities are increasingly taking into account the need for natural light and access to the outdoors.

In addition to the need for light, access to the outdoors is vital to the person's sense of mastery and control over his or her environment and, hence, his or her sense of well-being. One very interesting study found that when a patio door at a care facility was unlocked for resident use, residents didn't necessarily go outside for long periods of time, but they found great satisfaction in being able to open the door and look outside even briefly. This intervention also significantly reduced agitation (Namazi & Johnson, 1992). If this approach is used, however, the caregiver must remember to supervise the person to prevent wandering or other dangerous behaviors.

"This, doctor, is medicine for the spirit."

As she worked with other residents repotting plants, a nursing facility resident spoke the preceding words to her doctor. This statement underlines the positive therapeutic effects of working with plants, indoors and outdoors, which has been well documented in research and clinical experience (Bowlby Sifton, 1998; Hewson, 1994). In addition, for those who have spent their lives working in the outdoors or who have lifelong avocational outdoor interests, access to the outdoors is particularly vital for well-being.

The opportunity to be outdoors every day is essential to everyone's well-being and is particularly important for persons with dementia. Safe outdoor areas should be available, whether they are enclosed gardens, patios, or decks. Outdoor walking paths can be a great source of enjoyment and exercise. Walkways should be smooth, with definite borders that guide the person and avoid frustrating dead ends. Fences must be high enough that a person cannot climb over them. Chairs, benches, or other items that could be used for climbing should be removed from fence areas and securely fastened elsewhere.

By creating an interesting area within a fenced garden, the person will be less inclined to try to leave the area. Items of interest might include sculptures; birdfeeders or birdbaths; sundials; benches; and nonpoisonous, nonprickly plant displays. In congregate living areas or public parks, larger items of local interest (e.g., an anchor in a coastal area, farm equipment in a rural area) can be displayed. Large items of general interest can also generate engagement. For example, old cars have provided hours of meaningful activity in many care facilities (one old car was in a rooftop garden). Residents enjoy washing and tinkering with the car and even just sitting in it.

It must also be remembered that it is not enough to just simply have an outdoor area. Persons with dementia must be enabled to go out and make use of it. Making the area easily visible and obvious is important, but it may also be necessary to directly assist persons to go outside.

"Welcome to My Place"

At one unit where I worked, the old, awkward, institutional bathrooms needed to be made more suitable for persons with dementia. A local architect volunteered his skills to assist in redesigning the bathrooms, and the head nurse and I were thrilled with this opportunity. When we were assured that the women's bathroom was empty, we happily parade the male architect in. We were flabbergasted when Molly, usually a demure lady who always wore her hat and carried her purse, came storming in. She yelled at the astonished volunteer, basically saying that he had no business being there. The head nurse recovered quickly, took Molly's hand, apologized profusely, and said she was quite right. She then asked Molly's permission to have this gentleman look at the women's bathroom so that he could help redesign it. Molly calmed down and rather haughtily said that she supposed it would be okay.

We had committed a great faux pas by letting a man into the most private of places, the women's bathroom. Molly had advanced dementia, but she remained very aware of this. Although the bathroom is a shared space in most homes, its use is strictly private. This is a long-standing, highly guarded right within families that is usually especially protected by older adults.

When a person with dementia needs assistance with bathing and toileting, caregivers must be especially mindful of protecting privacy and dignity. Family caregivers may also find that they are embarrassed because helping with these activities is so much outside of their usual relationship with the person. Chapter 7 discusses these issues in more detail.

Privacy in the bathroom is fundamental. Beyond this, however, we all have a need for privacy and spaces that are just our own. Persons with dementia may be unable either to protect their privacy or to tell us about their need. Caregivers need to ensure that persons with dementia have privacy and help them to protect their space. If persons with dementia are unable to have physical privacy, they may create social privacy by withdrawing from others.

It is important to continue with the following accepted practices that support privacy:

- Keep the bathroom door shut and suggest that you will be just outside if help is needed.
- Always knock and ask permission before coming into someone's private space, such as his or her bedroom.
- Maintain traditional boundaries, such as railings around a porch or fences in the backyard.
- Respect the person's continuing needs for privacy, time alone, and a space that is his or hers. This space might be large, such as a bedroom, or much smaller, such as the person's favorite chair in the living room or his or her place at the table.

As dementia progresses and the person needs more assistance and is less able to state his or her privacy needs, these private spaces become especially important. Help the person to continue to use and locate these private places. In addition, consider the person's lifestyle patterns before he or she developed dementia; help a person who has always been private to continue to have as much privacy as possible.

Balancing the Need for Privacy with the Need for Socialization

As much as people need privacy, they also need to visit and spend time with others. The challenge for caregivers is to help a person with dementia maintain a balance of the two that is in keeping with his or her previous lifestyle. As with many other aspects of daily life, a person with dementia will have increasing difficulty getting started and organizing social activities, even though social skills generally form a continuing strength. Setting up the living environment to encourage being with others helps the person to overcome these challenges. Physical aspects that enable socialization follow; see Chapters 6, 7, and 8 for more details on encouraging social activities.

- Put a comfortable chair in a place where the person can watch others coming and going and respond to greetings (e.g., on the front porch, near the front window).

- Create a comfortable place near or in the kitchen so that the person can be part of the family's comings and goings. Just watching and occasionally responding is an important social activity. Check for signs of the person becoming overwhelmed if there is a lot of commotion, and guide the person to a favorite chair in a quieter location.

- If the person has always spent a lot of time socializing on the telephone, this activity should be encouraged by placing a familiar style telephone (e.g., one with a rotary dial with a separate handset as opposed to a more modern portable phone) in an easy-access location. If the use of stored automatic-dial numbers is introduced and practiced in the early stages of dementia, the person can often use these to call friends and family members well into the later stages of dementia. It is important to remember, however, that many persons with dementia find using the telephone challenging; for them, telephone use should be reserved for emergencies only (see Chapter 4.)

- For some people, a Dutch door (i.e., one that is divided horizontally) for the bedroom or kitchen provides a good balance between the need for privacy and the need to be part of the household and know where the caregiver is.

- Fabric door guards (held in place with Velcro) can serve the same function as Dutch doors. These can be purchased from catalogs (see the resources in Appendix B) or can be homemade. Make a double band of brightly colored fabric that is approximately 8" wide. Sew strips of looped Velcro across each end. Place strips of heavy-duty, adhesive-back, hook Velcro at waist height on either side of the doorway. (Adhesive Velcro sticks better if you carefully peel the paper strip off and heat the sticky area with a heat gun or hair dryer.) The fabric strip can then be fastened across the doorway when needed. In particular, using a fabric door guard can be an effective way to protect the privacy of residents in long-term care facilities. Another way to make a temporary door guard is to use a soft, colored rope or thick drapery cord such as those found in theaters to block off aisles. The rope or cord can be hooked into eye bolts on either side of the doorway. These cords can be made attractive by adding decorative tassels such as those used for draperies.

Sensory Stimulation without Stress

We all depend on our senses, perhaps even more than we realize, to let us know where we are and how to act and respond. And what a world of pleasure sights, sounds, touches, tastes, and smells bring to us! The sensory part of the brain is still very much intact for persons with dementia, but they sometimes have difficulty in understanding how to respond to this sensory information.

Understanding how to respond becomes even more difficult when there is too much sensory input. This is true of everyone. For example, I think about coming home tired after a demanding day at work when the house is full of the kids and their friends, the telephone is ringing, the dog is barking, the television is on full blast, and the kitchen is a disaster. Being tired, it is difficult to determine where to start to sort out all of this sensory information. The simple question, "What's for supper?" is then more than I can cope with.

For persons with dementia, even much less sensory input tends to cause sensory overload. So, although sensory experiences are vital for pleasure and provide hints for action, the amount of sensory input needs to be controlled to avoid over-loading them. This balance is sometimes referred to as "sensory stimulation without stress."

Chapter 6 provides much more information on making use of the senses, but some pointers about avoiding overload in the physical setting follow:

- Make use of familiar, comforting patterns and a variety of textures for wall coverings, furniture, and other decorating items. Emphasize the familiar, and avoid busy or abstract designs that could be too stimulating or confusing.

- Use familiar, rich-textured items such as shawls, afghans, and pillows to provide touch stimulation and comfort.

- Provide a variety of comfortable spaces with manageable sensory experiences. Examples include a seat on the patio; a seat by a window that looks out at a birdfeeder; and a seat in the kitchen to appreciate the sights, smells, and sounds of meal preparation.

- Make sure that the person has a pleasant and stimulating but calm place for retreat during busy activities that may become overwhelming (e.g., parties, family gatherings).

- Use of the aroma of favorite foods cooking (e.g., bread, stews, soups) not only to stimulate the appetite but also to create an atmosphere of comfort and reassurance. This is easily done with modern appliances such as bread makers and Crock-Pots (e.g., to simmer a commercial package soup mix).

Compensating for Losses

The following guidelines suggest ways in which the environment can be used to compensate for some of the losses in ability caused by dementia.

The Need for Home

There are ways to organize the physical setting that can help a place to feel more like home, more like a place where individuals with dementia would like to stay. This setup also provides reassuring, orienting information.

In addition to the previous tips on maintaining familiar places and faces, it is necessary to help a person with dementia find important locations (e.g., bathroom, bedroom). There are many ways to do this, so you may need to experiment to find what works best for the person you are caring for. It is important to balance these changes with the need for the living environment to look as much like a normal home as possible. Some suggestions follow.

- Mark the doorway in some noticeable and appealing way. Decorate it with fabric, wallpaper, or artwork. Painting the doorjamb the person's favorite color may work, especially if this color differs from that of the walls and other doors.

- Place a decorative banner, flag, or a three-dimensional object (e.g., a small table, a large vase, plant, a piece of art) near the doorway so that it is visible if the person looks down the hall toward the doorway.

- Create a "touch path" along the wall leading to the bathroom or bedroom. Some suggestions are a handrail, wooden molding, wallpaper border, or a carpet strip. Try to use something in keeping with the person's tastes, and reinforce use of the path by incorporating favorite colors or designs. To learn to use the touch path independently, the person initially will need some gentle direction and practice.

Finding the bathroom at night can be challenging for persons with dementia. Some people find it helpful if the bathroom light is left on or a series of night lights illuminate the hallway. For others, these approaches can add to disorientation problems. Motion-activated light switches (i.e., those that turn on when a person walks by) are available at hardware stores.

The Need for Reality Assurance

In addition to having difficulty with recognizing home, a person with dementia has difficulty with other orientation information (e.g., date, season, time, day of the week). Although there is no particular value in struggling to have the person remember or repeat such information, he or she (like everyone else) needs the reassurance of having this information available. Some ways to ensure that the environment can provide this information follow.

- Place easy-to-read clocks at eye level. Note that digital clocks are not as familiar as traditional clocks with faces. Clocks that chime on the hours can help to draw the person's attention. Talking clocks are also available, but these may confuse the person.

- Hang up a large-print calendar with the date indicated by, for example, crossing off the previous days. For some people, individual Page-a-Day type calendars with just the month and date are helpful. These are available at most office supply stores.

- Provide easy access to outdoor spaces and windows for orientation to the season and the time of day.

- Use familiar, adult seasonal decorations (e.g., for holidays).

As noted previously, persons with dementia often have perceptual problems, so they may not recognize people and

things in their surroundings. This makes it especially important to avoid decorations or items that may cause confusion.
A person with dementia may try to eat wax or artificial fruit,
water artificial plants, or walk into realistic wall murals of the
outdoors. Similarly, designs in flooring that look like dust
specks or holes may cause the person to try to clean up or
avoid the area, respectively. Mirrors or other reflective surfaces may be especially confusing because the person may no
longer recognize him- or herself. The person may be alarmed
at having a "stranger" in the bathroom with him or her, or the
individual may actually develop a relationship with the person
in the mirror. Large mirrors should be removed in the early
stages of dementia to avoid these challenges. Small mirrors
should be placed with sensitivity to the person's reaction to
them.

The Need for a Safe Place

Home safety for persons with dementia can be a concern
from several different angles: the physical changes associated
both with dementia and with aging as well as the changes in
judgment and perception caused by dementia.

Prevent Wandering

The top home safety concern of most caregivers is keeping the
person with dementia from wandering and getting lost or hurt.
As a result, some practical environmental steps are discussed
next (see Chapter 9 for more suggestions on preventing and
responding to wandering). However, bear in mind that wandering—or what might better be called "walking about"—is
not only healthy exercise but also expresses the need to explore
and investigate. When caregivers provide safe places for the
person to walk and explore, safety concerns are lessened.

Register with national safe return programs. In the United States, contact the national office of the Alzheimer's Association (800-272-3900) or your local chapter and ask about the Safe Return program. The program's registration form can also be downloaded from the association's web site at http://www.alz.org/SafeReturn. In Canada, contact the Alzheimer Society (800-616-8816) and ask about Safely Home—Alzheimer Wandering Registry. Information is also available on the society's web site (in English: http://www.alzheimer.ca/english/care/wandering-intro.htm; in French: http://www.alzheimer.ca/french/care/wandering-intro.htm).

The first step to preventing wandering is to provide plenty of exercise and stimulation during the day so the person feels content at home. This is especially important in helping the person to relax and rest at home in the evening. In addition, an emotional shelter—an accepting and interesting environment that says "stay here with me"—can also help prevent wandering. (Refer to the "Searching for Home" section at the beginning of this chapter.) Providing interesting opportunities for looking at and doing things at home also helps to prevent frustration and the wish to leave for stimulation. It is important to put away coats, boots, car keys, and so forth. Such items may trigger the person to go outside.

Secure the doors but in a disguised way that won't frustrate the person and give him or her the sense of being locked in. Some suggestions follow:

- Extra locks, slide bars, or dead bolts at the top and bottom of the door and two-step locks and keypad locks that are camouflaged to blend in to the surroundings (e.g., painted the same color as the door). For safety reasons, such as quick escape in the event of a fire, these devices must be easily managed by the caregiver.

- Use child-proof door handle covers (available at toy stores or in children's departments of large retail stores).

- Camouflage the whole doorway with fabric or artwork. Painting murals of nice scenes (e.g., flower gardens) that are attractive but clearly art, not the real thing, and that include the door, frame, and surrounding wall are very effective. (Painting the door frame the same color as the surrounding walls helps the door to "disappear.") At the same time, be sure to remove anything that will contrast with the mural and draw attention to the door, such as individual pieces of artwork, curtains, mirrors, or other decorations.

- Install devices that will let you know when the person is at an exit. Simple devices include bells on the door handle or above the door or an inexpensive welcome mat that plays a tune when stepped on. More complex devices include alarm systems with motion detectors.

Share your concerns with neighbors and local business owners. One caregiver reported that this type of community involvement also provided an excellent opportunity to educate others about dementia. Show others a photograph (as necessary) so they will recognize the person if they see him or her wandering.

Have the person wear an identification bracelet or necklace with your contact information. To encourage use of this item, try presenting it as a special gift.

Keep a current picture of the person handy for identification if he or she wanders off. In addition, keep a few unlaundered clothing items in a plastic bag in the freezer. These can be used for scent identification if tracking dogs need to be involved in a search effort.

Another concern is wandering into areas of the home where there are safety risks or where the person may disrupt the activity of other family members. Some of these suggestions may help:

- Provide stimulating sitting or work areas where the person will be reminded to stay and do things. Work station ideas are addressed in this chapter's "Set Up a Work Station" subsection and are discussed further in Chapter 6.

- Use half doors in areas such as the kitchen or bedroom so that the person can still look in or out of the room and see other family members.

- Create brightly colored fabric "cues" and use Velcro to affix them across doorways on an as-needed basis. These may be all that is needed to cue the person not to enter a particular room or to stay in his or her bedroom. Yellow plastic safety tape may also work. **Note that children's safety gates are not recommended, especially at stairways. The person usually sees these as unnatural obstacles and may try to climb over them and subsequently fall.**

- Make the most dangerous areas off limits by using some of the previously described locking or camouflage techniques. Some areas that eventually should be off limits are basements, attics, workshops, garages, and laundry rooms. If these areas have been valued places for work and activity, it is important to set up safe alternative areas to work on favorite activities (e.g., an area to fold laundry).

Provide Opportunities for Guided Wandering

Provide a safety-proofed area for pacing and wandering in the home or yard. Indoors, this could be a path that leads around the house. A circular or return route is best. Some house designs have a natural circular route (e.g., one that runs through the kitchen, along a hall, through the living room, and back to the kitchen). The person you are caring for will probably take advantage of this path independently. Ensure safety by checking for loose rugs or carpeting, uneven flooring, clutter, too much furniture along the way, or unstable furniture that the person may try to use for support. (See previous suggestions given in this section for additional information.) Handrails or short grab bars along the path will encourage the person to follow this route and increase safety. Although the path should be clear of obstacles, it should also pass by safe and interesting objects, such as pictures or mementos that entice the person to explore. A chair at an inviting and interesting place on the route encourages the person to sit and rest. Further encouragement to sit and rest can be provided by having tape-recorded music or other interesting objects at rest points. Try to avoid having dead ends that may frustrate the person (e.g., locked doors). As noted previously, touch paths can encourage walking in safe places.

Outdoor wandering paths should follow the same principles: They should be circular so the person isn't frustrated by dead ends; they should have even surfaces and be free of obstacles and other dangers, such as prickly or poisonous plants; and they should offer points of interest and places to rest. As noted previously, fountains, birdfeeders, statues, yard ornaments, and benches can be used for outdoor places of interest and rest. See the subsection titled "Access to the Outdoors" for more information.

General Safety Suggestions

Special consideration should be given to the kitchen, bathroom, and stairways. Beyond that, remember that out of sight is out of mind. Remove and lock up all hazardous materials, such as tools, knives, cleaning supplies, medication, poisonous plants (e.g., poinsettia, dieffenbachia), firearms, small appliances, car keys, alcohol, and foods and condiments that may be harmful if eaten in large quantities. Remove heavy or fragile objects, especially from high shelves, that may break or cause injury if dropped. Remove other items that may cause harm if the person forgets their proper use (e.g., pet food, cat litter trays).

Place safety catches on cabinets, drawers, windows, and closets. Various types of inexpensive safety catches are available at hardware stores. Gates can be secured by using two gravity latches, as the person probably will not be able to use two latches at once. Access to drawers can be limited by notching the bottom edges so that two actions are required to open the drawer: lifting up and pulling out. Most hardware stores have simple stops that can be installed on windows so that they don't open all the way. Access to a closet can be prevented by installing a slide bolt at the base of its door and painting it the same color as the door. To avoid frustrating the person, it is important to provide easy access to a junk drawer or other receptacle for safe materials that the person may sort, rearrange, and carry about (e.g., greeting cards, playing cards, papers, envelopes).

It is important to take steps to prevent scalding. Turn down the temperature of the hot water heater. Also, install inexpensive antiscald devices for taps and showers or replace showerheads with those that contain an antiscald mechanism.

Even and bright lighting, without glare, is essential. The aging eye needs as much as three times the amount of light for good vision. In addition, persons with dementia may have perceptual problems, making good lighting especially important. Ensure that potentially dangerous areas, such as the top of the stairs, are well lit. In addition, use lighting to eliminate shadows, which can be frightening and may be misinterpreted. Lighting is also discussed in the vision section of the main heading "Adaptations for Age-Related Changes."

Make sure the person cannot lock him- or herself in the bathroom or any other room with a locking door. If the bathroom door has an interior push-in lock, keep a key nearby (but out of sight) or put tape across the door latch. Also, remove slide bolts or hook and eye locks. Most home supply stores have two-way door locks that can be opened from either side.

Remove sink stoppers to prevent a flood if the water is left on. Some caregivers actually turn off the valve on bathroom sinks to prevent this problem. Inexpensive flood detector alarms can be purchased at most hardware stores. These devices sit on the floor, and the alarm sounds when they come in contact with water.

Add decals to sliding glass doors. This will increase visibility and help prevent the person from walking into them.

Disable the stove by removing knobs or fuses or by installing a control switch. This is not automatically necessary, especially if the person has never used the kitchen. Nonetheless, it must be considered, particularly if the person spends any time at home alone. The entire stovetop may also be covered with an aluminum cover so that the person will not see it and potentially become interested in using it.

Buy small appliances (e.g., electric kettle, iron) with automatic shut-off switches. In addition, appliances can be plugged into timer switches so that they can only be used at certain times—for instance, not at night. In general, small appliances should be left unplugged. Ground fault interrupters (GFIs) are an excellent addition. These electrical outlets shut off in cases when electric shock is a possibility. Popping a GFI's test button effectively disables the outlet, thereby allowing the caregiver to limit access to the outlet. Another way to limit access is to place safety cover plugs in electrical outlets.

When possible, remove sharp-cornered objects or furniture, and pad the corners of countertops. Foam pipe insulation makes an excellent and inexpensive padding for the hard edges of tables and countertops. Furthermore, leave doors completely open or closed. This will help prevent the person from walking into the edge of a door.

Emergency Plans

It is important to rehearse emergency plans in the event of a fire, a health crisis, or a fall. This is essential even in the earliest stages of dementia, as the person may panic in an emergency. A well-rehearsed plan and a list of emergency contact numbers posted by the telephone increase the person's ability to follow through with the practiced pattern.

These plans become even more essential as dementia progresses, especially if the person spends any time at home on his or her own. A person with dementia who lives alone needs special attention in this regard. Caregivers can arrange telephone checks and ask caring neighbors to check on the person. It may be helpful for the person to wear an emergency call system device and a medical emergency notification bracelet or necklace (if applicable). The earlier these systems are put in place and, hence, the person can learn to use them, the better. You may have more success with getting these systems in place by presenting them with statements such as "This is something you can do for me so I won't worry."

ADAPTATIONS FOR AGE-RELATED CHANGES

Many persons with dementia will also experience physical changes that are associated with aging. It is now known that many conditions once associated solely with aging, such as reduced physical capacity, are in fact related to lifestyle factors (e.g., diet, exercise) than to aging itself. However, some changes are part of normal aging. These changes—for example, in vision and hearing—may have an even greater impact on the person with dementia, so it is important that caregivers make compensatory changes. Some of these age-related changes and suggested compensations are outlined next.

Sensory Changes

Among persons older than 65 years, 75% have a significant impairment of one or more sensory functions.

Vision

Acuity (the ability to distinguish fine details) and accommodation (the ability to adapt the focus of the eye to objects at different distances) both begin to deteriorate when people are in their forties. For most persons, however, these changes can be corrected with proper glasses. The size of the visual field begins to decrease after age 60. Dark adaptation (moving from bright light to dim light or darkness) takes longer as one ages, as does the ability to recover from glare. Perceptual abilities—such as figure–ground discrimination (e.g., being able to see a green toothbrush on a green counter) and visual-spatial discrimination (being able to tell the relative distance and size of objects)—decrease with age. The ability to distinguish colors, particularly those in the blue/green wavelength, decreases with age and affects men more than women.

Adaptations

Persons with dementia are also likely to have perceptual deficits, making the following adaptations all the more important.

- Increase the available light by using task-focused lighting (e.g., a floor lamp beside the person's reading chair) or increasing the wattage of the bulb. Fluorescent lights are not recommended, as the older eye is disturbed by their subtle flicker.

- Eliminate glare—for example, from highly polished surfaces such as floors. Low-gloss floor waxes are available. Sheer curtains or blinds on windows and shades on lamps also help to reduce glare.

- Use color contrast to enhance visibility—for example, on the edges of steps or to distinguish the toilet from its surroundings. Colored electrical tape works well for this. Contrast between food colors and the serving plate is also important.

- Avoid colors in the blue/green spectrum; pastel colors that are hard to distinguish; and potentially confusing patterns or designs on flooring, wall coverings, placemats, and other household decorations.

- Introduce simple but effective changes such as making sure that glasses are clean, positioning lamps and work material appropriately, enhancing other sensory cues, and using large-print materials.

Hearing

The most common hearing loss associated with aging is presbycusis, which interferes with the ability to hear high-pitched sounds and thereby causes difficulty understanding speech. Aging also presents more difficulty with localizing the source of sounds, a decreased ability to mask background sounds (e.g., the hum of the refrigerator), and increased problems hearing while talking on the telephone.

Adaptations

- Decrease or eliminate background noises.
- Gain the person's attention before speaking; face him or her and enunciate your words carefully.
- Use nonverbal cues, enhance other sensory cues, write down key words, and make extra associations with names to clarify what you are saying.
- Ensure proper screenings for hearing loss; sometimes wax removal can vastly improve hearing.

Communication guidelines for persons with dementia are found in Chapter 4. The following suggestions are of particular note for persons with dementia and hearing loss.

- When it is necessary to repeat something, use the same words. This guideline contrasts with the habitual rephrasing that is advised for speaking with people who have hearing loss only. If the words are changed, a person with dementia may think that there are two different messages.
- Lower your voice pitch and speak somewhat more loudly, but do not shout; shouting further distorts sound and can convey anger.

- Persons with dementia and hearing loss are especially prone to feeling excluded or even paranoid due to the extra complications of cognitive misperceptions. Make sure you always include the person in conversation.

Smell

Marked changes in the ability to smell begin at about age 60, with up to half of people older than age 80 unable to smell at all. These changes have serious consequences for safety, as these people may not detect warning smells such as smoke, spoiled food, or escaping gas. Smell also affects appetite. Often, what we think of as the sense of taste is really the sense of smell. Older people with a poor sense of smell may also have hygiene problems, as they may be unaware of offensive body odors. There is some evidence that persons with Alzheimer's disease experience a greater than usual loss of the sense of smell.

Adaptations

- Increase home safety measures. Use smoke detectors. Regularly date and discard leftover food.
- Enhance other sensory cues and social activities during meals to make eating more appealing through other senses.
- Serve hot foods and slow-simmering foods, as these have an increased aroma. When serving cold foods, simmer soup mix on the stove to increase the person's appetite.

Taste

The sense of taste is most affected by aging with regard to the ability to sense sweet and salty flavors. This may explain why some older people use excessive amounts of salt and sugar.

The ability to sense bitter and sour tastes remains more intact, which also contributes to food having a less appealing taste.

Adaptations

- Enhance the gustatory aspects of meals by using extra flavorings and seasonings, favorite traditional foods, and a colorful presentation.
- Enhance the eating environment, making it as familiar and homelike as possible.
- Use natural appetite stimulants, such as savory appetizers, social gatherings, and exercise. Unless prohibited for medical reasons, a moderate amount of alcohol (e.g., one small glass of wine per day) is a good appetite stimulant.
- Help the person with dementia maintain good oral hygiene. Poor oral hygiene interferes with taste and can also cause pain and discomfort when eating.

Guidelines for encouraging the person with dementia to eat and for feeding persons who are dependent are found in Chapter 7.

Touch

The skin is the body's largest organ; as such, it provides vital feedback from the environment. Fortunately, touch and other somatic sensations are less affected by aging than the basic sensory systems and can be used to compensate for losses in vision, hearing, and so forth. There is some age-related loss in fine tactile discrimination, especially in the palms, fingertips, and soles of the feet.

Adaptations

See Chapter 4 for guidelines on the use of caring personal touch.

Pain

Pain is the body's alarm system, warning of a problem. Hence, the decreased awareness of pain that accompanies aging can be problematic; for example, older persons can be unaware that they've become ill or developed skin breakdown. This is a particular concern for persons with dementia due to problems with communication.

Adaptations

- Take special precautions against skin breakdown. The person's seating and lying positions should be changed every 2 hours to prevent skin problems.
- Watch for unusual presentations of infection—for example, if the person suddenly takes to his or her bed or suddenly becomes more confused.

Temperature

An older person, particularly one who is frail, often becomes especially sensitive to temperature extremes. He or she may feel cold at normal room temperature and find hot weather particularly disturbing. These changes are related to changes in blood circulation, a decreased number of sweat glands, and lowered body temperature. It is important to note that for an older person who is frail, hypothermia can occur even at normal room temperature; in turn, hypothermia can lead to apathy and lowered responsiveness.

Adaptation

- Take special precautions with older persons who are frail and live alone. It may be necessary to raise the standard room temperature by as much as 10 degrees Fahrenheit.

Kinesthesia, Proprioception, and Vestibular Function

Kinesthesia is the experience of the sense of movement. Proprioception is awareness of the body in space and in relation to objects in the environment. Vestibular function is related to the sense of balance. There is some evidence of age-related decline in these systems. Of particular interest is the possible relationship between these changes and the risk of falling. The increased incidence of falls in older adults is also thought to be related to changes in neuromuscular control. The following adaptations are precautions to avoid falls.

Adaptations

- Assess the environment for safety. For example, lighting at the top of the stairs is important, as the majority of falls occur in this area.
- Avoid distractions, such as pictures, on the stairwell walls. If the person becomes distracted, he or she may lose his or her balance.
- Allow plenty of time for movement.
- Carpets are a safer and easier walking surface than bare floors, and they also cushion falls.
- Ensure that the person has properly fitted, safe footwear.
- Position pictures, signs, and so forth at eye level. Doing so keeps the person from leaning the head back to look, which can lead to dizziness due to compression of blood flow to the brain.
- Install handrails and grab bars. These should be securely fastened into wall studs in any place where the person may reach for support (e.g., in hallways, stairways, and dressing areas; next to the bathtub, bed, and toilet). At the same time, unsteady items that the person may reach

for to support him- or herself (e.g., rocking chairs, wheeled furniture, towel racks, soap holders, toilet paper holders) should be removed. Many older people who are frail have become adept at "furniture walking"—holding onto items of furniture as they walk around the house. If this has become a pattern for the person with dementia, it may be safer to ensure that these hand holds are secure (i.e., very stable pieces of furniture or grab bars) than for the person to learn to use a walker or a cane.

- Take extra precautions in the bathroom. In addition to the top of the stairs, the bathroom is one of the most common places for falls in the home. There are a wide range of inexpensive safety aids for the bathroom, such as grab bars, toilet safety frames, tub transfer benches, and handheld showers, which make it possible for the person to shower while sitting down. The help of a qualified professional (e.g., occupational therapist, physical therapist) is important for deciding which of these items would best suit your needs and the needs of the person you are caring for. Nonetheless, every tub should have a nonslip bath mat with suction cups on the back. In addition, towel bars, soap dishes, and toilet paper holders that are not fastened securely into wall studs are dangerous because they are not sturdy enough to support the person's weight and often pull out of the wall, leading to a fall and injury. These items should be replaced with grab bars that are fastened into wall studs.

- Provide eating utensils that have normal or extra weight (as opposed to lightweight or plastic ones) to increase proprioceptive input.

- Encourage the use of rocking chairs, as rocking helps to improve balance.

Bones, Joints, and Skeletal Muscles

Research has shown that changes long thought to be related solely to aging are more related to lifelong patterns of exercise and activity.

Adaptations

Exercise is the single most important adaptation to compensate for losses in the function of the bones, joints, and skeletal muscles. Exercise programs, even with people who are in their nineties and very frail, make major changes in strength and endurance, improve respiratory and circulatory function, and enhance cognitive functioning (Cress et al., 1999; Fiatarone et al., 1990; Taaffe, Duret, Wheeler, & Marcus, 1999). It is truly never too late to make positive changes in health by beginning an exercise program (please seek a doctor's advice before any exercise program is started). See Chapters 3 and 8 for suggestions on movement activities.

Seating and Positioning

The brain damage caused by dementia eventually affects physical abilities, making it increasingly difficult for the person to walk, get in and out of a chair, and engage in other physical abilities. As these changes take place, it is vital to provide every opportunity to help the person continue to be as mobile as possible.

Adaptations

- Help the person to go for walks, even short ones, several times per day.
- Provide chairs that are easy for the person to get in and out of. The best chairs have solid arms that allow the

person to use his or her hands to get up; a firm, level seat that is approximately 16 inches from the floor, and a straight back. Nevertheless, the person may have a favorite chair that does not meet this description. Changing to another chair may cause too many problems, so adapting the favorite chair is a possibility. A chair or sofa can be made higher by adding blocks under the legs or putting it on a stable platform. Inserting dense foam and a piece of plywood under an easy chair or sofa cushion makes it firmer and higher. Easy-lift electric chairs are expensive but may be helpful to some.

Various types of raised toilet seats are available in home health supply centers. These can be a great help in allowing the person to stand up from the toilet independently. Choose a model that fits snugly and securely onto the toilet. A toilet safety frame fastens onto the hinges of the toilet seat. It is easy to install, doesn't require much space, and effectively turns the toilet into an arm chair. These are available at drug store home health centers or from the catalogs listed in Appendix B.

- Help the person to practice the easiest way to get up from a chair. Because of memory problems, it is important to use the same directions every time (you may want to write these down to remind yourself):

  1. Slide forward to the front edge of the chair.
  2. Bend your knees at right angles so your feet are directly underneath and flat on the floor.
  3. Push down with your hands on chair arms.
  4. Lean your body forward so that your nose is over your toes.
  5. Push forward and up with your hands and legs.

If the person uses a walker, ensure that he or she does not use the walker handhold for pulling up, as it can easily tip backward and lead to a fall. Rather, the person should push up with his or her arms (as noted previously), and the walker should be positioned right in front of the person for him or her to take hold of once standing. The caregiver can stabilize the walker.

Please note that for your own safety and the health of your back, you should not twist, turn, or try to pull the person to help him or her stand up. An occupational or physical therapist can suggest the easiest and safest way to help the person move.

- Consult with an occupational or physical therapist for advice on whether and how to use mobility aids such as canes or walkers. One challenge is helping the person learn to use these supports. When the person is no longer able to walk, a qualified occupational or physical therapist must fit him or her with a proper wheelchair. Many of the models now available are comfortable and help the person to take part in daily activities (e.g., meals) or to go on outings. A regular sling-seat wheelchair is suitable only for brief transportation needs and is very uncomfortable for long-term use. Sitting in such chairs for more than a couple of hours can cause skin breakdown.

Sleep

There is evidence that sleep patterns change with age. Most notably, normal aging causes people to sleep for shorter periods at night, but daytime naps may compensate for this. Stage IV sleep, the deepest and most satisfying part of the sleep cycle, is disrupted, particularly in males. These two changes often combine to cause an older person to feel less rested. There is also evidence that sleep disorders, such as sleep apnea, tend to be underdiagnosed among older people.

Adaptations

- Suggest more frequent, shorter periods of sleep. The usual response to feeling less rested is to go to bed earlier to get more sleep, but this further disrupts the sleep cycle.
- Help the person with dementia to practice good sleep practices. See Chapter 7 for more details.

CONCLUSION

This chapter has offered some guidelines and suggestions for developing a supportive and safe environment that can enable persons with dementia to "be the best they can be." Although there are many practical things that can be done, it is also important to keep in mind that changing the environment alone is not enough. The psychosocial environment—that is, the interactions with people within the physical environment—and the availability of meaningful activities are critical components that work together with a supportive environment to enhance quality of life. Chapter 6 shares information about enhancing quality of life through engagement in meaningful activities.

6

Maintaining a Familiar Lifestyle

But we can't help the way we are—we know there is something terribly wrong with us, and we seem to be losing touch with even who we are, all our feelings and our ability to express ourselves. We need all the help we can get. Don't hide us away—involve us, let us experience the joy of living, with the help of your memory, your abilities, and your patience. (Boden, 1998, p. 53)

Life is such for many people that they work to live. A job is simply that—a job. It means a paycheck and food on the table, a way to keep the rest of their life—the part that has real meaning—ticking along. Then there are those folks who live to work. Their job is more important than any other part of their life. Most of us are somewhere in between these two extremes, perhaps struggling to keep a healthy balance.

Although he never really thought about it, John didn't have any such struggle. His work as a carpenter, family life, and daily routines in the small town where he lived

Portions of this chapter previously appeared in Bowlby Sifton, C. (2000f). Well-being and doing: Enabling occupation with persons with dementia. *Alzheimer's Care Quarterly*, *1*(2), 7–28; adapted by permission.

formed a flowing pattern. This is not to say that John's life was perfect or pain free; the rhythm of his daily routines was changed and interrupted by the usual happy (e.g., marriages, births, vacations) and sad (e.g., sickness, loss, money troubles) circumstances that are part of living. However, because John was blessed with work that was a vocation, he could always count on returning to the patterns that he knew: the solid comfort of a hammer handle in his hand, the sweet smell of lumber, the ring of a saw blade. His workshop and tools were so much more than how he earned his living; his work gave him purpose, meaning, and an order to his days.

When John was diagnosed with Alzheimer's disease at age 60, his workshop became even more important. In a world that was becoming less familiar and more difficult to manage, the reassurance of his tools and his shop was a great comfort. He might, for instance, take tremendous pleasure and satisfaction in spending several hours sorting and organizing his drill bits. To the outside observer, however, the drill bits appeared to be in as much of a jumble when he finished as when he started.

As his disease progressed, John had increasing difficulty with the planning and organization needed for skilled carpentry. As word spread, he lost customers. Fortunately, there were some exceptions, people who could recognize that John still held immense skill in his hands, if not in his head. One such wise person understood that John was the only carpenter in the area with the skills to restore the woodwork in his heritage house. He organized the tools and supplies that John needed and then set himself up as John's apprentice. He showed John the awkward movement of a poorly fitted door. Although John could not say how to fix it, when his tools were placed in his hands, he went right to work. In this manner, every door in the house was restored to fit like a glove, just like they had 200 years before. The mind has forgotten what the hands remember. *For John, this was true.*

When there were no customers, thankfully John still had his workshop. Going there and simply puttering about, touching and rearranging his tools, helped to restore the familiar pattern of his life. It brought John tremendous ease and comfort.

Living with Alzheimer's disease had, of course, also disrupted the life rhythm of John's wife, Yvonne. She had a lot to cope with, such as determining how to manage on their now meager funds. When Yvonne saw all of the problems that John had doing simple things around the house, she worried that he would hurt himself while he was puttering about in his workshop. She decided to sell John's workshop and his tools, which would also help with her money worries. This seemed a logical and practical solution to her situation. Little did she know that this decision would lead to many more heartaches.

John simply couldn't believe that his workshop, his lifeline, was gone. Every day he would pedal his bike down to his old shop only to find, all over again, strangers there and none of his beloved tools. John was beside himself with grief and anger. These feelings didn't leave him when he returned home. None of Yvonne's careful explanations made any sense to him. Finally, John's gentle hands, that had never hit anything other than a hammer on a nail, lashed out in anger at the person who had sold his tools, who had robbed his life of the last shreds of meaning.

The life pattern for John and Yvonne was permanently broken at that point. John was placed in a nursing facility. Soon after, he responded to no one or nothing around him.

 Sam, like John, also had a life vocation. He loved to work with engines and machinery. Unlike John, he had never managed to make a living from his interest and skill. His wife Marion dismissed his interest and gave up hope in Sam and his ability to support their family. She got a job to support the family, worked hard on her own accord, and suc-

cessfully launched three children into the world. She also developed her own interests and friends and left Sam to his endless tinkering.

When I met Sam, he was in the later stages of dementia. Marion didn't seem to realize this, but by then she and Sam had a years-long habit of staying out of each other's way. Marion did not pay much attention to Sam's caregiving needs, but she also did not interfere with his tinkering. Engine parts and pieces were scattered around their porch and living room. Sam often needed clean clothes and a bath. His hands were coated with engine oil as he happily worked to reassemble about a dozen old motors.

UNDERSTANDING THE MEANING OF "DOING"

There is no doubt that both Sam and John were distressed by the losses and challenges that Alzheimer's disease had brought to their lives. One the one hand, however, Sam managed to continue with an occupation—an activity that brought meaning to his days—and the signs of his distress were less obvious. Marion did not help or support Sam in continuing this activity, nor did she help with his personal care, but she did not stand in his way. On the other hand, John was robbed of doing the things that brought him meaning and satisfaction, and he was very distressed. Although Yvonne acted with the best of intentions, her practical decisions entirely missed John's need to fill his days with meaningful activity.

Persons with dementia, like all of us, need activity that brings meaning and purpose to their days; they need to be involved in the web of life. **Meaning and satisfaction come from the doing itself, not necessarily from the final product or even from an objective, practical need for the doing.** Meaning lies in a person's satisfaction with the doing, with having his or her hands occupied in familiar ways.

John and Sam both knew what they needed to do and continued with it. The experiences of these two gentlemen dramatically illustrate the powerful positive impact of doing (or the negative impact of not doing) on the well-being of persons with dementia. Unlike John, however, many people have a less obvious and less dramatic response to "not doing." These individuals' *apparent* loss of interest in doing anything can often be a big challenge for caregivers. They need support and encouragement to continue with doing, to be engaged in the web of life. Ways to provide this support are discussed in the "Maintaining a Familiar Lifestyle" section of this chapter and in Chapters 7 and 8.

Doing Is the Core of What it Means to Be Human

Neither Sam's nor John's caregiver really understood the importance of continuing with lifelong interests. The fact that Sam was able to continue to do was more a matter of his wife's disinterest and of happenstance than of understanding his needs. In most cases, happenstance does not work out well. Conversely, John's wife did what *she* thought was best. This also did not work out well. To avoid both of these pitfalls, caregivers must understand the unique needs of the person who they are caring for. Often, the best way to reach an understanding of others—to stand in their shoes—is to start with the person one knows best: oneself. So, I am going to ask you a personal question: "Why do you do things?"

As a busy caregiver of someone with dementia, you may answer, "Because I have to." This is absolutely true—I know because I was a caregiver, too. Your day is so filled with things you have to do—making meals, cleaning the house, helping the person dress or bathe, answering the telephone, doing laundry, and so forth. It probably makes you tired just thinking about all of the things you *have* to do. I would bet that the idea of doing absolutely nothing for awhile sounds too good to be true.

But stop a minute and imagine. What if you had absolutely nothing to do 24 hours per day, 7 days per week, 52 weeks of the year? Does this also sound too good to be true? Probably not! In fact, it sounds boring to most people because we all need something to do. Doing is the core of what it means to be human. For example, we tell others who we are by describing the kinds of things we do—I'm a mother, a gardener, a sports fan, a teacher, a cook, a knitter, and so forth. Have you ever thought about how typical greetings center around doing? For example, "How are you DOing?" or "How DO you DO?"

Think about the things that you like to do for fun or to relax, even if you don't have much time to do them now. What might you do? Listen to music? Watch television? Go for a walk? Go to church? Numerous activities are important to each person for different reasons.

There are also the basic things that we have to do for ourselves on a daily basis, such as combing our hair, getting dressed, and bathing. We tend to take these commonplace activities for granted. But have you ever been sick and had to depend on other people to do these things for you? How did that feel? Maybe for a while you enjoyed the "room service." Yet, there comes a time (usually sooner rather than later) when you really want to do these things, in your way, for yourself. Is anybody else really able to comb your hair or brush your teeth when and how you would like? Can you imagine being forever deprived of the privilege of getting a cup of tea or taking a shower when you want one?

Returning to the question "Why do you do things?" I suggest that we do things for a host of reasons. We do things for fun, for pleasure, because we have to, because it is part of who we are, and because taking care of ourselves is part of what it means to be an adult.

Doing Is Life Itself

Whatever the particular reason for doing, humans are by nature doing creatures; doing is life itself. When we are doing, we are involved in the web of life; doing confirms our worth as persons. Doing—or activity or occupation—includes everything we do during the course of a day. Major activities—such as buying a car, going to work, and shopping for groceries—and the thousand daily rituals—brushing our teeth, looking out the window, saying hello—are all part of the rhythm of our days, all part of the web of life. When we are well and active, attending to these daily personal rituals, such as doing laundry, may be taken for granted and may even be a nuisance, interfering with what are often viewed as really important occupations, such as going to work. However, when an illness or a disability interferes, these personal, routine occupations tend to take on great significance.

Aging Persons Who Continue to Do Are Healthier

The more scientists study aging, the more they learn about how important it is for older people to keep doing things that they have done all of their lives. Older people who maintain a familiar lifestyle—doing things for fun and taking care of themselves—are healthier, happier, and cognitively sharper. Conversely, having nothing meaningful to do leads to illness. For more information, see Bowlby Sifton (2000f).

The really good news is that it is never too late to make gains in health from exercise and activity. For example, research studies have found that even very frail people in their nineties experienced tremendous improvements in strength, stamina, breathing, and other functions after they took part in a simple light exercise program (Cress et al., 1999; Fiatarone et al., 1990; Taaffe et al., 1999).

David Snowdon's (2001) study of the aging process in a community of almost 700 teaching nuns is another fascinating example of the role of activity in successful aging. These women agreed to participate in testing and study during their life and to brain autopsy at death. They were all in their eighties and beyond, but for the most part also led very active lives. They continued to be involved with their families and community and to maintain physical and mental activities. Sister Mary, who lived to be 101, is an excellent example of successful aging. She retired from active teaching at age 84; afterward, she continued to teach family members and other sisters, maintained a keen interest in world events, and remained physically active. She also continued to have normal scores on cognitive tests. When she died, however, the autopsy results were surprising. Her brain was riddled with plaques and tangles, the key markers of Alzheimer's disease. This study and others suggest that those who are involved in activities build a rich network of pathways in the brain that serves as an insulating effect against the damage caused by Alzheimer's disease.

We All Need Something Meaningful to Do; We All Can Do Something

I just take one day at a time, I try to enjoy life as it is. I go with the flow and try to do the things that I still can do. If I wasn't busy, I just couldn't get along, they might as well put me out to pasture. I just take my time, and plan everything out, it may take me a lot longer, but so what? (Bowlby Sifton, 2000a, p. 1)

Verbally or through their actions, persons with dementia are always telling us that they need meaningful things to do. Being able to continue to do, to maintain a familiar lifestyle is critical. As damage to the brain gradually robs them of the ability to do more complicated activities (e.g., paying the bills, driving a car), continuing to participate in simpler daily routines becomes especially important. It is essential to their sense of themselves, to being involved in life. Try putting yourself in their shoes, and imagine what it might feel like to have nothing to do, hour after hour, day after day, week after week.

Left to their own devices, persons with dementia are often astonishingly creative at finding things to do. Examples include shopping, rearranging, organizing, walking, greeting others, folding, smoothing, sorting, and exploring textures in clothes and surfaces. Persons who fold and refold the same worn tissue; pat and rub a table, a tray, or clothing; repetitively clap; or pace the same worn path are expressing the need to do, the need to be occupied, in the only way they know how. Sometimes these attempts may not be viewed positively by others. Quality of life for all can be improved and challenges can be reduced when caregivers support and direct the need to do, finding meaningful replacements for created activities that caregivers don't find positive. One such example follows.

Rosie's husband Al had been a letter carrier. She was frustrated by the fact that Al constantly moved and reorganized the papers in her desk—important personal documents and any other bits of paper that he could find. Rosie kept reminding him to leave these things alone, but Al continued with this behavior and became agitated and distressed. At the suggestion of day program staff, Rosie set up a mail-sorting station and a simple delivery route for Al. Every morning, Al would go to his work station and spend many happy hours sorting and organizing a collection of junk mail and flyers, which he would then distribute around the house and to some understanding neighbors. When Al moved to a long-term care facility, Rosie told his new caregivers about his delivery route, and they were able to set up a similar job for him.

The Person with Dementia Lives Most Fully in the Present Moment

I want to carry on drinking in the beauty of this world and feel the love of my family and friends. Even if I might not remember these experiences very long, I still want to have them. Surely remembering an experience doesn't constitute the sole enjoyment of that moment. (Boden, 1998, p. 145)

The preceding quote from a person with dementia reminds us of the heightened value of the moment. This topic was detailed in Chapter 2 but is mentioned here because it is central to understanding doing as it is experienced by persons with dementia. The meaning lies in the moment, which may be quite different from how those without dementia experience activity. Living with memory loss means that the person lives most fully in the present moment; the present moment becomes the most important moment. The future cannot be imagined, and the past is dimly recalled or forgotten; right now is the time that matters most. The person with dementia has a remarkable ability to savor now, to celebrate the present moment. It is perhaps an ability that caregivers can learn from to enrich our own lives.

It is certainly something we need to bear in mind when we try to support continued involvement in doing. Living in the moment means that it is not so much the outcome or end product of doing but the process of doing that matters most.

Time and efficiency notions need to be put aside to capture the simple pleasure of the doing itself. It may, for instance, take the person much longer to peel the vegetables for supper than it would to do it ourselves. However, the key consideration is whether this activity brings the person pleasure and satisfaction. The same can be said about the person who derives great pleasure from redoing the same task (e.g., sorting a drawer, folding laundry). Caregivers should allow for this extra time in planning the day's activities.

Elizabeth found that her sister, Amanda, brought her own meaning to the task of folding and sorting the towels and washcloths. Because Amanda had always worked in an office, she developed a "filing system." She sorted the items into various categories: those with tags and those without, colored items and white items, large items and small items. Constantly reorganizing her filing system happily occupied Amanda for many hours. The next day, Elizabeth would present Amanda with the same collection of disordered towels and washcloths, and Amanda happily went to work again. It took Elizabeth some time to relinquish her meaning for this activity (i.e., to get the laundry sorted) and to appreciate that Amanda's own meaning kept her happily engaged in the moment.

The Person with Dementia Needs Caregiver Support to Continue with Doing

Unfortunately, it becomes increasingly difficult for persons with dementia to do things conventionally or independently. Damage to the brain leads to problems with planning and carrying out activities. Fortunately, there are practical ways to get around these problems.

This may sound like one more task for you—the already-too-busy caregiver—to do, but this isn't the case. It's not so much about things to do *for* the person with dementia but about how you can do things *with* the person with dementia. By supporting the ability to do, caregivers support the person's self-esteem and offer a present moment that is as rich and as meaningful as possible. In this way, caregivers can reach out and touch the whole person and help him or her to stay connected with life.

Doing Provides a Treatment for Some of the Symptoms of Dementia

Nona had worked in an office all of her life and was very skilled at organizing and tidying. She was particularly concerned that things always look neat. When she moved to a long-term care facility, she continued this work. She found the many notices taped on the facility's wall to be untidy, so she conscientiously removed the tape and stacked all of the papers neatly. Staff members, of course, found this frustrating. They tried to explain this to Nona, but she kept on with her work. As a result, the maintenance department was asked to construct a glassed-in notice board. Nona was very distressed and agitated when she found that she was unable to do her work. Her distress entirely disappeared when a creative staff member posted old notices for Nona to remove and organize.

Experience with persons such as Nona, John, and Sam—combined with mounting research—shows that persons with dementia who have something meaningful to do are much happier and display fewer challenging behaviors. **In other words, doing helps reduce or even treat some dementia symptoms.** For more details, see Bowlby Sifton (2000f).

Because most dementia symptoms are changes in behavior, care can become overly focused on how to cope with challenging or negative behaviors. By turning this concern around and asking instead how caregivers can support doing (i.e., positive behavior), we take a positive, proactive approach to dementia care. For instance, Nona's work project reduced her agitation far more effectively than other attempts based on reasoning, scolding, or distracting.

In addition to providing an essential treatment for the person with dementia, this change in perspective can lighten caregiving burdens. This certainly was the case in a story shared by Dr. Carolyn Baum of the Washington University Medical School (Bowlby Sifton, 2000f). One very wise and patient caregiver encouraged her husband, a retired plumber, to continue with his lifelong practice of bringing his plumbing work belt with him to the breakfast table. After breakfast, he would strap on his belt and go to work "fixing" the plumbing around the house. He spent many happy hours taking apart and putting together the taps and drains. Everything went well until he attempted to fix the "plumbing" on the gas stove. Fortunately his wife intervened before anyone was hurt, but she decided that it was no longer safe to continue with this practice. After she put away his plumbing belt, it didn't take very long for her gentle husband to become uncharacteristically aggressive, both verbally and physically. Life became so difficult that she thought that she would have to place her husband in a nursing facility. However, with the support and encouragement of a memory disorders clinic care team, she decided she would make one more effort to restore her husband's familiar life pattern. One Saturday, a group of friends came in and created a safe plumbing workshop in the garage. Her husband went back to work and was able to remain happily at home for some time.

Care that Supports a Familiar Lifestyle Is the Best Possible Care

As more is learned about caring for persons with dementia, it is becoming very clear that care that supports a familiar lifestyle—that is, focuses on the person and encourages continuing with meaningful activity—is the best possible care. You, as a caregiver, have the best opportunity to provide this "treatment" for the person you are caring for. In fact, you are the best treatment now available for dementia and Alzheimer's disease. At the same time, you just might have more time to do some of the things that you would like to do.

Doing Brings Meaning to the Moment

Although doing is essential to the well-being of the person with dementia, the activity needs to be meaningful. Busy work (activity that has no personal meaning) is insulting and frustrating. The goal is to find activities that fill the moment with meaning, not just to pass the time. The nature of these activities is uniquely personal and is tied closely to a familiar lifestyle. These ideas are explored further in the following sections.

PERSON-CENTERED CARE

Change and doing new things can be especially frightening for persons with dementia. Refusal to participate in something signifies fear of failure and the unknown more often than disinterest. For example, although participating in a day program may help both the person and the caregiver, it initially can be difficult to get the person to go to the program center. Once he or she becomes familiar with the place, the people, and the expectations, going to the day program becomes an accepted and anticipated part of the routine. The following examples present two solutions to this challenge that reflect the different life experiences of the persons involved.

Joanna has always held her doctor in high regard and follows his every word. When she becomes anxious and confused about doing something, such as starting a day program, her daughter doesn't argue. She simply says, "That's fine, Mom. You call Dr. Miller and tell him that you aren't going today." With this cue, Joanna recalls that this is what her doctor wants her to do and goes along happily.

In addition to dementia, Audrey has a chronic illness. As a result, she has had a lifetime of experiences with doctors, some of which were negative. She continues to resent these unhappy experiences and usually refuses to see the doctor, let alone follow his advice. She does, however, put great stock in the care and advice of her oldest daughter, Sara. So, when Audrey becomes anxious and confused about going to the day program, her husband reminds her that Sara will be disappointed if Audrey doesn't go.

Both Joanna and Audrey are now happy and enthusiastic day-program participants. To reach this stage, however, their caregivers used two different approaches. This makes sense because Joanna and Audrey are two different people, with different experiences and different life stories.

It always amazes me to realize that we humans are more alike at birth than we ever will be again. What an astonishing and wonderful variety of experiences fills the following years and shapes each one of us. The wide variety of experiences that we each have between childhood and old age means that we are even more unique in our old age than we were as children. When you add to this the changes and differences associated with dementia, the mix becomes still more complicated. As noted in Chapter 3, we can make more general statements about a small child and the ways to care for that child than we can about an older person and the ways to care for that person when he or she is ill.

To paraphrase the words of the physician and healer Sir William Osler, the most important question is not what disease the person has, but what person the disease has. Dorothy Seman—wise caregiver, friend, and colleague—told me of this invaluable reminder. I try to make it the center point of caregiving.

Understanding as much as possible about the person's life story is the most important guide to compassionate and creative care. Despite general guidelines for care, each person with dementia is unique, and each care situation is unique and may call for unique approaches. Although it may be possible to devise a particular diet and dosages of insulin for a person with diabetes, there are unfortunately no recipes or standard care plans for persons with dementia.

This is old news to caregivers. For example, going for a drive after supper helps your friend's mother to sleep better, but it causes your husband to become agitated and upset because he can't drive anymore. Or last week, laying clothes out in the order in which they are put on worked very well, but this week your mother keeps putting her underwear on top of her slacks.

At the same time, when you are in the midst of providing day-to-day care and are so anxious for solutions to the challenges that you face, it is easy to become overwhelmed. It can seem impossible to come up with creative, person-centered solutions. This is the tremendous challenge of dementia care and requires caregivers to muster all of the skills and tools they can. But don't lose heart, because you already possess the single most important tool in meeting this challenge: You know the person—his or her likes and dislikes, habits, values, and life story—better than anyone else. This information is at the center of meeting care challenges. You can record and share this information with other caregivers by using the All About Me form in Appendix A.

Furthermore, although there are no "recipes," there are guidelines such as the ones in this book that can be individualized. Later in this chapter, the section titled "Hands to Health: How to Support Doing" offers suggestions for using such guidelines to maintain a familiar lifestyle and meet some of the challenges of caregiving. In addition, the section titled "Capturing the Simple Pleasures" offers suggestions for concentrating on the person, not on the task or the challenge.

Focus on the Person Doing the Activity, Not the Activity Itself

Although this chapter is about the essential role of activity for the person with dementia, the person doing the activity, not the activity itself, is the most important thing. It is not the outcome of the activity—for example, getting the cookies made or lunch finished—but the person's involvement that matters most. As caregivers, we are taking care of people, not getting tasks or jobs done. The many activities of day-to-day care make it easy to lose sight of this difference. We need to frequently ask ourselves whether we are acting as a caregiver or as a caretaker. *Caregivers* provide opportunities for the person to continue to be involved in daily living activities; *caretakers* see that these daily living tasks are done in the most efficient way. In so doing, caretakers may do the task for the person and, thus, deprive him or her of the pleasure of doing for him- or herself.

CAPTURING THE SIMPLE PLEASURES

Environmental psychologist M. Csikszentmihalyi (1988) has studied and researched what makes experiences or activities pleasurable. He talked to hundreds of people with widely different backgrounds and uncovered eight universal elements of enjoyable or optimal experiences, or *flow experiences:*

1. The person has the skills to succeed at the task.
2. The person has the ability to concentrate on the task.
3. The task has clear goals.
4. The task provides immediate feedback.
5. Engagement in the task is so effortless yet focused that everyday worries are forgotten.
6. The person feels in control of his or her actions.
7. Sense of self fades during the task but flourishes after completion.
8. Time perspective shifts; hours may seem like minutes.

These eight elements have been reframed as seven questions (the seventh and eighth elements have been combined into one question) in the following sections to guide caregivers in helping the person with dementia to have enjoyable experiences, to capture the simple pleasures of daily living.

Can the Person Succeed?

When Erma couldn't use her oil paints anymore, her caregiver tried to get her to color in a children's coloring book. Erma became very angry and threw the crayons across the room. This caregiver, like many of us at times, was unable to find a task that was just the right challenge—an activity that avoids being so simple that the person is insulted or so difficult that the person fails. The just-right challenge is an activity that guarantees success. Think about an activity that you find difficult. For me, an example is anything to do with making a hammer and nails connect. I would become pretty angry and discouraged if I had to repeatedly struggle to pound a nail, especially if other adults were watching. Unfortunately, decreasing abilities due to brain damage means that persons with dementia have many experiences with failure. Caregivers who try to discover activities at which the person can succeed support pleasure by avoiding still more experiences with failure.

Discovering the just-right challenge usually takes some trial and error. Most of all, we need to understand the person—his or her likes and dislikes, as well as his or her strengths and weaknesses. In Erma's case, adult posters that can be colored with markers *may* work. Or Erma may enjoy looking at art books or some of the paintings that she created in the past, sharing comments and memories with her caregiver. Or it may be necessary to avoid reminding Erma of her loss and to devise a whole new activity.

Reviewing the continuing strengths of persons with dementia (described in Chapter 3) may help in finding activities that are the just-right challenge. The section in this chapter called "Adapt the Task and/or the Environment" provides guidelines for adapting favorite activities for success. A professional assessment by an occupational therapist may also help.

Family caregivers should be sure to note information about successful activites on the All About Me form (Appendix A) so that it can be shared with all caregivers.

Is the Person Able to Concentrate on the Activity?

Due to brain damage, persons with dementia will have increasing difficulty concentrating and paying attention. To compensate, it is important to have an environment that is as free of distraction as possible. For example, although sharing in family mealtime has important benefits, the person with dementia may find it difficult to concentrate on eating in this setting. Families may need to make an effort to have calmer mealtimes. This is detailed in Chapters 5 and 7. Later in this chapter, the section titled "Hands to Health: How to Support Doing" provides suggestions as well.

Physical discomfort also interferes with the ability to pay attention. Because persons with dementia have difficulty verbally communicating what they are feeling and thinking, it is important for caregivers be mindful of other signs of physical and emotional discomfort. If the person seems unwilling to participate, restless, or anxious, he or she may be saying that creature comforts have not been met.

Using the communication guidelines in Chapter 4, work with the person to determine the following:

- Is the person hungry, thirsty, too hot, too cold, or tired?
- Does the person need to go to the bathroom?
- Are the person's shoes or clothes too tight?
- Is the person seated uncomfortably?

As the person faces increasing frailty and physical disability, proper seating becomes especially important. Often, difficulty with eating or restlessness can be overcome by having a comfortable chair or a proper wheelchair. An occupational therapist should be consulted to determine which chair or wheelchair is best. Also, please note that among hundreds of assessments to date, geri-chairs have never been found to be the best seats! I am not sure who these chairs were designed to fit; they do not fit any older person I know. Try one out yourself sometime—you'll likely start feeling restless and move around a lot while trying to get comfortable.

Pain is a particular comfort concern. Because of communication problems, persons with dementia may not be able to indicate when they are in pain. In addition, the effects of aging often mean reduced sensations of pain. This is a concern because pain is a warning sign that something is wrong. Caregivers need to watch for other warning signs such as increased activity (e.g., agitation) or decreased activity (e.g., sleepiness, listlessness, refusal to get out of bed) or a relatively sudden increase in confusion or disorientation.

Because most persons with dementia are also older adults, they may be experiencing pain from osteoarthritis. As they become frail and spend more time sitting, moving can become even more painful. One study researched occasions when caregivers had been hit by persons with dementia (Talerico & Evans, 2000). The study found that approximately 95% of the times that these residents hit came after the persons had been moved. When these individuals were given a mild pain reliever such as aspirin a half hour before they were moved, hitting was reduced by 75%.

Verbally expressing emotional discomfort can be even more difficult for persons with dementia. Fortunately, their ability to use nonverbal expression is excellent. Caregivers can become skilled at seeing signals of fear, anger, anxiety, displeasure, or a sense of being ill at ease by watching the person's face and body language. These nonverbal expressions often mirror what the person is feeling but is unable to express in words. Please see Chapter 4 for more information on nonverbal communication.

Does the Activity Have Clear Goals?

With regard to persons with dementia, consideration of activity goals should be further broken into two questions: 1) Do the goals of the activity have meaning for the person? and 2) Does the person understand the goals of the activity and the activity itself?

Do the Goals of the Activity
Have Meaning for the Person?

Because a person with dementia needs the help of caregivers to plan and organize activities, it can be easy for caregivers to impose their goals on the person. It's not surprising, then, that the person may resist or fail to find the activity pleasurable. For example, caregiver goals about the method for and importance of bathing may not be shared by the person. In turn, he or she may balk at bathing. To avoid this pitfall, it's necessary to consider the person's previous interests and daily routines. For instance, offering a reason for bathing that is important to the person (e.g., getting ready to go to church) can help the person to become involved. Family caregivers are in the best position to know these previous interests and routines and can guide other caregivers by keeping the All About Me form (Appendix A) updated.

Does the Person Understand
the Goals of the Activity and the Activity Itself?

Continuing social skills are an important strength of persons with dementia and help to protect dignity. However, the presence of these skills can also lead the person to act as if he or she understands something when he or she has no idea what has been asked or what is expected. Due to memory loss, the person usually does not remember what was said earlier, either. Even leaving the room to get an item of clothing can be enough time for the person to forget that you are helping him or her to get dressed. Every time you engage the person in an activity, **it is important to explain everything as if it was the first time.**

Providing constant reassurance and abundant repeated information throughout all steps of an activity helps with understanding. The person may need frequent reminding about the goal of the activity (e.g., "We are going to have the potatoes that you are peeling for supper"). This is especially true when the activity has several steps (e.g., getting dressed) or is for some event or person that is not present. For example, if the person is sanding blocks for a grandchild, it would be helpful to have a picture of the grandchild, and some finished blocks nearby. Frequent explanations avoid assumptions about what seems obvious (e.g., that the meal on the table is for the person to eat). In one situation reported by Mary Lucero, caregivers put bubble bath in the bathtub, and when the person saw this "foaming cauldron," she said, "My dear, I cannot possibly chop enough vegetables to make that much soup."

It is especially important for paid caregivers to introduce themselves every time they interact with a person who has dementia. Even if paid caregivers see the person often, difficulty with memory and recognition may lead the person to think, for example, that a total stranger is trying to take his or her clothes off (when the reality is that a paid caregiver is trying to help the person bathe).

Does the Activity Provide Immediate Feedback?

We all need positive feedback. Sometimes, this comes from the satisfaction of the activity itself, such as reading. Other times, we may anticipate future outcomes, such as graduation and getting a job. Persons with memory loss are challenged by such long-off rewards and may have difficulty judging how well they are doing with a particular activity.

Some activities, such as listening to music or cooking, have immediate rewards built in, making them excellent activity choices. For other activities, such as craft or woodworking projects, frequent positive feedback from caregivers is vital for enjoyment and encouragement to continue with the activity.

We all have the need and the right to experience pleasure during the course of our day. As a person with dementia faces increased disability, he or she is less able to find pleasurable things to do independently. It is up to the caregiver to find ways to bring pleasure to the person—ways that enrich the present moment. What brings the person you are caring for pleasure? A song, a hug, a favorite snack, a short conversation, a cup of tea or coffee? Retelling a favorite experience, sitting beside him or her and holding hands, looking at favorite pictures? There are dozens of simple activities that don't take very long and can bring the person so much pleasure. By preceding a challenging activity (e.g., bathing) with short, pleasurable activities (e.g., a conversation), you can provide pleasure and encourage the person to participate.

Is the Person Fully Engaged in the Activity?

Descriptions of flow experiences usually suggest involvement with the activity to the point that everyday worries vanish; it is as if nothing else exists but this particular experience. For most of us, everyday activities do not require this level of focus and involvement. However, when dementia enters the picture, what may have been a simple activity (e.g., brushing one's teeth, folding laundry) may require enormous focus. Intense focus is often seen when a person with dementia creates an activity, such as sorting items in a drawer or trying to figure out the combination on a door lock. If caregivers offer activities that are structured for success, they can tap into this potential to help the person become completely engaged in an activity and set aside everyday worries.

Does the Person Feel in Control?

Mrs. MacDonald had a midmorning appointment with a medical specialist who she had seen many times.[5] She was so concerned about keeping this appointment that she repeatedly asked her caregivers how she was going to get there and who was going to take her. Because this appointment was so important to Mrs. MacDonald, caregivers were sure that it would be no problem to have her ready on time. However, they were surprised to find that despite frequent reminders to hurry along, Mrs. MacDonald was still working on her hair and makeup minutes before she was supposed to leave. Exasperated care staff suggested that it might be necessary for one of them to accompany Mrs. MacDonald to the appointment because she was being "difficult."

Mrs. MacDonald was not fully dressed and was still busy fluffing her hair when Veronica, the van driver, came to the door of her room. Instead of joining the "hurry up" chorus, Veronica wisely stepped into Mrs. MacDonald's shoes for a minute. She said, "I understand what you are doing. I do it myself every morning. You need to be sure that everything is just right, don't you?" When Mrs. MacDonald agreed, Veronica said, "Can you do what you need to do in 6 minutes? We really do have to leave then, because you know we can't keep this doctor waiting."

Given this opportunity to do things her way, Mrs. MacDonald was ready to leave in less than 6 minutes. The "difficult behavior" that challenged her caregivers disappeared, and she and Veronica had a pleasant outing.

---

[5]A previous version of this story appeared in Bowlby Sifton, C. (2000e). Meeting needs. *Alzheimer's Care Quarterly*, *1*(4), v; adapted by permission.

Adults are used to feeling in control of what we do during a day. We make hundreds of decisions every day—from small ones, such as which television program to watch, to big ones, such as whether to sell the house. Making these decisions strengthens our sense of being independent, capable adults. It supports our dignity and worth. Caregivers are well aware, however, that even in the early stages of dementia, the person begins to have difficulty making decisions and organizing the activities of his or her day. Difficulty with complicated decisions, such as planning finances or making judgments while driving, appears first. Eventually, even seemingly minor decisions, such as what to wear or what to order in a restaurant, become too challenging. This is a result of damage to the brain.

To protect their dignity, persons with dementia may cover their decision-making difficulties in several ways. They may use social skills by saying things such as, "Whatever you like is fine." Or they may withdraw from activities altogether. As noted previously, this seeming lack of interest is often due in part to fear of failure. Most caregivers have probably had the experience of asking the person something such as, "Would you like to go for a walk?" and getting an emphatic "No" in response. Overwhelmed by anxiety over what is expected and fear of failure, it probably seems much safer to say no. See the section titled "Barriers to Participation" for more details.

Persons with dementia may also become defiant and angry and insist on doing things that they are not really able to do (e.g., use the stove). Angry and resistant behavior may be the person's desperate attempt to hang on to some control in any way that he or she can. This, of course, is the most dangerous response and the one to avoid for everyone's safety. Caregivers can go a long way in preventing these challenges by giving the person as much opportunity as possible for choice and control.

 Before he developed dementia, Raymond always did the laundry. As the dementia progressed, he had increasing trouble sorting the clothes and remembering the steps involved in doing the laundry. He became so frustrated with his failures that his wife Gloria decided to save him the frustration and took over his job. Instead of being relieved, Raymond actually became very angry and often shouted at Gloria, which he had never done in all their years of marriage. One day, after hanging some items on the clothesline, Gloria made a quick trip to the store. While she was out, it started to rain and Raymond wisely brought in the clothes. Raymond was trying to be helpful, but his next decision was a very dangerous one. He turned on all of the stove burners and had just started hanging the clothes nearby when Gloria returned.

How might this story have been played differently? If Gloria had helped Raymond sort clothes, giving him cues for the next steps, he could have still participated in his job. He probably would have felt more in control, less robbed of his self-esteem, and less angry at her. This situation is not analyzed to lay blame on Gloria or others in similar situations, however. Taking over when the person starts having difficulty doing something independently is a natural response and is usually done with the best intentions. We are used to thinking that either a person can do something or they can't.

Coaching adults to do something that they used to do independently is a new skill for most of us. It is crucial to search every activity for opportunities to give the person a sense of control. Having control is not the same thing as being independent. The person who can no longer take a bath can still wash his or her face or at least hold the washcloth. Even simple activities contain opportunities for the person to participate and to feel more in control. For instance, choosing a cookie from a plate feels quite different from being given a cookie; passing an empty dish when a meal is done offers more control than having it taken away. Asking the person if he or she would like the caregiver to come back later to help with a required activity (e.g., a bath) gives the person a sense of control. Note that the choice offered does not include whether or not to participate in the activity.

Can the Person Lose Him- or Herself in the Activity?

In a long-term care facility, one staff member and the recreational therapist decided to plan a summer outing for residents with advanced dementia. All of the residents required total care, and many were unable to walk. The two organizers persisted in planning a trip to the local ice cream shop, despite the doubts of most direct care staff. For instance, one concerned staff member wondered how staff would manage to give everyone ice cream, as most of the individuals with dementia needed to be fed.

Once at the ice cream shop, trays of cones were ordered and passed to each person. What a transformation took place: hands that couldn't lift a spoon managed to reach for one of those cones; drooped heads lifted to attention; closed eyes opened and sparkled with merriment; speechless lips chorused "Thank you," "Mmm," and "Wow, that's good." All of these persons became fully immersed in the joys of eating an ice cream cone and, in the process, skills thought to be long forgotten were awakened. This joy and interest continued during the bus ride back to the facility. While driving through the countryside, many individuals nodded in recognition at the sights and voiced appreciation for the chance to see favorite local places again.

Persons with dementia have a remarkable ability to live in the moment, to lose themselves in whatever is happening at that particular time. In fact, they have already achieved one of the key features of an enjoyable experience. By supporting this ability, you can increase enjoyment for the person and yourself. Conversely, feeling threatened or insecure can undermine this ability. Whenever possible, the goal of care should be to eliminate situations where the person feels threatened and to maximize opportunities for the person to lose him- or herself in the pleasure of an activity. This can give persons with dementia the chance to be part of something larger than themselves, which does wonders for self-esteem.

Another feature of flow experience is a shift in the sense of time. When a person is fully involved in a desirable activity, time seems to have no meaning and worries are suspended. For me, this is working in the garden. For others, it may be listening to music, reading, or engaging in a sports activity.

The brain damage caused by dementia eventually leads to an impaired sense of time, which may explain, in part, the ability of persons with dementia to lose themselves in the moment. Whatever the reason, persons with dementia have a natural capacity to experience a state of enjoyment and involvement that most people must work hard to achieve. Caregivers who take advantage of this capacity by providing opportunities for meaningful activity help persons with dementia to capture the simple pleasures, to celebrate the precious present.

INVOLVEMENT IN FAMILIAR LIFESTYLE ACTIVITIES

 Elsie was a loving, gentle person who never had a harsh word for anyone. She was cherished by all who knew her. She was also known to her friends and family for her lifelong positive outlook, for making the best of the

hand that life had dealt her. To top things off, she was a fabulous cook. Her molasses cookies were legendary!

When she was widowed at a relatively young age, Elsie moved from her home in a rural area to an apartment in a large city. Although she missed her husband tremendously, she astonished everyone by flourishing in this very different life. She made new friends; loved her new home; and made bushels more of those cookies for church bake sales, grandchildren, and neighbors. Because Elsie was so social and enthusiastic, it was some time before her family realized that she was not doing as well as she let on. The tip-off was the terrible disarray of her bank account and bill payments. After numerous appointments with specialists, Elsie was diagnosed with Alzheimer's disease. Elsie's daughter took over regarding financial matters, and Elsie got someone to help with housework and meals, so she carried on with her life in the city for a couple more years.

Eventually, however, Elsie's family became concerned about her safety and health. Family members decided that it would be best if Elsie moved to a boarding house near her son, who lived in a faraway rural community.

Elsie missed her apartment and friends in the city, but with characteristic cheer, she settled in to still another different life. She maintained that a few months later, she would move to a "senior's apartment" to be near her daughter, who lived in an island community.

The boarding house was very nice, but Elsie's son was concerned that his previously active mother spent most of her day sitting. She didn't seem to keep up with any of her hobbies, such as doing crossword puzzles and reading. He encouraged her to attend a day program where I worked, and Elsie's sweet charm was a delight to staff and fellow participants. When asked, she helped program staff make a community lunch and was a happy participant in all of the planned activities. When not involved in these activities, however, Elsie just sat and watched.

Everybody at the day program was eager to sample Elsie's famous molasses cookies; we were waiting until she got her new glasses so she could read the recipe. After her glasses arrived, the days went by and Elsie always had something else to do that interfered with the time needed to make those cookies. I began to suspect that Elsie could no longer manage this complicated activity without some help.

One day after coffee time, I put my arm around Elsie. I said that I had the recipe and ingredients for her molasses cookies and would really like her help to make a batch. She looked a little reluctant, but she was pleased by compliments about her cookie-making skills and agreed to help. I bowed to Elsie's expertise, saying that I would be her "gofer." She glanced at the recipe and, looking perplexed, she sweetly asked what I thought we should do first. I suggested that we measure out the ingredients one by one. Elsie was hesitant and consulted me about each cupful. This was a long process, but when the measuring was finally accomplished, Elsie took on a more confident air. She made quick work of mixing the batter and dropping it by spoonfuls onto the cookie sheets. She nervously watched each batch and sought advice about whether they were done.

Everyone gathered around while the delicious smell of molasses and ginger filled the air. Elsie smiled rather nervously as we bit into the warm cookies. Her hesitant smile gave way to beaming as we heaped her with praise and asked for seconds. She was smiling even more broadly a few hours later when she handed her son a package of her homemade cookies—the first batch she'd given him in many months.

Elsie had always been very active. Unfortunately, the effects of Alzheimer's disease had made it increasingly difficult for her to do her usual activities, from managing her finances and her meals to continuing with hobbies such as baking and knitting. Although her son was concerned, Elsie's inactivity at the boarding house wasn't a pressing problem because Elsie used her lifelong social skills to adapt and didn't seem too distressed. However, when she was encouraged and supported in a favorite activity (cookie baking), she absolutely flourished. Elsie could no longer manage all of the complicated steps involved in making cookies. However, with help measuring ingredients and reading the recipe, she was still able to make cookies. She got tremendous satisfaction from doing this familiar and meaningful activity and from having something to offer her friends and family. She felt valued and needed; her well-being was enriched.

Elsie also got a great deal of satisfaction out of helping to prepare the community meal at the day program, and she could have done the same at the boarding house. Unfortunately, although the person who ran the boarding house was kind and caring, she didn't understand the importance of finding a way to get Elsie involved in preparing meals. She said that she would sometimes ask Elsie if she would like to participate and Elsie would say, "Oh I'm just fine, dear. I don't want to get in your way."

Elsie's story illustrates the positive effects of being involved in familiar life activities and the challenges that caregivers face in thinking of ways to keep the person involved and to maintain a familiar lifestyle. The remainder of this chapter and the following three chapters offer many hints and suggestions to help meet these challenges.

BARRIERS TO PARTICIPATION

To begin to answer the question "What do you want to do today?" I would like to return to Elsie's story. Understanding how to invite persons with dementia to do something is key in getting them involved, in maintaining a familiar lifestyle.

When the boarding house manager asked questions such

as, "Would you like to help me prepare supper?" Elsie replied "Oh, I'm just fine, dear. I don't want to get in your way." In similar situations, the following questions and answers are common.

Caregiver:	"What would you like to do today?"
Person with dementia	"Nothing" or "Whatever you would like to do."
Caregiver:	"Would you like to go for a walk?"
Person with dementia:	"No."

Do these responses sound familiar? Do you, like most caregivers, find it both sad and frustrating that the person in your care, who was once busy and active, no longer *seems* interested in doing anything? The person who used to be a proud homemaker no longer bothers to wash her own clothes. The dedicated gardener lets weeds overrun the yard and stares out the window all day long. Even when suggestions are made, the person *seems* to prefer to do nothing. He or she *seems* to have no interest in daily activities that used to mean so much. This is puzzling, especially given the overwhelming human need to do, as previously discussed. The following subsections explore why a person with dementia might decline to participate in activities.

Comfort with the Present Moment, Discomfort with Anticipating Future Moments

Understanding comes more easily if we are able to stand in the shoes of the person with dementia; those shoes are firmly planted in the now, so the person lives most fully in the present moment. If this particular moment is rich and satisfying for the person, we need to ask ourselves if the pattern really needs to be changed. We need to try very hard not to put our own values on what it is that the person should or could be doing. Persons with dementia have a remarkable capacity to just be—to feel well, whole, complete, and content in their own inner emotional world. For example, the previously active gardener may be totally lost in the beauty of the rose beside her. Caregivers may have difficulty understanding that in some cases "being is doing." As a result, we may unwittingly disturb the person's pleasant contentment by imposing our own agenda for more active involvement.

Determining the difference between such contentment and genuine boredom brought on by inactivity calls for an intimate understanding of the person's world, past and present. By using an understanding of past interests and responses and by paying close attention to facial expression, body posture, and other signs of well-being or discontent, caregivers can assess the person's current need for activity and respond accordingly.

With someone like Elsie, this can be particularly challenging. All outward appearances implied that she was quite happy to just "be." However, knowing something about her past skills and interests gave me a window into how her days might be enhanced, how she could experience even greater joy and well-being through involvement in a favorite pastime.

Caregivers should also bear in mind that a negative response to a suggested activity may not spring from contentment but from difficulty understanding anything happening outside of the now. This situation again underlines the importance of focusing on the pleasure of doing an activity (process) rather than on the final product (outcome).

Fear of Failure

Because of damage to his or her brain, a person with dementia may not have had many recent successful experiences. In fact, he or she may have experienced numerous failures. Elsie, for instance, was having trouble managing her meals and making cookies long before she came to the day program. Making cookies may have seemed daunting because she had not had any recent successes with her kitchen activities. She may have been worried that she couldn't actually do what was expected when people asked her to make cookies. Like most of us, she wasn't keen on making mistakes, at failing and being embarrassed in trying to do what might seem like such a simple task. All around, then, it was safer and less embarrassing to find excuses for not making cookies.

Persons with dementia probably feel much safer in simply saying "no" when faced with possible failure. This response is a way of protecting dignity and self-esteem. It is easier not to participate than to risk failing and being embarrassed. As an adult, have you ever been in the situation of feeling less than capable and confident? If so, you will probably understand the person's feelings. Being a new adult learner, especially if others are present who are more skilled, can be very stressful and embarrassing. The level of embarrassment is probably even greater if the person is trying to do something that they used to be good at.

One of the earliest warnings that Alice was having problems was when she began to have trouble turning the heel on a sock when knitting, an activity that she had done dozens of times. She became so embarrassed and frustrated that her many knitting projects got put away "for the summer." Understandably, she couldn't seem to face the risk of failure again. However, Alice was motivated to get out her needles again by my 8-year-old daughter Miriam, who wished to have her favorite hand-knit "Gramma" outfit lengthened. Alice spent all morning determining how to add some rows to the outfit's plain knitted skirt. When Miriam innocently asked how the project was going, Alice angrily threw the skirt and the needles across the room, astounding everyone. Alice was so frustrated and humiliated at being unable to do this previously simple task that she later refused to go on a planned trip to visit her much-loved sister. Thinking about it now, I can only guess that she was unwilling to risk a public failure yet again.

Difficulty Making Choices

If we think about it from the person's point of view, saying "no" to the general question "What would you like to do today?" becomes even more understandable. The brain damaged by dementia causes problems not only in doing the steps of familiar activities but also in initiating activities and in making choices and decisions. As a result, this sort of open-ended question must seem totally overwhelming. As the possibilities for failure and embarrassment are huge, it is much easier to just say "no."

Like many family caregivers, I found it very challenging to get Alice started on an activity. Doing so can be especially difficult if the person is also social and pleasant. It was puzzling to me that a previously active person such as Alice didn't seem to have any interest in looking after her garden, inviting people over, or knitting. At first I tried suggesting—well, truth be known, this eventually crossed over into haranguing. I'd say, "Have you called that nice lady from church to come over for coffee?" or "Have you started on the scarf that we got the yarn out for?"

Finally, I got the point that Alice just couldn't do these things on her own anymore and settled into the idea that she needed more structure and support. Her son and I helped her to attend a day program one day per week, which she loved and called her "classes." A wonderful family friend took Alice to Bible study and helped her to feel comfortable with the group and to participate in the discussions. We were fortunate to get a wonderful housekeeper, Jean, who worked three mornings per week and understood that she was helping in *Alice's* house. They did the housework and meal preparation *together.* Jean was Alice's caring companion and went far beyond the call of duty. For instance, Alice and Jean would assemble a casserole on Friday mornings. Then, even though Friday afternoon was Jean's time off, she would telephone Alice and remind her to put the casserole in the oven so it would be ready later when we all came over for supper.

Alice spent a lot of time with us on family outings: church, our children's music recitals, family meals, and so forth. I finally learned not to offer these occasions as options but to gently say something such as, "We will pick you up at 10:30 for the drive to the valley." She had always loved to be included in all these occasions and continued to do so once I figured out how to ask. In the early days, I said things such as, "We are going for a drive to the valley tomorrow—would you like to come?" and she usually replied with something such as, "I am too tired for such a long day."

The biggest challenge in maintaining a familiar lifestyle came when I realized that Alice was no longer bathing properly. My first attempt to get her to have a bath was really disastrous. She had always been a very particular person and, as a registered nurse, even the hint that she wasn't clean understandably caused a major upset. With some firm direction from her son, Alice did get in the bathtub, but none of us felt very good about the process. In the end, the best solution was to enlist the help of Jean, someone outside the family circle.

Inability to Understand What Is Expected

Caregivers often find that even when they narrow down the choices, questions such as "Would you like to go for a walk?" still elicit a "no" response. In this case, refusal may be related to continuing concern with failure and difficulty understanding what is expected. Although this question may seem absolutely clear to us, it may represent a vast number of unknowns to the person with dementia: "Am I expected to walk by myself?" "Where will I go?" "What if I get lost?" "How will I find my way back home?" "Where is my coat and how will I get it on?" "What is the weather like?" "What if that nasty dog is outside?" When plagued by so many fears and uncertainties, it seems so much easier to say "no."

The Effects of Brain Damage

Persons with dementia have a remarkable capacity to pull out all the stops and muster their many remaining strengths to present themselves with dignity and competence. This capacity is not only laudable but also should be cultivated and supported by caregivers (see Chapter 3).

At the same time, caregivers need to be aware that strengths such as excellent social skills or long-term memory can cover but not compensate for lost skills such as the ability to take initiative or plan activities. Persons with dementia may not take the initiative to continue with familiar activities or respond when asked because they have lost the ability to plan and carry out activities on their own.

Depression

Persons with dementia, particularly those in the early stages, are highly susceptible to depression. Among persons with dementia, 30%–50% also have clinical depression. Because the symptoms of dementia can often cover the symptoms of depression, caregivers need to be especially alert if withdrawal or loss of interest in activity is persistently accompanied by other symptoms of depression (e.g., sleeping too much or too little, loss of appetite, excessive weight gain or weight loss, extreme fatigue, feelings of hopelessness). If these symptoms are present and persist for more than 3–4 weeks, a physician should be consulted immediately. Depression is treatable but unfortunately is often overlooked in persons with dementia.

WAYS TO ENCOURAGE PARTICIPATION

If asking questions in a straightforward way leads the person with dementia to say no, how should you ask? Finding an answer to this question begins by going back to Chapter 2 and thinking about living in the moment. The person, at the moment, feels afraid of failure, unsure that he or she can do the activity, and uncertain about what is expected. To compensate for these challenges, our invitations need to be full of reassurance that we will be there to help, to be very clear on what exactly we are going to do, and to address fear of failure by including reminders of the person's past successes.

An invitation is much different from telling or asking someone. An invitation offers respect to the person and opens the door for opportunity. This tone, in itself, sets the stage for a positive response. For example, we can say, "I would be very happy if you would join me for lunch; we are having your favorite chicken casserole" instead of "Lunch is ready," or we can say, "It is such a lovely day; I am going to walk to the park on Beacon Street and would be delighted if you would come with me" instead of "Let's go for a walk."

As independent adults, we don't have to think too much to appreciate which sort of message is more welcoming and more likely to be positively received. As caregivers of persons with dementia, we need to be especially mindful that opportunities for engagement in activity—any sort of activity, whether self-care or leisure—are presented as warm invitations that respect adult dignity and welcome participation.

By applying an understanding of the reasons behind the person's seeming lack of interest or reluctance to participate, caregivers can offer invitations in ways that encourage participation. Some suggestions are discussed in the ensuing subsections.

Honor Individual Dignity

The goal of invitations is to help the person continue with a familiar lifestyle—that is, to support lifelong interests, habits, and values. Invitations that are based on an intimate understanding of the person's lifelong preferences honor individual dignity. Caregivers can then offer invitations and adapt these activities and the environment in ways that have personal meaning and ensure success.

When we offer an invitation that is grounded in an intimate knowledge of the person's life story and compensates for fears and concerns, true acknowledgment of dignity also includes accepting a valid "no thank you." It is a mistake to imagine that we know better what the person needs or wants than he or she does.

Nonetheless, it is important to respect the person's need for opportunities to grow and have new experiences. Just because a person has never previously gardened, gone fishing, or cooked doesn't necessarily mean that he or she may not enjoy the opportunity to do so now. The skill lies in using our understanding of the person and presenting activities in a meaningful and achievable way.

Expect a Positive Response

How you pose the question makes a huge difference in how the person responds. If your invitation includes a gentle expectation that the person will agree, the person is more likely to say "yes." The old adage "It's not so much what you say but how you say it" is especially true in communicating with persons with dementia. Persons with dementia develop great skills in reading the nonverbal, emotional part of language, perhaps to compensate for the losses in verbal language.

In the preceding story about Elsie, if the boarding house operator had said something such as, "Elsie, I would really appreciate your help with peeling these carrots while I prepare the potatoes for supper," Elsie would have been more likely to agree. From this invitation, Elsie would have known exactly what was expected of her, that her caregiver would be right there, and that her help was valued and appreciated. Although Elsie still may have been a little unsure, she likely would have been reluctant to turn down someone who needed help. Other suggestions follow for asking the person to do something in ways that expect a "yes" reply. These invitations are enhanced by using nonverbal messages such as speaking in a warm tone of voice, gently taking the person's arm, or using other techniques described in Chapter 4.

- "Lunch is ready; let's walk to the kitchen together."
- "I would be really happy if you would come for a walk with me to take these cookies to our friend Harriet."
- "I need your help with setting the table."
- "I have a nice warm bath ready for you; I will walk with you to the bathroom."
- "You are so good at gardening; I would really like your help with picking the tomatoes."
- "We are getting ready to play cards and would be happy if you would join us."

These kinds of invitations expect a positive response, reduce fear by letting the person know that you will be there with him or her, and avoid giving orders that insult adult dignity. How would you feel if you were told to take a bath or to go to the bathroom? Even though persons with dementia may no longer remember to do these things by themselves, they don't forget that they are adults and never lose touch with a sense of dignity and self-protection. This middle road between giving orders and asking can do a lot in getting the person involved in activity. However, it does take a lot of practice.

Provide Opportunities for Making Manageable Choices

An invitation that includes choices encourages a positive response and participation. However, individuals begin to have difficulty making choices in the early stages of dementia. Caregivers can help overcome this problem by using an understanding of the person to offer manageable choices, usually between two different things. For instance, you can say, "Would you like a ham sandwich or a tuna sandwich for lunch?" (instead of "What would you like for lunch?") or "Would you like to listen to Perry Como or Lawrence Welk?" (instead of "What music would you like to hear?").

It is also important to think carefully about the sort of choices we offer. For instance, the choice is not "Would you like to have lunch?" There is no option about whether to eat lunch. Similarly, as noted previously, although bath time can be challenging and it is important to offer the person choices, the choice is not whether to have a bath. Instead the choice can be about real options by asking questions such as "Would you like your bath now or after breakfast?" or "Would you like to put on your green shirt or your red shirt after your bath?" One creative paid caregiver encouraged the person to take a bath by having available a lovely basket of soaps and shampoos from which the person could take her pick. The person became so interested in these lovely items that she forgot her anxiety about taking a bath. Workers in some long-term care facilities have successfully used this approach to transform bath time into a "spa experience." This is not an expensive program because supplies come from staff, volunteers, and family members who are asked to save free soaps and shampoos from hotels.

Provide Reassurance and
Support Success During the Activity

Invitations that are based on understanding and empathy for the person and are offered in a warm and caring manner, encourage the person to get involved. To keep the person involved, it is important to continue to provide reassurance and praise. This is so important that it is detailed in the following extensive section.

HANDS TO HEALTH:
HOW TO HELP WITH DOING

The previous sections have provided information on the importance of maintaining a familiar lifestyle, of enabling meaningful activity. As you are only too aware, a person with dementia has increasing trouble doing things independently. Without help from others, the person often spends a lot of time doing nothing. The following guidelines, which can be used for all types of activities, will help you to keep the person active. As with all areas of dementia care, there are no rules or recipes—just suggestions that you can use according to the needs and strengths of the person you are caring for.

See Chapter 7 for more details on using these guidelines for daily life activities and Chapter 8 for more details on using them for leisure activities.

Make Use of Continuing Abilities

In the face of the many losses and disabilities that accompany dementia, it can be easy to lose sight of the fact that the person also has many remaining abilities. These abilities can be used to encourage doing and compensate for some areas of difficulty. For example, the person may not be able to independently prepare lunch for friends; however, with help, he or she can do some parts of the meal preparation (e.g., set the table, arrange the flowers, prepare the vegetables). In addition, greeting his or her friend at the door and acting as the host or hostess makes use of ongoing social skills. As another example, the person may not be able to speak in sentences, but he or she may be able to sing along with familiar music, which is a relaxing activity during bathing or at bedtime. For more details on these strengths and how to use them in daily care, see Chapter 3.

Be Consistent and Follow Lifelong Routines and Habits

We are all creatures of habit; we have hundreds of personal rituals that we have developed over a lifetime. Generally, we follow a certain routine when we get up in the morning; from here until bedtime, the day is filled with ways of doing things that are usually unconscious but very important. Included are larger things, such as the time we prefer to get up or the foods we like, right down to small details, such as the method we use for brushing our teeth. These are uniquely personal habits. We tend to feel most comfortable and at ease when we can continue with these habits. Most of us can adapt but we still carry out our preferred routines as much as possible. For example, because I travel a lot for business, I have grown accustomed to sleeping in different beds in hotels. Usually, I sleep well because I carry on my bedtime routine of reading the newspaper in bed for a few minutes. In fact, on most nights, I read little more than the headlines before I fall sleep. There is no particular logic or benefit to this routine, but maintaining it helps me to sleep no matter where I travel.

The progression of dementia makes it more difficult to do daily and other activities and to maintain valued personal routines. Persons with dementia must increasingly rely on caregivers not only to help them do the activity but also to help them continue doing it in the same way that they always have. Supporting personal habits and routines also triggers doing familiar activities. It helps the person to be more independent and to feel much more comfortable and at ease. It can be tempting to dismiss these routines as unnecessary fussing; however, they are vital. They provide the framework for daily life and support well-being. Imagine how devastated you would feel if you couldn't have a cup of tea in your favorite chair in the morning (or whatever personal routine you particularly value)? What follows is just one example of the powerful impact of maintaining familiar routines.

When George retired, he continued to dress in a shirt and tie, just as if he was going to the office. When he developed dementia, he began to have difficulty buttoning his shirt and tying his tie. However, his wife knew how important this was to him, so she did it for him. When she could no longer manage his care, he and a large collection of his favorite shirts and ties moved to a nursing facility. The busy staff members thought it would be much easier to dress him in polo shirts. He resisted this, but they managed to dress him. Most mornings, George was rather upset and agitated, not only with getting dressed but also in general. This was thought to be caused by his move into a care facility and the progression of his dementia. Although both of these factors probably played roles, one staff member noticed that George was quite calm when his wife came to visit and helped him dress in a favorite shirt and tie. On her next morning shift, this staff member decided to try dressing George in a shirt and tie. She and others were astonished when George not only didn't resist help with dressing but also was cheerful and calm most of the morning. When George's lifelong routine for dressing was respected, he was happier, and providing his care became much easier.

At all stages of dementia, care should be guided by personal lifelong routines to encourage doing and enhance well-being. Family members and significant others know the person and his or her routines better than anyone else. This information is invaluable in caregiving. It is even more critical when there are multiple caregivers or paid caregivers who do not have this intimate personal knowledge. The All About Me form (Appendix A) provides an outline for this personal information. As care needs change, new information should be added. In the early stages of dementia, the person can and should contribute a great deal to this form as well.

Organize Necessary
Materials and Equipment in Advance

Olga was trying her best, but it was becoming increasingly difficult to provide the care that her mother needed. She finally decided to get help from a paid caregiver for a few hours per week. One of the things that Olga found

most difficult was helping her mother shower. Olga had the home aide take over this task. Usually, Olga took full advantage of this time to take a break outside of home. One day, she was late leaving the house and was astonished when the home aide walked Olga's mother into the bathroom and got her under the already running shower without a word of protest. A few days later, Olga set out clean clothes, a towel, and the necessary toiletries; started the shower; and found that her mother happily got in the shower, just as she had for the home aide.

Whether we are helping the person with dementia bathe or working with him or her in the garden, the person needs and deserves our full attention. Having things planned and prepared in advance as much as possible allows us to give our full attention to the person. As Olga found, this encourages participation because it provides extra cues for the person about what is going to take place.

Help the Person to Get Started with the Activity

The person with dementia often appears to have lost interest in doing things. This can be especially troublesome to family caregivers, because they have always known the person as an independent, self-directed adult. As noted previously, this seeming loss of interest is partly due to one of the most challenging of the disease symptoms, difficulty getting started. It may be helpful to think of this like a broken starter on a car. We as caregivers need to act like a starter. Once started, the habitual memory of familiar activities often helps the person to continue. For example, the person may be able to feed him- or herself if assisted with hand-over-hand guidance to make the first few hand-to-mouth movements. He or she may be able to wash his or her hands and face if his or her hands are guided to the warm water and the washcloth. For other less familiar or more complicated activities, such as getting dressed or feeding the dog, the person may need help getting started at each step of the activity.

Provide Hints or Cues

Most of adult communication is based on words. Losses in verbal communication make it increasingly difficult for persons with dementia to understand word cues or suggestions for activity. Even something as basic as "Here is your lunch" can be difficult for persons with dementia to follow. When they don't respond, it is easy to assume that they are unable to feed themselves. However, several types of cues make use of the person's continuing nonverbal communication skills and compensate for decreasing verbal skills. All of these ways of communicating should be explored. Nonword hints or cues are helpful for familiar, overlearned, repetitive activities, such as eating, brushing one's hair, or raking the leaves.

Nonverbal cues or hints—such as drawing attention to the smell and appetizing appearance of food, the feel of a spoon in one's hand, or a taste of the food—can be used to encourage the person to start an activity. Demonstration, such as making eating motions, is another helpful method of cuing. Physical guidance may also be needed, such as hand-over-hand guidance to gently direct a spoonful of food to the person's mouth.

These same levels of cues or hints can be used for all sorts of activities, including familiar leisure activities such as misting the house plants. In this case, the following cues might be provided:

- Say, "Here is the mister bottle to spray the plants" (verbal cue).
- Gesture toward the plants and spray them (demonstration).

- Put the mister in the person's hand and point out the plant (nonverbal cue)
- Put your hand around the person's hand and gently start spraying the plant (physical guidance).

Different parts of an activity may require different types of cues. For instance, only a verbal cue may be needed for putting on a sweater or jacket, but putting on a shirt may require demonstration and a nonverbal cue. The person may need physical guidance and/or physical assistance to get started in putting on his or her pants.

Nonverbal cues or hints are also important for helping the person to get involved in less familiar or more complex activities, such as baking or doing a craft project. However, it is unlikely that the person will be able to continue independently; he or she will likely need further hints and reminders for each step. See Chapter 4 for further information on these communication techniques.

People respond to different types of hints. For instance, one person may only need to see his or her jacket as a cue to put it on; another person may need to feel the jacket. When you discover which cues or hints work best with the person you are caring for, record them on the All About Me form (Appendix A) and try to use these same hints every time. It is especially important to share these hints with other caregivers, such as respite care workers.

Break the Activity into Several Steps and Give Guidance as Necessary

Although we may think of brushing our teeth or preparing our coffee as one activity, these basic activities are made of many steps. There are, for instance, as many as 35 steps in the activity of our brushing teeth! Persons with dementia often forget the order of these steps, lose the cognitive glue that holds the many steps of an activity together, and get lost before the activity is finished. The person may see brushing his or her teeth, for instance, as several different activities (e.g., uncapping the tube of toothpaste, squeezing the toothpaste on the toothbrush). However, if the activity is broken down into steps and the person is helped to do one step at a time, he or she can usually succeed. For brushing one's teeth, the steps (accompanied by nonverbal cues, as needed) might sound like this: "It's time to brush your teeth. Come with me to the bathroom and I will help you. Here is the toothpaste. Take the top off. Here is the toothbrush. Squeeze some toothpaste onto the brush. Put down the toothpaste. Put the brush in your mouth. Now brush your teeth." **It is important to use the same steps and the same directions every time.** Otherwise, the person may think that this is a whole different activity.

Begin the Activity at the Step Where the Person Can Succeed

Busy caregivers do not have the time to take the person through all 35 steps of brushing his or her teeth, one step at a time. Yet, it is possible to start partway through the activity and eliminate a number of steps. For example, beginning with toothpaste already on the toothbrush eliminates many steps, but the person still has the chance to participate. As another example, the person may enjoy baking but have difficulty measuring the ingredients. If the caregiver measures everything in advance, it is possible for the person to begin by stirring the wet ingredients into the dry ingredients.

The steps of an activity may also be spread out over time. Caregivers may find this approach challenging to use if they value finishing what is started. However, the fragile attention and energy levels of persons with dementia may not allow them to do an entire activity at once. For instance, a person with dementia may really enjoy watering the houseplants or making a favorite recipe but needs to take rests and spread the activity out over the day or even more than one day. With advanced planning, many activities lend themselves to this sort of breakdown. Obviously, busy caregivers need to decide which tasks need to be finished on the spot (e.g., helping to prepare supper). However, with advanced planning, even these activities can be spread out over time. If a person with dementia enjoys preparing vegetables for the evening meal but gets fatigued before finishing, his or her caregiver can finish the task so that supper is served on time. Alternately, the preparations can be started in the morning (when the person usually has more energy) and worked on in brief periods over the course of the day. Several persons with dementia once helped me make pumpkin pies for Thanksgiving. Everyone participated at some level, and we did one step per day for several days. It was a long process, but they enjoyed every step and their satisfaction with the final product was well worth it.

Adapt the Task and/or the Environment

There are many ways to adapt or change an activity so that the person can succeed. However, it is important to introduce changes slowly and to keep the activity as familiar as possible to make use of the person's habitual memory. Consult an occupational therapist for specific recommendations.

Caregivers can *grade an activity*—that is, change the way an activity is done according to the person's skills (e.g., giving a sponge bath instead of a tub bath, cooking finger foods instead of a casserole). A sponge bath requires fewer physical skills than a tub bath. It is also possible to grade an activity according to the level of participation. The person may be involved in every step of the activity, may do only one or two steps, or may be involved by being present and watching or commenting while others do the activity. Someone in the early stages of dementia will probably be able to carry out the whole activity of baking cookies—shopping for ingredients, following the recipe, baking the cookies, serving them, and eating them. An individual with moderate cognitive impairments may require assistance with selecting and measuring the ingredients but will likely be able to mix, shape, and serve the cookies as well as help clean up. A person who has severe cognitive impairments will be able to mix the dough (perhaps with hand-over-hand guidance), drop spoonfuls of dough on a cookie sheet, appreciate the aroma of baking cookies, and eat the cookies. This last step—eating the cookies—is something that everyone can do! It is also important to note that sitting and watching is an activity. Some may enjoy the activity of being in the family kitchen while baking or meal preparation takes place.

We can also change the things or materials used for the activity so that the person can succeed (e.g., provide pull-on clothes instead of ones with buttons and fasteners, buy eating utensils with bigger handles). There are thousands of ways to adapt activities so that the person can succeed. For persons with poor vision, use larger letters, coarser yarn, or outline guides or templates for activities such as writing. For persons with poor grasp in the fingers or hands, use larger handles and fatter pens and stabilize items with clamps or nonskid material. Chapters 7 and 8 provide further suggestions. In addition, Appendix B lists resources for adapted equipment to use in self-care and daily activities, but you may find similar items more economically priced at your local pharmacy or hardware store. For example, handles can easily be built up for better grip by using inexpensive foam tubes meant for insulating water pipes. Rubberized mesh matting, often used on cupboard shelves to keep dishes from moving in campers, can be used under plates or mixing bowls or on door handles to make a nonskid surface. A damp washcloth can also be used for this purpose. There are also many ways to change the environment to make tasks safer and easier for the person with dementia (e.g., hidden security locks on outside doors, labels on kitchen cupboards). See Chapter 5 for suggestions on adapting the environment.

Explain Everything, Every Time, to Compensate for Memory Loss

Although persons with dementia have remarkable abilities, it is best to assume that every moment is brand new. Do not assume recall from one moment to the next. For more on communication, see Chapter 4.

Reduce Distractions and Ensure Privacy

To be successful in activities, persons with dementia need to concentrate on the task at hand. Damage to the brain makes it increasingly difficult to screen out background noises and to pay attention to an activity. As dementia progresses, it takes less to distract the person, even the refrigerator's hum or traffic noises coming through an open window can be a distraction. During difficult tasks, it is especially important to keep distractions to a minimum. Turn off the radio, attend to the person, and do not converse with others. Do the activity in an area where disruptions are least likely. Serve meals one course at a time and as dementia advances, provide only one eating utensil.

Allow Plenty of Time

Because of damage to the brain, it takes much longer for the person with dementia to do things. The whole sequence of doing—understanding what is to be done, starting the first step, making the necessary movements, and so forth—is slowed down, rather like running a movie in slow motion. Caregivers who are accustomed to moving quickly through a series of tasks can find this challenging. Again, there is a need to step into the world of the person with dementia and remind yourself that the joy and the pleasure is in the moment, in the process of doing the activity and not in the final outcome. One person might be fed lunch in 10 minutes and another may take an hour to eat independently, but both will have a meal. The question is, which person experienced more pleasure and satisfaction?

Although it may be faster (for you) to get the person dressed or to feed him or her, what's the rush? Doing such activities independently helps the person to feel better about him- or herself and is an important occupation. If you rush the activity, not only can the person become agitated but also you then have to think of something for him or her to do.

STIMULATING THE SENSES

We all understand and respond to the world around us through millions of sights, smells, sounds, feels, movements, and tastes. The smell of the stew on the stove welcomes us home and tells us that it is supper time. The green grass and the singing birds tell us it is spring. It is a blessing that for persons with dementia, the part of the brain that takes in the senses usually continues to work quite well. These experiences, such as hearing a favorite song or tasting freshly baked bread, bring pleasure in themselves.

Beyond the sheer pleasure of sensory experiences, sensory stimulation is essential for brain functioning. We all need sensory stimulation until we die. Experiments have demonstrated the powerful negative effect of *not* having sensory stimulation (Zubek, 1969). Healthy, young college students spent various periods of time in sensory-deprived environments where they couldn't move around or talk to anyone; they had nothing to do and nothing to look at. After leaving these environments, the students had difficulty solving simple problems, were apathetic and unmotivated, and had poor concentration and uncoordinated movements. All of these individuals eventually returned to normal functioning. However, the longer they stayed in the sensory-deprived environment, the longer it took to get back to normal.

For obvious reasons, such experiments are now illegal. However, we can benefit from the knowledge gained by applying the information to the situation of persons with dementia. It is interesting to note that the losses the students experienced were quite similar to some of the symptoms of dementia. Although we know that sensory deprivation does not cause dementia, it can worsen the symptoms of dementia.

Brain damage makes it increasingly difficult for persons with dementia both to notice and to interpret the stimulating sensory world around them. Persons with dementia, especially those in the later stages, need help to be able to respond to sensory experience. Without this help, they become more isolated from the sensory world and receive less sensory input, thereby decreasing responsiveness. Unless caregivers intervene, this situation can continue in a downward spiral, making the symptoms of dementia even worse. In addition, most persons with dementia are older and may well have age-related losses in hearing, vision, taste, touch, and movement. Persons who live in institutional environments are at an even greater risk for sensory deprivation due to understimulation or overstimulation, both of which are more common in these settings.

When there is too much stimulation, such as a lot of commotion at a family meal, persons with dementia may become upset or withdraw. They become overwhelmed and cannot determine how to manage. Have you ever had a long, problem-filled day at work when you're tired and just want to go home, but the telephone keeps ringing and everyone's asking you questions? The overload makes it hard to cope; the simplest things can become huge problems.

Because of brain damage, it takes much less to overload and overwhelm persons with dementia. As dementia progresses, they are less able to cope with overstimulation and have more trouble understanding normal sensory stimulation. When persons with dementia are overwhelmed with more stimulation than they can interpret, their responses often don't make sense, either. This is shown Figure 4.

One example of overstimulation is a family meal. Say hamburgers are the main course. There is a lot of talking and laughing as people pass around the condiments for their hamburgers. Jim, who has dementia, looks perplexed, then reaches for the condiment in front of him (ketchup) and starts shaking it all over his plate and the table. Another example is tray meal service in a long-term care facility. All of a meal's courses come out on one tray. As a result, it is common for persons with dementia not to eat or to do things such as trying to eat a napkin or putting scrambled eggs in their tea.

Thus, although stimulating the senses is really important, care must be taken to avoid incorrect stimulation or overload. The goal is stimulation without stress. When this goal is achieved, the person has a pleasurable experience and is stimulated to respond to the world around him or her in a way that makes sense. This is shown in Figure 5.

There are hundreds of ways to use the senses to provide pleasure and to help the person to respond to the world—that is, to do things. These opportunities bring pleasure, encourage doing, and may even help the brain to continue to grow. Widespread evidence shows that in response to stimulation, the human brain continues to grow throughout old age (Diamond & Hopson, 1999). Although the number of brain cells does not increase, dendrites (the connections between these brain cells) grow in response to stimulation. As discussed in Chapter 3, this helps to explain why autopsies of some people's brains evidence severe damage from Alzheimer's disease even though the people showed few symptoms of the disease while alive.

As dementia progresses and the person is less able to interpret and respond to the sensory world, it becomes more important to structure sensory experiences. The point of structuring these experiences is not to isolate the experiences as separate activities but to make them available as an integrated part of the daily routine. In institutional settings, this can take the form of a specialized group run by a skilled clinician.

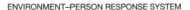

ENVIRONMENT–PERSON RESPONSE SYSTEM

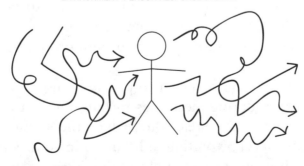

Confusing, disorganized environmental input   Confusing, disorganized responses

Figure 4. Illustration of overstimulation. Too much stimulation can lead to responses that do not make sense.

ENVIRONMENT–PERSON RESPONSE SYSTEM

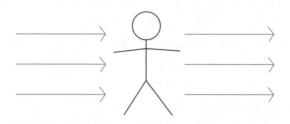

Orderly, understandable environmental input   Orderly, functional responses

Figure 5. Illustration of stimulation without stress. The person has a pleasurable experience and is stimulated to respond in a way that makes sense.

Consider what might happen during mealtime with Jim's family if stimulation is reduced to a manageable level. The family members talk more quietly among themselves and the person next to Jim focuses on Jim's needs. Because Jim only uses ketchup, this person moves away everything else. She then picks up the hamburger, invites Jim to smell it, and reminds him that it is a hamburger. He responds with pleasure, so she gives Jim the ketchup bottle. The feel of the bottle and the smell of the hamburger stimulate Jim to squeeze some ketchup on the hamburger. The stimulation of this activity and verbal encouragement lead him to take a bite. The hamburger tastes good to Jim—a response to stimulation that makes sense and helps Jim to be more engaged in the world around him.

Similar steps can be taken to provide sensory stimulation without stress during mealtimes in long-term care facilities. The most important step is to reduce the stimulation to a manageable level by putting only the main course in front of persons with dementia and reducing unnecessary noise in the dining room. Chapter 7 provides much more information on the important topic of eating and dining in long-term care facilities. See Chapter 5 for more information on sensory stimulation without stress.

Steps for Keeping Stimulation Manageable

Get the Person's Attention

Persons with dementia have difficulty paying attention or even noticing things that seem to be right in front of their eyes. They also have difficulty independently starting activities. You can help a person with dementia who has these difficulties by catching his or her attention. Appealing to sense of smell is a good way to get attention, but so is using the senses of touch, taste, and movement, as shown in the following example.

Bill used to like to peel an orange for his mid-morning snack. As his dementia worsened, his wife Annette noticed that he began to just let the orange sit on the table beside him. One day, she decided to help draw his attention to the orange. She scored the skin for easier peeling, touched Bill's hand gently, and said, "Good morning, Bill. I brought you an orange for your snack. Doesn't it smell good?" While saying this, she put the orange in Bill's hand and gently guided it up to his nose so he could smell it. The stimulation—the touch of the orange in his hand, the movement of his arm, and the scent of the orange—got Bill's attention. He put the orange down on the plate that Annette had placed on his lap, then peeled it and relished every bite.

Perhaps touch and smell stimulation would not have been enough to get Bill's attention. If so, Annette could have given him a taste of an already peeled orange.

Focus on One Sense at a Time

Most things in the world around us stimulate many senses. In Bill's story, for instance, the orange had a smooth and perhaps cool feel, a bright color, and a delicious taste. To make all of this stimulation manageable for persons with dementia, it is important to focus on only one sense at a time. In this case, Annette chose to focus Bill's attention on the smell of the orange. Sense of smell is a good starting point because it is such a basic sense and occupies more space in the human brain than any other sense. In fact, it is the only sense that is directly wired from the outside world to the brain.

As the person becomes more alert from the stimulation, the focus can be changed to other more complex elements, such as color and sound. For instance, Annette might have drawn Bill's attention to the orange's bright color and mentioned other things that are orange. She also might have been able to help him remember things such as getting an orange in his stocking each Christmas. The increased attention from this stimulation could have been used to draw Bill's attention to the music on the radio. Of course, the grand finale of this experience would still be the taste of the orange.

Encourage an Active Response

The point of stimulating the senses in this organized way is to help the person respond and reach out to the world around him or her, to be stimulated to do things. In the preceding vignette, Bill was stimulated to respond in a complicated way—that is, to peel and eat the orange, thereby engaging in an activity that he used to like. However, there are many other less complicated but still important responses to stimulation: smiling, speaking, clapping to music, putting flowers in a vase, stirring cookie dough, and so forth. The point is to stimulate the senses that are connected with the activity. For example, drawing a person's attention to the smell of some flowers can stimulate the person to put the flowers in water.

A Word Regarding Paid Caregivers

By the time persons with dementia need paid help with personal care and other activities, they will also be having difficulty sorting out how to respond to the sensory world. Personal care activities are amazingly rich opportunities for using the three previously outlined steps—get the person's attention, focus on one sense at a time, and encourage an active response—to provide pleasure and increase responsiveness. Providing opportunities for manageable sensory stimulation becomes especially vital in long-term care settings.

The following example illustrates how sensory stimulation can be used in a long-term care facility to provide pleasure and to encourage a person with dementia to eat breakfast.

- Introduce the activity by using the person's proper or preferred name. As you speak to the individual, provide reassuring orienting information, such as, "Good morning, Mrs. Matthews. I have brought you some toast for breakfast on this sunny Wednesday in June."

- Use a verbal approach that encourages a positive response and nonverbal cues that communicate warmth and reassurance.

- Target one sense at a time, such as the toast's delicious smell.

- Reduce confusion and competing stimuli. Place only the toast in front of the person, not the whole meal.

- Provide verbal and nonverbal hints to encourage an active response. For example, provide hand-over-hand guidance to bring the toast to the person's mouth.

- Make connections with personal interests or habits. Say something such as, "Here is some delicious strawberry jam to put on your toast. What is your favorite kind of jam?" or "Did you ever make strawberry jam?"
- Give ample—but not excessive—positive feedback, using caring personal touch. Squeeze the person's hand or put your arm around his or her shoulder. Give verbal praise, such as, "Great! You have eaten the whole piece of toast. That will give you energy for the day."

USING REMINISCENCE ON A DAILY BASIS

Persons with dementia remember things that happened 50 years ago much better than things that happened 5 years ago or even 5 minutes ago. Although this can be frustrating, it is also a strength. Recalling the past—that is, reminiscing—can be used to bring pleasure, to support the person's sense of self-worth, to encourage involvement in activities, and to provide a pleasant distraction when the person is distressed.

All people, including children, look back over things that happened in the past. It is essential for emotional health. As we age, it becomes even more important to look back over good and bad life experiences, sort through them, sum them up, and come to terms with all that has happened. It is the main emotional task of aging, just as becoming an independent adult is the main task of a teenager. Reminiscing in this way is not the same thing as living in the past; rather, it is a healthy process of coming to terms with the past, with the life road traveled.

Persons with dementia also have this need to look back, to sum up, and to come to terms with life experiences. However, due to brain damage, they may need our help to do so. At the same time, recalling past life experiences can bring great pleasure and satisfaction. When we help persons with dementia to recall a special occasion or personal accomplishment, we also take them back to the emotions of that experience, to a time when they were competent and successful. This can be a great boost to self-esteem.

Reminiscence can be used on a daily basis by everyone who comes in contact with a person who has dementia. For instance, while helping the person dress, caregivers can also help the person to recall a favorite outfit from the past and where he or she might have worn that outfit.

Know the Person's Life Story

As dementia progresses, the details of past experiences become hazy. However, when caregivers trigger these memories with reminders about past special events or experiences, the memories usually come flooding back. Family caregivers, with their intimate knowledge of the person's life story, are in a perfect situation to use this information. Sharing this information with paid caregivers helps them to know your loved one's personal story. This adds to the caregiver relationship and is a tremendous contribution to quality of life. The All About Me form in Appendix A is one way to share this information. A life story poster or labeled photo album is another. When a paid caregiver comes to your home, it is helpful to point out treasured pictures and mementos. These become especially precious in long-term care facilities. At a quality facility, these mementos will be welcomed and staff will seek to learn about the person from family members.

A photo album with special pictures from the person's life is a great help for all caregivers. It is best to label the pictures. This album can be a wonderful focus for family visits, especially as the person loses verbal skills. Most persons with dementia never seem to tire of commenting on and looking at the pictures. This is also a wonderful way to share a person's life story with paid or nonfamily caregivers.

Use Opinion-Seeking Questions

Questions that have correct answers are difficult for a person with dementia. These sorts of questions should be avoided because they put the person on the spot and set up him or her for failure. Everyone can give an opinion, however; opinions are never wrong.

Asking the person's opinion can stimulate memory and get the person involved. By seeking the person's opinion, you give him or her hints and guarantee success. Examples of such questions include the following:

- "Have you ever seen anything like this before?"
- "Have you ever used anything like this before?"
- "Does this look familiar to you?"
- "What do you like best about spring?"
- "What do you like least about spring?"
- "What is your favorite food?"

Use Hands-On Physical Cues

The term *reminiscing* brings to mind sitting around and talking over old times. This certainly is an important aspect of reminiscing. Verbal reminiscing can be difficult for persons with dementia who have experienced verbal losses. Using actual objects, such as an old watch or school book, adds physical and sensory input that helps to stimulate verbal memories in amazing ways. Personal mementos and photographs are especially powerful at calling forth memories. Mementos or artifacts with action components, such as old-fashioned ice cream churns or crank telephones, are also very helpful in stimulating memories.

Use Music to Stimulate Memory

Music is another nonverbal pathway to memory. By using familiar and favorite songs, it is possible to bypass verbal losses and take the person to an experience associated with the songs. This is true for most of us—for instance, the first strains of the Beatles song "She Loves You" takes me right back to a dance at my high school's gym! Think about which songs can take you on memory journeys, and try to help the person you are caring for do the same.

Be Comfortable with Unhappy Memories

Life is hard and not all memories are happy. For example, there are many fun stories about the ways that people managed to live through the Great Depression, but there are also many sad stories of loss. It is unrealistic to focus only on the happy survival stories. The person's happiness is a caregiving goal, and sharing his or her tears can lead to greater happiness. Recalling and sharing unhappy times, as well as the happy ones, can help the person to be more at peace with his or her past. If the person constantly focuses on past sorrows, however, it is necessary to seek professional help.

Help the Person to Reconnect with the Present

The purpose of using reminiscence is not to encourage living in the past. This can lead to disorientation and confusion. After recalling the old days for awhile, help persons with dementia to reconnect with the present. For instance, if you have been reminiscing about first cars, make a link to present-day cars now: talk about how much they cost in comparison to people's first cars, favorite models of new cars, and so forth.

CONCLUSION

The pointers for using reminiscence brings this chapter on being and doing, on maintaining a familiar lifestyle, to a conclusion. It is a fitting ending because the main point of the chapter has been to share not only the importance of and techniques for enriching life now through activity but also how vital it is to know the person's story, to know a person's accomplishments and activities. Chapter 7 provides detailed information about enabling engagement in daily life activities.

7

Success with Daily Life Activities

PERSONAL CARE ACTIVITIES

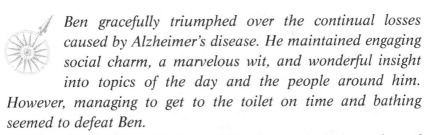

Ben gracefully triumphed over the continual losses caused by Alzheimer's disease. He maintained engaging social charm, a marvelous wit, and wonderful insight into topics of the day and the people around him. However, managing to get to the toilet on time and bathing seemed to defeat Ben.

It wasn't that Ben didn't try. His urine-soaked shoes showed that he often struggled to get to the bathroom but couldn't quite make it. He also tried to care for himself. For years, Ben had dealt with nonhealing sores on his arms by covering them with a pillowcase-type dressing. When Ben started attending a day program, he was struggling to continue this complicated process, using numerous rusty safety pins to keep the dressing in place. He also tried his best to trim his toenails, ending up with a pretty ragged and sore looking mess. Getting dressed was another challenge; he sometimes ended up with three shirts and no underwear. At the day program, he tried his best to take part in bathing and dressing, packing a grocery bag of clean clothing into the basket on his walker. Imagine a certified nurse assistant's surprise one day when she found that Ben's grocery bag contained the veg-etable scraps for the compost instead of clean clothes!

Until a year previously, Ben had struggled to take care of him-self in his own home. His children, who lived far away, were con-cerned and arranged for a live-in housekeeper. Ben cheerfully gave over his cooking and cleaning chores to the first house-keeper; unfortunately, he also gave over some cash and valuable antiques.

Rachel and Jeff, an honest and hard-working couple, later moved in. They were great with the housework and chores but couldn't understand Ben's self-care difficulties. The first time Rachel met with day program staff, she seemed baffled and annoyed by Ben's inability to get to the bathroom on time and seeming lack of interest in bathing. This meant many bedding changes and extra laundry for Rachel, and she was understand-ably frustrated. Rachel said when she asked Ben if he had to go to the bathroom, Ben always said no. The next thing she knew, Ben had wet himself again. When Rachel directly told Ben to go to the bathroom, he would angrily say "no."

Over the following months, program staff tried to explain to Rachel why Ben could not get to the bathroom independently. Staff also suggested ways that Rachel could help Ben get to the bathroom, get washed, and get dressed.

Unfortunately, there was little progress in Rachel's understand-ing, but a home care aide did come to help bathe Ben. One day program staff were hopeful when Rachel talked about watching a television program about Alzheimer's disease and reported that she thought that Ben might have it. However, almost immediately, she voiced another puzzled statement. Rachel could not under-stand why Ben kept asking when supper would be ready. She remarked, "It's enough to drive a person crazy."

Although Rachel had good intentions, she was in a caregiving situation that was beyond her skill level. On duty 24 hours per day and apparently unable to learn new ways, Rachel's distress with caregiving mounted. Staff members were unable to persuade Ben's family that the situation was breaking down and that they should seek other care arrangements. This held true even when Ben's daughter came to visit. She was prickly when a day program staff member suggested that her father was not receiving proper care. In turn, she blamed the day program staff for not being able to teach Rachel how to be a better caregiver.

Sadly, Rachel and Jeff treated Ben's memory loss as a joke. For example, Ben could not determine that a picture of his daughter Barb as a young woman was the person he knew as Barb. Ben tried to cover his confusion by saying that he had two daughters named Barb, whom Rachel and Jeff laughingly referred to as "Barb-Barb." They would quiz Ben on this topic in front of others as if it was parlor entertainment.

Rachel also could not understand the need to put away cleaning supplies, scissors, and other dangerous things. She could not believe that Ben might mistake bleach for liquid soap or a drink. Day program staff managed to get these things put away. They also replaced the rusty safety pins (for Ben's arm dressing) with stainless steel ones. Sadly, day program staff still were not successful in preventing a crisis.

One day, Rachel called the day program in great distress. Ben had wet himself again while sitting in a chair, and he wouldn't move. Rachel said that she was just going to leave Ben sitting there. Someone else could clean up Ben's messes, she said; she was not going to do it any longer. Day program staff persuaded a neighbor to bring Ben to the program, where he was bathed and cared for. When Ben's doctor was informed of the situation, he arranged for an emergency admission to the hospital until other care arrangements could be made.

Happily, Ben now lives in a pleasant and supportive nursing facility. Every day he signs the guest book with great enthusiasm, and staff members thank him for the compliments that he records in the book.

Ben's story offers many lessons about caregiving in general and about the activities of daily living in particular. These topics are explored in the following subsections.

The Basics of Personal Care Activities

Ben used his excellent social skills to compensate for his losses. Unfortunately, Rachel was so fooled by Ben's social skills that she thought Ben was just being lazy. Without help from others (e.g., caregiver support at the program), however, Ben was as powerless to stop having accidents as a person with Parkinson's disease is powerless to stop shaking. Rachel was also powerless in this situation, as she was in a caregiving role that exceeded her abilities.

The Activities of Daily Living Are Complicated

As dementia increasingly damages the brain, the person forgets how to organize and order the many steps of daily activities. The most complicated activities are the ones with which the person will first have trouble. This explains Ben's difficulty with getting dressed. Furthermore, like many others with dementia, he found bathing so complicated that he stopped trying. Bathing is usually the first self-care activity to pose problems for persons with dementia. However, this may go unnoticed for awhile because it is easier to hide than others, such as dressing, which are immediately obvious.

The Person Will Continue to Try to Do as Much as Possible

Most people with dementia will continue to try to do as much as they can. For example, Ben continued to try cutting his own toenails. Being independent in self-care activities—such as bathing, dressing, or going to the bathroom—is a mark of adulthood. When a person begins to have difficulty with these activities, it is undoubtedly very distressing and must feel like a loss of adult status. Naturally, the person will continue to try to be independent, to stand on his or her own as a capable adult.

As abilities decrease, increased help from caregivers is needed. However, this does not change the person's normal, adult need to be as independent as possible and to have control over private and personal activities. For example, when Ben was told to go to the bathroom, he was offended and refused to go. He needed to have control of this personal activity. Yet, when he was given a sense of control (i.e., when he was gently reminded to go the bathroom), he was very cooperative.

Treating the Person with Respect Is Essential

Persons with dementia must feel a terrible sense of loss about their failing abilities and decreasing independence. There is no reason for them to lose their dignity and respect as well. In fact, this is all the more reason to honor the person's dignity. When Rachel and her husband made jokes at Ben's expense, he was embarrassed and became increasingly confused and upset. If someone chatted with him about the photos of his new grandson, Ben became a confident and cheerful social companion.

Maintaining Lifelong Routines and Habits Helps the Person Do as Much as Possible

Maintaining lifelong routines can be compared to recalling a song from years gone by. Although we may remember the tune and perhaps some of the words, we would probably have difficulty singing the whole song on our own. However, if we hear the song played, we fall right into the rhythm and the

words seem to come unsummoned. The person with dementia may not be able to recall the notes or the complete lyrics
(i.e., the steps and the order) of a once-familiar activity, such
as getting dressed. However, playing out these activities in the
familiar rhythm of life habits helps to trigger participation.
Details that may seem of no significance to us and may have
even lost their once-practical value, can mean a great deal to
the person with dementia. For example, Ben's pillowcase
dressing did not serve an actual purpose but it was an important part of his personal routine. It helped him to feel capable
and in charge of his own care. Think about the little rituals
and preferences in your own routines—how much they mean
to you and how they help you to function.

Individuals Have Different Thoughts About Which Activities and Ways of Doing These Activities Are Most Important

Some people value being able to do as much for themselves as
possible no matter how big the struggle or how long it takes.
Others are happy to be taken care of or to have help with
housework. They would rather spend their time visiting with
friends or doing hobbies. As dementia progresses, although
people may have difficulty telling others about these lifelong
preferences, they remain very important. This is when the
personal information from a family caregiver is so important
(as suggested in the All About Me form in Appendix A). It is
important to balance the time spent in the various aspects of
life activities. The nature of this balance depends on the person's lifelong preferences.

There Are Ways to Help the Person with Daily Activities, but These Require Special Skills and Flexibility

Some people have a natural gift for providing care for persons
with dementia; however, for most of us, understanding the

special care needs of someone with dementia requires training. For very few people, such as Rachel, it seems to be very
difficult, if not impossible, to learn different ways of caring.
This is not a character fault; we all have different strengths.
Not everyone is cut out to provide care for people with
dementia. It is a special skill that some can learn and some
seem not to be able to learn.

The first step in learning to provide dementia care is trying
to understand that the person has a brain condition that
affects how he or she acts. The person is not being difficult
on purpose but is just trying the best that he or she can to get
by with a damaged brain. Before anything else, caregivers
need to enter into the moment with the person with dementia. As Leitha pointed out in the Preface, it's necessary to
"walk a mile in the other person's shoes." Please see Chapter
2 for more details.

Many things can be done to help the person with dementia
to maintain a familiar lifestyle and to be as independent as
possible in the activities of daily living. The general suggestions in Chapter 6 all come in to play. The sections that follow provide specific suggestions for particular activities.

Sexuality[6]

*Alberta says that she and Alan, who has early stage
Alzheimer's disease, have not had intercourse in more
than a year. This is a tremendous loss in their relationship and for her. However, she finds it better just to let
go of this particular aspect of their sexual relationship. On several prior occasions when Alan had tried to have sex, he was unable
to maintain an erection and both partners were upset and tearful.*

---

[6]Portions of this section previously appeared in Bowlby Sifton, C. (2000c). Caregiving
challenges: Sexuality and persons with dementia. *Alzheimer's Care Quarterly, 1*(2), 87–90;
adapted by permission.

Often now at bedtime, Alan says, "I suppose you have cramps, dear?" Alberta gracefully says "yes," and they share warm cuddles and caresses.

Sexuality is a normal adult function and a need. Humans are by nature sexual beings; expressing our sexuality is an essential part of life. As with Alan and Alberta, sexuality is often a topic of concern to persons with dementia and their caregivers. It is a private and personal activity and a topic that most people, particularly those of the older generation, do not feel comfortable discussing. Many older couples have never talked, even with each other, about their sexual relationship. Unfortunately, until recently, there has been little discussion—in print or in person—about ways to support the sexual needs of persons with dementia and their caregivers. Yet, sexuality is such an important aspect of life.

When one partner develops dementia, sexual expression changes just as most other aspects of the relationship change. Both partners still have needs, but previous practices may no longer be satisfying or possible. If the relationship (sexual and otherwise) has already been difficult, it can be even more challenging to cope with these changes. Because sexual intercourse involves many complex brain and body interactions, the person with dementia may no longer be able to perform, although he or she may try. Women may experience decreased vaginal lubrication, and men may have difficulty maintaining an erection. This is embarrassing and frustrating for both partners.

Conversely, due to damage to the frontal areas of the brain, a small number of persons with dementia may experience increased arousal. This can become embarrassing and difficult for the partner, especially if the person has lost some sense of social control. The person may request sex in public from his or her partner or others, masturbate in public, or make inappropriate sexual comments that are completely out of keeping with the person's behavior before the onset of dementia. All caregivers are called on to remember that the person has a brain condition that causes such changes in behavior. The person is not a sex fiend but someone with a brain condition and an unmet need. Realize that the person may:

- Have unmet needs for caring and affection or for understanding him- or herself as a sexual being
- Miss the love and companionship of a spouse or partner
- Come from a culture where or time when making such sexual comments were acceptable
- Not have privacy for sexual expression
- Be so upset with the losses and changes he or she is experiencing that expressing sexual prowess becomes extra important

In addition, understand that brain damage may cause the person to:

- Not realize that he or she is in a public place and should not carry out private activities such as masturbation
- Have difficulty getting to the bathroom (taking off clothing or unzipping pants in public can actually mean that the person needs to go to the bathroom)
- Use inappropriate means to address discomfort (trying to remove clothing may be an attempt to get comfortable)
- Have difficulty expressing sexual needs in appropriate ways
- Think that the provision of personal care is actually a sexual overture from the caregiver

- Lose previous social inhibitions and controls (e.g., the person may have always thought, "What a gorgeous woman—would I ever like to get her in bed"; brain damage may cause the person to say that out loud and perhaps even to act on it)
- Think that you are a lover or partner from the past

Meeting your partner's sexual needs when you are also a caregiver can be very difficult. Many say that although they care deeply for their partner, becoming his or her caregiver has taken away their sexual desire for the person. Caregivers need to be reassured that these feelings are natural and they need not feel guilty.

When one partner has dementia, the ways that couples express their sexuality inevitably change. You are not alone. You are also not alone in your need to receive and give affection, to express your sexuality. It is a universal human need. However, ways to continue with expressions of sexuality and affection are unique to your relationship. Try to adapt and change past practices so your partner can participate and respond. Nurture other affirming relationships. Often a burden shared is a burden lifted. Talking about sexuality concerns with a trusted friend, another caregiver, or an understanding professional can help to relieve feelings of guilt and may lead to some positive changes. For more information on taking care of yourself and your needs, please see Chapter 1.

Intercourse is but one aspect of expressing sexuality. There are many other essential ways of expressing and experiencing sexuality in a relationship. Feeling cherished and respected and sharing these sentiments through touches, hugs, and close times together is the foundation of a healthy expression of sexuality. These aspects can be explored and enriched. Although Alberta misses love making, she has found satisfaction through hugs, cuddles, holding hands, and sharing quiet times with Alan. Alan has responded to her openness about continuing their sexual relationship in these ways. Alberta cherishes his touches and warm smiles.

Unfortunately, again it is usually the caregiving partner who needs to take the initiative. The person with dementia may not take initiative because of fear of failure or loss of ability. For the most part, the partner will only be disappointed if he or she waits for the person with dementia to express his or her affection first. However, the person with dementia does understand the genuine expression of affection from another and almost always responds in kind.

With the partner as the initiator, some couples are able to continue with familiar patterns of togetherness and intimacy. For instance, one man with dementia had always washed and brushed his arthritic wife's hair. When he could no longer organize this activity, they still sat on the couch together, and when she handed him a hair brush, he lovingly brushed her hair.

Yet, some caregivers have been further challenged by how to communicate the intent of these caring actions to the person with dementia. Some persons with dementia may think that these expressions of affection are an invitation to intercourse and feel either incompetent if they can't perform or rejected if they attempt to initiate sex and are turned down. Solutions to these complex communication issues are unique to each couple. In these cases, the help of a sensitive and caring friend or professional may be needed. Beyond empathetic support, some couples may benefit from referral to a qualified sex therapist. Unfortunately, such therapists, especially those who also understand dementia, remain scarce.

For caregivers who are not partners, the topic of sexuality can be particularly challenging. Adult children, who are often not accustomed to thinking of their parents as sexual beings, may be embarrassed by the topic, let alone any changes in their parent's behaviors. A daughter who may look like a younger version of her mother is understandably shocked if her father makes sexual comments to her. It is important to emphasize that there is brain damage; the father may see his daughter as the wife he fell in love with years ago. In the event that a parent with dementia makes such a remark, the immediate response depends on the situation. Stepping back and firmly saying something such as, "Dad, I know you miss Mom a lot, and I am sorry. I am your daughter Susan, and I will take care of you as best I can." It may then be best to suggest a favorite activity—such as a walk, a game of cards, or a snack—as a diversion. To prevent this from happening in the future, the daughter may try not to act or talk in any way that would trigger her father to respond this way. However, she should continue providing daughterly expressions of affection and respect. Other preventive measures that caregivers should implement include the following:

- Ensure that the person has ample opportunity to feel cherished, special, and valued.
- Help the person to express emotions and feelings.
- Always explain who you are and what you are doing, especially when doing personal care activities and invading personal space.
- Treat the person with dignity and respect.
- Avoid situations that may be misinterpreted (e.g., providing care while sitting close to the person on the bed).
- Ensure that the person has privacy.

If inappropriate sexual comments or gestures do occur, however, keep the following in mind:

- Reject the behavior, not the person. It is best to say something such as "John, please don't talk to me that way. I find it embarrassing and hurtful." Depending on the person, the caregiver should either leave the situation or divert the person's attention to another activity.
- Never treat sexual comments as a joke or encourage inappropriate sexual banter.
- In congregate care situations, switch care assignments, if possible, if one particular staff member always seems to trigger this response.
- Gently redirect the person to a private space if he or she is masturbating or undressing in a public place.
- Have a medical review to determine if the behavior is caused by illness or medication.

Another challenging situation can arise when the person with dementia at a long-term care facility develops a relationship with another resident. This can be particularly hurtful if the person's spouse is still alive. There is no right or wrong way to respond, as long as it is done with sensitivity to the needs of all partners. Things to think about include the following:

- Does the new relationship meet the needs of both persons with dementia in a respectful way, or is one possibly being taken advantage of?
- Are staff responding with respect?
- Are there other ways to meet the person's need for love and affection?

Meeting Needs

The act of sex is only one way that we experience ourselves as sexual beings. Being touched and hugged and being spoken to with respect and affection are even more important. Continuing or developing special times together—for example, looking at family pictures, listening to music, dancing, and sitting together on the couch while watching television—are all important ways that partners can continue to express sexuality.

A person with dementia also benefits from the expressions of affection and caring touch from others. The primary caregiver usually knows how to best offer caring touch and can be a model for other family members and caregivers. In addition, sexuality is closely connected with self-esteem. All of the losses and disabilities that a person with dementia is experiencing, mean that he or she especially needs to be buoyed up. Ways that are described in this and other chapters—such as recalling past accomplishments, having meaningful things to do, and having opportunities to give to others—can be used to support the person's self-esteem. The person needs to get a strong message from others that he or she is valued, worthwhile, loved, and cared about for who he or she is at this moment. Complimenting the person, on anything from her lovely hair to his important accomplishment in the past, is one of the best and easiest ways to support the sense of self.

A Word Regarding Paid Caregivers

As outsiders to the family and personal culture, concerns about sexuality are especially tricky for paid caregivers to handle. Professional caregivers must be careful not to impose their personal values and norms about sexuality on persons with dementia and their family caregivers.

If inappropriate sexual behavior does occur, it is essential for a paid caregiver to seek understanding and to keep the event in perspective. The degree or frequency of inappropriate sexual behavior can easily be exaggerated because it tends to cause a great deal of stress and embarrassment for all involved. It is helpful to try to understand the behavior both from the point of view of the person and with regard to the effects of brain damage.

Bathing

Bathing is generally the first daily personal care activity that the person with dementia will find difficult. This is understandable because it is a difficult activity made of many steps. It is also a personal and private activity that is closely tied to being an independent adult. Both the person and the caregiver may be embarrassed once taking a bath independently becomes challenging for the person. The person with dementia will likely be embarrassed and frustrated. You will likely find that help with bathing represents a real crossing over into a new role. Whatever your previous relationship (spouse, adult child, or friend), it was as adults—a relationship that seldom involves helping with personal activities such as bathing. Many caregivers find it easier and more comfortable to use paid caregivers, if possible, for assistance with bathing.

Suggestions for Helping the Person to Continue with Bathing

Maintain Lifelong Bathing Routines

Help the person organize his or her normal bathing time. Some people shower first thing in the morning; others prefer a warm bath at night before bed. If the person has always taken a sponge bath, this can continue if he or she is willing to let you help.

By sharing as much information as possible about personal bathing habits, family caregivers can be a tremendous help to paid caregivers. Most people have amazingly detailed routines that are based on years of habit. Maintaining lifelong habits promotes comfort and helps the person to participate. Think about the following questions to help the person to continue with personal routines:

- What time of day did the person usually bathe?
- What type of bathing did the person do (e.g., sponge bath, shower, tub bath)?
- How often did the person bathe?
- Did the person take his or her clothes into the bathroom and dress there or return to the bedroom for dressing?
- What type of soap and shampoo does the person prefer?
- Does the person use powder or body cream?
- For men: Did the person shave before, during, or after bathing?
- For women: Did the person shave her legs and underarms? If so, when and how was this done?

Protect the Person's Privacy

Give the person as much private time as possible. At first, the person may just need help getting everything ready (e.g., preparing his or her clothes, towels, and bath water). As more help is required (e.g., with undressing or washing), find ways to cover the person, such as using towels or having the person wear an old bath robe while bathing. Because you are invading personal space, always let the person know why you are there and what you are doing.

Ensure the Person's Dignity

No matter how much help the person may need, he or she should always be treated with respect and as an adult. Bathing is perhaps the best activity for you to stand in the other person's shoes and think about how you would like to be treated.

Provide Opportunities for Personal Control and Independence

There is always a chance for personal choice and control, even when a person requires full assistance with bathing. Even a person with advanced dementia can hold a washcloth, thereby receiving a sense of control and participation. Caregivers also can enable control by giving the person a choice between two things (e.g., clothing items, different towels).

Make Bathing a Pleasurable Experience for the Person

Bath time is the perfect opportunity to bring pleasure through the senses. Is the bathroom itself pleasant, colorful, and warm (in both temperature and appearance)? Use big, fluffy, comfortable towels in the person's favorite colors. Provide pleasant scents from soaps and lotions, taking precautions for allergies and sensitivities as necessary. Provide favorite calming music.

Prepare Bathing Materials in Advance

Because bathing is so complicated and may be stressful for you and the person you are caring for, it is especially important to have everything organized in advance. Lay out clothing, towels, soap, and so forth. Draw the bath water or have the shower running to avoid delays, and give the person an extra hint about what is taking place.

Separate Bathing and Hair Washing

In some cases, hair washing may be causing distress at bath time. Hair washing can be approached many different ways:

take a real or simulated trip to the beauty parlor, wash hair at the sink, use a special basin to wash it while the person is lying in bed, or use dry shampoo products. Short, thin hair can be washed with a washcloth and rinseless soap.

No matter how much effort caregivers put into these suggestions, bathing can become a challenge. If this happens, applying the steps of problem solving may help you focus on the situation and the possible solutions, not just on your frustrations (see Chapter 9).

Toileting

This chapter's opening story shared how Ben had difficulty getting to the bathroom on time. The brain damage caused by dementia eventually makes it difficult to follow through on the numerous steps involved: attending to the signal that the bladder is full, finding the bathroom, removing undergarments, and so forth. However, in most cases, helping the person to get to the toilet every 2 hours can help prevent accidents, which is what the day program staff did for Ben. If this has no effect or if the person suddenly becomes incontinent, take the person to his or her doctor. There could be an infection or other physical problem.

Challenges with toileting mean that the person with dementia is at risk of developing a urinary tract infection. To prevent this, it is important to help with proper toileting hygiene and to be sure that the person drinks a lot of fluids. Cranberry juice is especially good, as its acidity helps prevent infections from developing. Like any other physical illness, a urinary tract infection is of particular concern because persons with dementia are often unable to tell caregivers about their symptoms. Watch for other signs of infection and immediately call them to the attention of a doctor. Increased restlessness or agitation, frequent attempts to go the bathroom, foul-smelling urine, and signs of pain and discomfort when attempting to urinate may indicate a urinary tract infection.

Establish a Regular Bathroom Routine

Set up a schedule for toileting that matches the person's life-long pattern and help the person to follow it. This can help prevent incontience. Remind the person or assist him or her to the bathroom every 2 hours. Give special reminders first thing in the morning, after meals, and before bedtime.

This is a very sensitive issue, and the manner in which reminders are given makes a huge difference. Some people may take offense at suggestions that they need help getting to the bathroom. Make suggestions quietly and privately; protecting dignity and being respectful are key. The following wording can be used while gently taking the person's arm and walking toward the bathroom:

- "Let's head to the bathroom before we go for our walk."
- "I will help you walk to the bathroom."
- "Come with me to the bathroom."
- "Let's go this way and get washed up for breakfast."

Once in the bathroom, proceed toward the toilet, using mostly nonverbal clues. If necessary, help the person to take down his or her undergarments. Once the person is seated on the toilet or standing in front of it (as the case may be for men), he or she can be offered privacy.

You may need to remain with persons who have short attention spans so they will stay seated. Use conversation or activities such as looking at a magazine or photos as a diversion. Keep favorite items in the bathroom just for this purpose. The person may also need help in using toilet paper afterward. Sometimes, just handing the person the paper is enough; other times, he or she may need your assistance in wiping. Keep disposable rubber gloves on hand. The person is more likely to need help if he or she is not at home. In public washrooms, use the wheelchair-accessible stall so that you have room to offer this help.

For some people, it is helpful to use the terms they may have previously used when referring to the bathroom. Common alternative expressions that have been used include the head, the loo, the john, the can, the little girl's room, or even going to see a man about a horse. However, always be sure to protect dignity by using these expressions in only the most adult tone.

Offer Plenty of Fluids During the Day

Drinking water and juices is a good health practice in general. It also helps with continence, as it keeps the bladder healthy and increases the feeling of having a full bladder. The person may need reminders to drink. Remember that drinks with caffeine (e.g., coffee, tea, cola) are actually diuretics. They empty the system of fluid and increase the frequency of having to go the bathroom. Grapefruit juice is also a diuretic. Reduce fluid intake closer to bedtime and try to avoid fluids altogether 2 hours before bedtime.

Make Sure the Bathroom Is Easy to Find

People who urinate in wastebaskets, closets, and flowerpots may be unable to locate the bathroom or identify the toilet. A clear sign or a brightly painted or decorated door may help. Because these kinds of decorations don't help the person identify the bathroom when looking down the hall, some kind of three-dimensional sign or decoration that sticks out from the wall may help. Install a night light to guide the way, but be sure that the night light doesn't cause extra confusion. Put a lid on the waste basket, lock closet doors, and remove other items that may be confusing.

Make the Bathroom a Pleasant and Easy-to-Understand Place

Simple and inexpensive decorating changes, such as softer lighting from a lamp (rather than an overhead light), warmer colors from paint or a wallpaper border, potpourri, curtains, plants, pictures, and a book and magazine rack can change the bathroom from an uninviting place to a pleasant space. Because the person with dementia may associate the bathroom with failure and humiliation (due to difficulties with bathing and toileting), creating a pleasant atmosphere can make a big difference in changing these negative associations.

At the same time, care should be taken not to overstimulate the person with too-busy décor. It is especially important that the toilet and sink are obvious and easy to find. Due to changes in perception, a light-colored toilet on a light-colored floor against a light-colored wall may simply disappear. Contrasting colors will help. For example, outline the toilet with colored tape and use a different-colored toilet seat or seat cover. Although good lighting is important, lighting that is too bright and reflects off shiny surfaces can be problematic because of changes to the aging eye and perceptual changes caused by dementia. Some people may find the glare so disorienting that they won't go in the bathroom at all. Shiny floors and countertops should be avoided. Mirrors, especially large ones, can also be a problem. The person may no longer recognize him- or herself and become frightened and disoriented by seeing "another person" in the bathroom.

Toilet paper roll holders and towel bars that may be used for grab bars should be replaced with actual grab bars. Other

safety equipment, such as raised toilet seats and bath benches, may be helpful, but if they are unfamiliar, they may cause
confusion. They should only be added if absolutely necessary,
and repeated practice in use is required. An occupational
therapist can advise on this and other safety equipment.

Provide Easy-to-Remove Clothing

Pants and skirts with elastic waistbands and loosely fitting
undergarments make it easier to prepare to go to the bathroom. It can become a challenge for a man to manage a zip-
pered fly. Sports pants with elastic waistbands are a socially
acceptable alternative. Males with dementia may have difficulty urinating while standing up and/or managing the flies
on their pants and underwear. Yet, because of habit and
prostate problems that can come with aging, it may be important to help the person to continue standing. Providing a grab
bar near the toilet at the proper height can help. Others may
have more success with using a urinal.

Always Have a Change of Clothes
Handy, Especially When Going Out

Accidents cause everyone embarrassment, especially the person with dementia. Having clean clothes at the ready helps to
reduce embarrassment. Assist the person and offer reassurance. There is no point in scolding, as incontinence is a disease symptom. Scolding will just cause further humiliation
and add a negative tone to your relationship.

Watch for Signs that the Person
May Have to Go to the Bathroom

Restlessness, pacing, and fidgeting with clothing may indicate
that the person has to go to the bathroom. The signs are par-

ticular to each individual and, thus, must be shared with other caregivers.

Use Incontinence Products

Incontinence products, such as adult briefs and mattress and chair protectors, are available in most drug and department stores. There is a wide variety of these products; finding the most suitable one may take several tries. The least noticeable and most socially acceptable items are small pads that fasten to underwear and are used for stress or dribbling incontinence. There are several brands that are like disposable briefs or underwear, which again are socially acceptable. These have the advantage of being easier for the person to manage independently. They also come in several weights. Home care or home health store staff are often a good source of advice for deciding which product would be best. Some even provide free trial samples.

Protecting dignity is key, and the names used for these products make a big difference. They can be called briefs or underwear. There is never a need to humiliate the person by calling them diapers.

If the person is unsteady or has difficulty walking, a commode chair can be handy to have in the bedroom. A commode chair can be kept in an out-of-the-way place on the main floor if the bathroom is upstairs. The disadvantage is that it is not familiar and the person needs practice to learn how to use it.

Use washable chair covers or cover cushions by placing plastic underneath the covers. If you fear a favorite chair or rug will be damaged, remove it.

Bowel incontinence may cause the most embarrassment, but in many ways, it is easier to maintain bowel continence, especially if the person had regular habits. Follow the person's habits by taking him or her to the bathroom at the usual time for a bowel movement. A healthy diet with plenty of fiber (e.g., from bran, fruits, vegetables, whole grains, and seeds—especially flax) and fluids helps keep the person regular. Exercise, even just walking around the house, is also important. Diet and exercise are always better than laxatives or other measures, as the bowel can become dependent on these means. If the person has problems with irregular bowel movements (i.e., too many or too few), consult his or her physician.

Maintaining continence at night is another challenge. Again, it is important to know the person's lifelong habits. If the person always had to get up at night, it is good to check on him or her just before the usual nocturnal waking time and help the person to the bathroom. This approach disturbs the caregiver's sleep, however, so you may prefer to protect the bed and use special, extra-absorbent nighttime incontinence products. Keeping a commode chair and/or a urinal near the bedside can be a help. As long as the person doesn't have skin problems, there is little to be gained by waking a sleeping person to change him or her. If the person does experience incontinence during the night, it is extra important to help him or her wash properly in the morning.

Dressing

My mother-in-law Alice always took pride in her appearance and enjoyed getting dressed up. She loved clothes, and she loved to look nice. When she developed Alzheimer's disease, she continued to try to look her best but sometimes couldn't get it all together. One Sunday morning when we picked her up for church, she was all dressed in a beautiful suit with no blouse underneath. Because the jacket didn't have buttons, she knew something was wrong and had tried to fix the situation by using safety pins. She knew there was a problem, so it was easy to suggest that she could look even more lovely by wearing a blouse that I'd help her put on.

As Alzheimer's disease progressed, dressing presented another challenge for Alice. She almost always wore the same two outfits. She liked the beautiful new clothes that I helped her to pick out when we went shopping, but they just stayed in her closet. As her favorite outfits became worn and shabby, I upped the campaign for Alice to wear her new clothes. She kept saying that she was saving them, and after far too long, I realized that this issue was my concern, a problem that I was creating. Alice was perfectly happy in her favorite outfits; they were reassuring. I needed to stop being embarrassed about what others might think.

Like everyone, persons with dementia like to try to look their best. Sometimes caregivers need to fill in the blank spots when the person's efforts don't quite meet the mark. However, our efforts to help need to be based on what matters most to the person. For instance, like Alice, the person may take a liking to a particular item of clothing, such as a pair of pants. Buy several pairs to ensure that there is always a clean one. Remove seldom-worn clothing from the closet.

Help the Person to Maintain Old Habits

As with every activity, following the person's previous routines is very important. If the person usually dressed after breakfast, try to continue this routine. Introduce as little change as possible. In addition, avoid delays or interruptions in the morning routine. These can cause the person to forget the activity in which he or she is involved.

Remember that Dress Is Connected with Self-Image

Try to help the person to continue with the style of dress that he or she preferred. For instance, Alice never really took to wearing pants. She always felt much better about herself when wearing a dress or a skirt, even though doing so was more complicated and didn't seem very comfortable to me. Whatever is appropriate and familiar is usually best.

In addition, frequently compliment the person about his or her appearance. This supports self-esteem and encourages the person to continue trying to look his or her best.

Create a Feeling of Privacy

Privacy is especially important if the person needs help with dressing. Shut the bedroom or bathroom door and pull the curtains or blinds.

Encourage the Person to Participate

There is always a way for the person to be involved. For example, he or she can finish pulling up a pair pants after being helped into the leg holes. Or, he or she can simply hold onto an item, such as a belt, while you are assisting with another article of clothing. In this case, you would give the cue (e.g., "Would you please hold this belt for me?").

Remember that Choice Is Essential

Providing choice helps the person to feel in control of the activity. However, persons with dementia may be overwhelmed by the difficulty of opening the closet door and deciding what to wear. Caregivers can help to narrow the choice by picking out two favorite items and offering a choice between them. For people who have always been interested in coordinated outfits, hanging coordinated tops and bottoms on the same hanger may help the person make independent choices.

In the morning, lay out the person's clothing in the order that each item must be put on, ensuring that all articles of clothing are right side out. This will give the person hints on what to do first. Unless it is a lifelong pattern, laying clothing out the night before is not recommended; the person may think that it is time to get dressed instead of time to go to bed.

If necessary, help to begin the activity by, for example, starting the person's arm in one shirt sleeve. This may be the only cue that is needed for the person to finish putting on the shirt. Complicated buttons can be replaced with Velcro fasteners or zippers if fine motor coordination is becoming a problem. However, if a person has never used Velcro before, it may create a problem rather than solve one.

Keep clothing in the same location that the person has always used, and keep his or her dresser drawers organized in the same manner. It can be very helpful for persons in residential care environments to have their own dresser from home, with the drawers organized just as they always were. Keep the room as clear from clutter as possible to lessen confusion.

Labeling dresser drawers and closets may be helpful for some people. Be sure to do this sensitively to avoid offending the person. Involving him or her in the activity of creating and affixing the labels can help. This could be a decorating project, with the person and the caregiver making use of attractive labels. Perhaps the project would be more acceptable for the person if a grandchild was involved in getting suitable pictures for making découpage labels.

Some persons with dementia find it satisfying to work at reordering and reorganizing dresser drawers. However, this may interfere with the caregiver's attempts to keep items for daily dressing organized and easy to find. If this is the case, try having a drawer or two—or a whole dresser—filled with items (e.g., socks to sort) that the person can freely reorganize. Keep daily items in less accessible or locked drawers that are opened only when the person needs them.

Provide comfortable, easy-to-manage clothing. Use skirts or pants with elastic waistbands to facilitate ease of use, especially for toileting. Try to find such clothing in styles and colors that the person prefers.

Putting on a bra can become too complicated for the woman with dementia, and helping her can be embarrassing for you and her. There are various solutions here, depending on the person. Some women may be perfectly happy and comfortable wearing an undershirt or a camisole. It helps if these items are introduced positively, perhaps as a gift, and selected according to the person's tastes. For example, some women may respond to the comfort and coziness of a soft undershirt. Others may be more interested in a pretty, feminine camisole. For those who may be physically or socially uncomfortable without a bra, it may be possible to change the style of bra—for example, a front-closing bra or a looser fitting one made of softer fabric.

Adaptive clothing manufacturers can be of help with wrap-around dresses, skirts, and nightgowns. Please see Appendix B for catalogs that provide such resources.

Shoes and stockings can also present challenges. Knee-high stockings or socks may be easier than nylons for women to manage, but make sure they are not too tight at the top. Tube socks solve the problem of finding the heel. Some persons may have adapted to challenges with putting on shoes by wearing loose fitting slippers or socks. However, this is a safety risk, especially as the person develops problems with balance and coordination. The person should wear supportive, comfortable shoes that are easy to get on and off. If new shoes need to be introduced, offer the person choices within a suitable range, and try to make the occasion a positive and fun experience. New shoes should be broken in gradually by having the person wear them for a few minutes longer every day.

Velcro fasteners can be convenient for the person and/or the caregiver. Elastic shoelaces can be used to turn any lace-up shoe into a pull-on shoe. These have the advantage of maintaining a familiar style. The disadvantage is that either the caregiver will need to help or the person will need to learn a new method for putting on shoes. In some cases, it is easier just to help with tying shoes. For some people, there may be a particular challenge around issues of style. For instance, women who have always worn heels may not only want to continue with this but may actually have a shortened Achilles tendon that makes wearing flat shoes painful. In this case, change to lower heels gradually, starting perhaps with wedge heels. Stylish pumps that the person helps choose are a good alternative. Donning party shoes for special occasions is ' important to some individuals, and this should be continued. Chances are that once the person gets used to the feel and comfort of more "sensible" shoes, she will be quite happy.

Address Attempts to Undress

In a few cases, the person with dementia may keep trying to take off his or her clothes. The first response is to try to figure out the reason behind the behavior. The person may be uncomfortable (i.e., clothing is too tight), may be hot or cold, or may need to go to the bathroom. This may also be the first sign that the person is getting sick, and his or her physical health should be checked.

It could also be that the person needs more control over selecting the clothes that he or she wears. Offering the person manageable choices and frequently complimenting the person's appearance throughout the day can help to overcome this challenge.

If these causes are ruled out, it could be that the person is bored and is providing self-stimulation by doing something

with his or her hands. Try introducing items for self-stimu-
lating, repetitive activities, such as a purse or wallet with
interesting items inside (see Chapter 8 for further suggestions). Conversely, the person could be distressed by an environment that is overstimulating, and this is how he or she is
responding to this stress. Modifying the environment can
help.

It may be that none of these solutions will help and caregivers will need to do some creative problem solving. For
example, in one long-term care facility, caregivers tried many
responses to this challenge, but the only thing that really
worked was telling the resident that the facility's rabbi wanted
her to leave her clothes on. In some cases, one-piece jump
suits or clothing fastened in the back may be needed. If the
person was getting stimulation from unfastening clothing,
remember to present him or her with other interesting things
to do (see Chapter 8).

Grooming

Grooming activities—taking care of hair and teeth, shaving,
and putting on makeup—are the final touches of looking and
feeling good. As with all other personal activities, everyone
has his or her own habits and routines; because these routines
are complicated, they can become difficult to maintain as
dementia advances.

Maintain Lifelong Habits and Routines

Doing hair and makeup and shaving are incredibly important
and can be amazingly detailed, right down to the type of hairbrush or toothpaste used. It is best never to make assumptions
based on your own habits and preferences. We are all so different. For example, for many women, going to the hair-
dresser and having someone else do their hair is a treat; for

me, it is torture. I have a sensitive scalp and can't tolerate any-one brushing my hair. Furthermore, I dislike the whole experience—for instance, the smell of the chemicals used for permanents makes me sick. If my future caregivers don't know this, it will be a problem. Yet, Alice found going to the hair-dresser relaxing and uplifting. Family caregivers need to think hard about these details and share them with other caregivers. (See the All About Me form in Appendix A.)

Help the Person to Feel Involved and in Control

Doing hair and makeup and shaving are intensely personal activities, which makes it especially difficult when help is needed. If you have ever experienced dependence yourself, you are probably well aware that no one else can really ever comb your hair or brush your teeth just the way you would like it done.

In every activity, for every person, there is a way for them to feel in control, to make decisions. Encourage and support the person to do whichever parts of the activity he or she can manage. For example, let the person towel dry his or her hair after it is shampooed, rub on after-shave, or brush his or her hair. When hands-on physical help with grooming activities is needed, holding a hair brush, toothbrush, or razor in the person's hand, even if he or she is unable to use it, gives a sense of control and personal involvement. The person can participate by passing items (e.g., a comb, a piece of jewelry) to the caregiver. Even these small acts bring a feeling of involvement. The person can also make choices about which brush to use, which type of after-shave to use, or which color of lipstick to wear.

One way to help the person do such activities is to break the activity down into several steps and give the person directions, one step at a time. Use short simple directions, and use the same words and order every time. This can be difficult, so it can help to write down the exact directions on a cue card. Of course, it can take far too long for you as a busy caregiver to guide the person through all of these steps, one at a time. However, you can start at a step partway through. As noted previously, a lot of tooth-brushing steps can be skipped by starting with the toothpaste already on the brush.

When assisting with routines, it is important to **be generous with compliments.** This supports self-esteem and encourages the person to continue to be involved.

Encourage Reminiscence and Call Attention to the Senses

When assisting females with dementia, doing their hair and makeup is a perfect opportunity to help them recall favorite outfits, hairstyles, or dress-up occasions. This type of reminiscence is also a great boost for self-esteem.

Grooming activities are also rich sensory opportunities. Caregivers can use sensory stimulation techniques (see Chapter 6) to draw the person's attention to the smell of the after-shave, the feel of the hand lotion, or the color of the hairbrush and then to encourage participation. Using reminiscence and focusing on the senses helps to turn the grooming activity into a pleasant personal time with the caregiver and will encourage future participation.

Eating

Eating is unique among self-care activities. There is no doubt that it is essential for maintaining life. But beyond this, there is no doubt that eating is a vital, life-sustaining activity from a social point of view. There is much more to the experience of eating than just taking in calories and nutrients. In most societies, people gather together and share food not just for special celebrations but also as an essential social activity of everyday life. In many families, the main meal is a time for sharing the day's activities and news, for catching up with each other. For most people with dementia, the evening meal was a central social time in their pasts. Although busy schedules, take-out food, and eating on the run mean these patterns may be changing in modern households, sharing food together continues to be an important social time for most older people.

As dementia progresses, the person will begin to have difficulty eating independently. Unfortunately, this can lead to the person's exclusion from mealtimes with others. This is a devastating loss of an irreplaceable social time. The process of sharing food together with others is at least as important as the end product (i.e., nutrients from a finished meal). In addition, without the familiar social cues of eating with others, the person's feeding skills may further decline and cause a further decrease in appetite.

It is much better to do everything possible to adapt mealtimes to suit the person's needs. This keeps the person connected with an essential life activity and important people. It also usually means that he or she remains independent longer and has a better appetite. Some suggestions follow for helping the person to continue being a part of the life-affirming activity of eating.

Support Personal Control and Opportunities for Choice

Sylvia came into the care facility's assessment unit with a very unusual problem. She would not swallow her food. Her husband had tried everything he could think of, and a thorough medical check had been done. There

was no physical reason keeping Sylvia from swallowing. She would take food in her mouth and then, after chewing it a bit, she would go over to the garbage can and spit it out. There was only a slight improvement when she was given small amounts on her plate or finger foods such as sandwiches. Stimulating her salivary glands did not seem to make any difference, either.

I wish I could say that I thought of the change that did make a difference, but, in fact, Sylvia showed me herself. Sylvia was part of a small dining group in a residential facility where the goal was to use a home-like dining environment to encourage eating and socializing. One day, Sylvia reached over and picked up an orange from the basket of fruit on the table. I watched with interest as she peeled and sectioned the orange. I watched with amazement as she put the orange sections in her mouth, chewed, and swallowed them. She ate the whole orange and did not spit any of it out! I was so excited by this response that I presented Sylvia with bread, a jar of peanut butter, and a knife. Sylvia made herself a peanut butter sandwich, which she also chewed and swallowed. Based on this experience, we were able to work with the dietician to come up with a healthy menu where Sylvia could somehow prepare her own food. As long as Sylvia could do this, she swallowed everything.

Some background on this unusual story is helpful. Years before, Sylvia's brother had choked on a fish bone and died. Of course, this was very upsetting for Sylvia, but it didn't really interfere with her life at the time. It is hard to know for sure, but it seems that when Sylvia developed dementia, she had some deep memory of her brother choking and she became fearful of the same thing happening to her. Her fear of choking led her to stop swallowing her food. However, involving Sylvia and giving her some control over the preparation of her food seemed to settle her fears.

This is a dramatic illustration not only of the importance of ensuring that the person feels in control but also of knowing the person's history. Our food preferences and ways and times of eating are highly individual and can have a big influence on appetite and consumption. By supporting lifelong food habits, caregivers can help mealtimes to be a celebration and encourage the person to continue to feed him- or herself. Sharing information about food habits and preferences with paid caregivers is vital to the person's well-being, especially as dementia progresses. Please see the All About Me form in Appendix A.

By using this information, caregivers also can support the person's dignity and independence by offering opportunities for manageable choices at mealtimes. There are dozens of possibilities—would the person like a ham sandwich or tuna sandwich? White bread or whole wheat bread? Tea or coffee? An important and long-standing element of choice and control at mealtime is serving yourself. If the meal is served family style, help the person to serve him- or herself from bowls and platters. If the household style has been to present the whole meal to each person on his or her plate, continue to consult, as you would have done in the past, about serving sizes and so forth. Other opportunities for choice are allowing the person to take relishes, pickles, and side dishes; a roll from a basket; or a cookie from a plate. These opportunities for choice are very important to people with dementia.

Joe, who had Huntington's-related dementia, showed me the impact of such simple choices. Joe was mostly nonverbal, and his uncontrollable movements made it very difficult for him to feed himself. He often refused to eat when staff tried to feed him. We were all concerned, as Joe was already very thin and needed more calories, not fewer, because of the energy used by the constant movement of his arms and legs. Although Joe was unable to participate in meal preparation, I invited him to our once-a-week breakfast club. This small group of residents worked together to prepare their own breakfasts, so I thought that the social atmosphere might help Joe's appetite. When John had finished making a huge plate of toast, he sat it on the table in front of Joe. To my amazement, Joe reached over and took a slice of toast and ate it with enthusiasm. He had equal enthusiasm for the next four pieces of toast that he took for himself!

Provide a Pleasant, Social, and Normal Mealtime Atmosphere

Alice always joined us for Sunday family dinner. She was at her social best on these occasions, and many of our friends who joined in these meals had no idea that she had Alzheimer's disease. Even when she lived in a care facility and needed a lot of help with her meals, Alice continued to be able to feed herself during these family meals.

Keeping family mealtime habits and patterns supports the social aspects of meals. It also provides vital hints or cues that it is mealtime. It helps trigger the lifetime habit of feeding oneself. As far as possible, the place where the meal is served, the way of serving, and the people present should continue.

When the person starts to have trouble eating independently, it becomes even more important to expose him or her to the social aspects of meals. Some changes may be necessary, but these changes should be guided by lifelong habits. For instance, perhaps the person has always had his or her evening meal on a tray while watching the news. It may become too difficult to manage a lap tray, so try a small portable table instead. The distraction from the television may be too much, so try quiet music or a videotape of a favorite calming program instead.

Reduce Noise and Confusion that May Interfere with Concentrating on the Meal

Although Alice had always loved to eat out and continued to enjoy it, the stimulating restaurant environment and the need to make choices sometimes became too much for her. One day, when her meal arrived, she looked at it with bewilderment and then finally removed her false teeth and handed them to me. Even though I had helped her to order by suggesting manageable choices and it was a small, quiet restaurant, she had become overwhelmed by the stimulation. She couldn't think how to respond, although she knew she was supposed to do something.

Calm stimulation such as the smell of the food and quiet conversation with the person encourages participation; too much stimulation can overwhelm the person, interfere with concentration, and lead to poor eating habits and unusual mealtime behaviors. In the later stages of dementia, even the stimulation of having more than one course on the table at a time or too many other items like salt, pepper, and condiments can be too much.

Turn off the radio and the television. Keep the conversation calm, social, and focused on the person. At family or group mealtimes, it can help if the person with dementia is seated next to an understanding person who is able to give his or her undivided attention. Keep extra silverware and other items to a minimum while still having a normal table setting. Serve only one course at a time. Avoid table linens and dishes with busy designs. As dementia progresses, only give the person one piece of cutlery.

Use Ample Caring Personal Touch and Other Forms of Encouragement

Quiet conversation about the food and the person's preferences is helpful, as is encouragement to eat. Research has shown that when verbal encouragement to eat is accompanied by a light touch—for example, on the arm or hand—the person eats even better (Eaton, Mitchell-Bonair, & Friedman, 1986).

Allow Plenty of Time for Eating

Enjoying a meal is one of the most pleasurable and anticipated times of the day. The whole experience is valuable, filled with meaning and richness. There is too much of worth here for meals to be treated as just another household task to get out of the way as soon as possible. As dementia progresses, the person may need more time to finish a meal, but what is the rush? Why hurry the person to finish this pleasurable activity, which is probably a highlight of the day? If the person is content sitting at the kitchen table while you do other things, the person is engaged in an activity that has great meaning and value to him or her.

Serve the Person's Favorite Foods

A meal is a time to tempt the person's interest in food by serving favorites. It is not the time to introduce major changes in diet. There are many valid health reasons for cutting down on ingredients such as salt, sugar, and fat. However, these changes should be introduced gradually and in keeping with the person's lifelong preferences. The person who has never liked eating breakfast or vegetables is not about to start now and shouldn't be expected to. If changes are necessary for health reasons, they should be introduced subtly and slowly. Some suggestions follow.

To reduce salt intake, don't use salt while cooking and improve flavor with spices and seasonings. Dishes that are cooked for a long time at a lower temperature (e.g., casseroles, soups, stews) have more chance to develop flavor. Remove the salt and pepper shakers from the table. The person may forget to ask for the salt, but if he or she asks, provide a shaker that contains salt substitute instead.

For a person with diabetes, adapt lifelong favorites to fit within a balanced diabetic diet. For example, if the person has always had desserts, provide diabetic desserts instead. Because people with dementia gradually lose the ability to make good decisions, don't keep forbidden foods (e.g., candy, doughnuts) in the house or else put them in a secure, secret place. One woman who had managed her diabetic diet well for years before developing dementia astonished her husband by eating a whole box of chocolates at once. Unfortunately, she got very sick.

Use Sensory Appeal

Food preparation and mealtime are wonderfully rich sensory experiences. Focusing on sensory experiences is a natural way to encourage participation. As dementia progresses, it is helpful to use the sensory stimulation techniques in Chapter 6 to interest the person in food. In brief, the basic steps of sensory stimulation are 1) draw the person's attention to the item (e.g., a hamburger), 2) focus on one sense at a time (e.g., the hamburger's smell), and 3) encourage a functional response (e.g., encourage the person to spread on the mustard or take a bite).

All good cooks know that presentation accounts for a great deal of food's appeal. Food that looks attractive and appealing on the plate or in a serving dish will be more readily eaten. Taking the time to present food in this way is worth the effort.

The smell of appetizing food is especially important in enhancing appetite and eating. A great deal of what is considered taste is actually smell. This explains why food seems to have no taste when you have a cold.

Serve Nutrient-Dense Foods

Examples of nutrient-dense foods are puddings and milk shakes; whole-grain breads and cereals; and high-protein, low-fat foods such as lean meats and certain cheeses. The nutrition of foods such as muffins, breads, soups, or casseroles can be increased by adding extra milk powder and/or eggs. Commercial high-protein drinks are sometimes recommended. Some individuals will drink these straight from the can, especially if the drinks are chilled, but others don't like the taste. In such cases, these drinks can be frozen like Popsicles or used in puddings or whipped frozen desserts by substituting the high-protein drink for the milk or other liquid ingredient in a recipe. Instant breakfast products are another concentrated source of energy.

Use Nonintrusive, Adult Adaptations to Encourage Independence

Eventually, the person will start to have trouble eating independently. This is the time to use the many techniques suggested in Chapter 6 to help the person continue to participate. Although this may seem time consuming, it is worthwhile in terms of the person's self-esteem and quality of life. Research also established that it actually takes less caregiver time to encourage the person to feed him- or herself than it does to feed the person (Nolen & Garrard, 1988). Some-times, all that is needed is some help getting started; then, the over-learned habit of feeding oneself kicks in. Put some food on the utensil and use hand-over-hand positioning to guide the person's hand to his or her mouth. Sometimes, this is only necessary once; on other occasions, a few initial attempts may be needed or it may be necessary to repeat this cue a few times over the course of the meal. Encourage other ways that the person can be independent, such as spreading butter or condiments or adding milk and sugar to tea. Special dishes and utensils might help, but these should look and feel as normal as possible. Examples are plates with rims to help with loading utensils with food, thicker-handled cutlery, and covered spouted mugs (e.g., travel coffee mugs). An occupational therapist can offer specific suggestions on using adapted eating equipment.

Encourage Participation in Meal Preparation

A dozen times each day, Tony asked when supper was. Yet, when it was actually supper time, he wouldn't stay seated very long and needed a lot of encouragement to eat. When his wife followed the example of a home care aide and had John help to prepare the vegetables, he asked about supper less often and ate better.

Involving the person in meal preparation tasks such as setting the table, preparing vegetables, or mixing ingredients makes an important connection with the coming meal and can help the person to be more interested and involved. This can be particularly important for persons who once enjoyed cooking. Getting the person involved in making a favorite meal can provide a special connection.

Switch to Nutritious Finger Foods
or Drinkable Meals if Necessary

When the person is no longer able to use cutlery, there are many types of foods that he or she can still manage. Sandwiches, vegetable pieces, meat and cheese chunks, or pieces of fruit are all good choices. These foods are also good for a person who walks around and finds it difficult to sit at the table. As noted previously, enriched drinks can be made into desserts that may be easier to eat. Drinkable meals (e.g., puréed soups, clear broth, milk shakes, instant breakfast drinks) are also easier to manage.

Serve Hot Foods to Stimulate Appetite

There is nothing like the smell of something cooking to stimulate appetite and let the person know that it is mealtime. When not serving hot foods, simmering soup mix on the stove or in a Crock-Pot can also do wonders. For instance, a long-term care facility's kitchen ventilation system was broken. For the few days when the kitchen was not vented outside, the aroma of cooking food wafted through the facility, and there was a noticeable improvement in the residents' appetite and interest in meals.

Guidelines for Feeding Persons Who Are Dependent

As noted, cognitive, motor, and coordination problems will eventually make self-feeding impossible for most persons with dementia. If the person seems to be having difficulty swallowing, the caregiver should have a physician check for an active gag response. **If the person does not have an active gag response, he or she is at risk of choking and aspirating (inhaling) food into the lungs. In this case, feeding should only be done by a caregiver who has been trained by a professional** (e.g., an occupational therapist, a speech-language pathologist, a dietician, a nurse). For persons at risk for choking or aspirating, thin liquids should be avoided. They are actually harder to swallow because they offer less resistance than slightly thickened liquids, such as milk shakes and puréed soups. Gelatin, as well as a commercial product called Thick-It, may be used for thickening. A dietician should be consulted for appropriate foods and nutritious recipes.

Always maintain an upright sitting position with the back straight and the neck flexed slightly forward. **No one should ever be fed while lying down.** In addition, feed slowly and avoid overloading the spoon or the person's mouth. Take the timing cues from the person, and wait until he or she has swallowed before offering the next spoonful. Using a smaller spoon is also helpful.

Tell the person what is coming or provide other sensory cues, such as a touch on the hand. Avoid wiping the person's mouth or chin while feeding, as this may be confused with giving food.

Treat the person with compassion, caring, and dignity. Continue to maintain a warm, social, adult mealtime atmosphere. Furthermore, provide comfort and reassurance by gently holding the person's hand while feeding him or her. This also serves to reduce the possibility of the person interfering. Some people who are unable to eat independently feel part of the activity and are reassured by having a spoon to hold. Continue to encourage as much independence as possible—for example, by using hand-over-hand guidance to help the person butter bread or add milk to tea.

Avoid stimulation of primitive reflexes, if present (see Chapter 3). Those who have cared for children will be familiar with certain reflexes, such as the grasp reflex, which initially help the infant to survive and respond to the world. As the infant develops more mature and controlled movements, these reflexes disappear. The damage caused by a neurological disease, such as Alzheimer's disease, affects movement, and these early or primitive reflexes may appear again.

The grasp reflex is triggered by a light touch on the palm; if present, it causes the person to grasp tightly onto whatever touches the palm. The root reflex is triggered by a light touch on the cheek and causes the person to turn her or his head toward the touch. The tongue thrust reflex is triggered by a light touch on the bottom lip and causes the person to thrust his or her tongue forward. If the grasp reflex interferes with feeding or other activities, give the person something to hold onto. In this way, the grasp reflex can be used to help the person to hold onto a spoon or other item.

Stimulate swallowing by offering flavored ice cubes to suck on or by lightly massaging the saliva glands under the chin. Also, serve foods that are well moistened and smooth (i.e., avoid nuts, chunks of vegetables, or other food pieces with different textures). Serve soft, familiar adult foods (e.g., mashed potatoes, casseroles, puddings, scrambled eggs, porridge, pancakes).

A Word Regarding Paid Caregivers

This is not the time to introduce major dietary changes. Respecting and understanding the person's lifelong food preferences and eating habits is absolutely vital. To ensure adequate nutrition and participation in this essential life activity, paid caregivers must learn about preferences and habits from family members or others who know the person well.

If the person no longer lives at home, keeping up meal routines from home becomes even more vital. It can be a challenge, but the outcome is so worthwhile. The person eats better and is happier, and there is less work for the paid caregiver. Sometimes, paid caregivers get into an "assembly line" mode and forget about simple things that can help the person to eat better and to enjoy the mealtime experience. For example, in one very caring facility, two people who needed to be fed were seated at some distance from the table because there was concern that they would knock over their beverages if seated close to the table. This had been done for so long it had become a habit. Because there was hardly anything to remind them that it was mealtime, these two individuals sat like passive zombies and often needed extra stimulation to open their mouths for feeding. A new staff member moved the beverages to the back of the table, pulled the chairs up to the table, and gave each person a spoon to hold onto. She talked to them about the food being served and used other normal mealtime conversation. There was no need to prompt these individuals to eat.

Here are some suggested guidelines for helping the person to feed him- or herself in a paid caregiving situation.

- The person should be seated at a table, and there should be as many familiar cues as possible that it is mealtime (e.g., homelike dining room and table setting, familiar foods, kitchen aromas).

- As with any caregiver, paid caregivers must respect life-long eating habits. A special issue here concerns people who have lived alone for years before coming into a care facility. There are benefits to the social atmosphere of a dining room, but such individuals may find the whole experience too different and overwhelming, especially if the institutional dining room is large and noisy. These residents often do better in their own room, if possible, or in a small dining room.

- Persons need the full attention of paid caregivers. This is a time for the caregiver to socialize quietly with the resident, not to catch up on the news with co-workers. Extra chatter among staff can decrease the already poor attention of persons with dementia.

- Meals should be served one course at a time. If the facility has tray service, the eating habits of people with dementia will usually be vastly improved just by removing one course at a time from the tray and offering it to the person.

- The person with dementia probably lived through the Great Depression, when many individuals faced the real possibility of food shortages. When someone with this difficult life experience comes into a care facility, he or she may become concerned about not being able to pay for the food being served. A book of meal tickets may help people who are troubled by this, so that they can "pay" every time they eat. Sometimes, all that is needed is frequent reassurance that there is no charge; certain people may find it comforting that the government or a family member is paying for their meals because they have worked so hard all their lives. Others may find any suggestion of charity an insult.

Sleeping

"Sleep which knits up the raveled sleeve of care."

Shakespeare's poetic understanding of the importance of sleep to restore and repair is especially true for persons with dementia. Trying so hard to manage day to day with a damaged brain takes huge amounts of energy. You have probably noticed that the person gets tired very easily and can manage much better when he or she is well rested. Like all of us, when the person gets overtired, he or she is much more easily upset and distressed. If you can think about a time when you have been sick, you will probably remember that even simple, ordinary activities seemed like huge, tiring tasks. This must be what it is like, on a daily basis, to live with dementia.

Unfortunately, for numerous complex reasons, dementia can also interfere with the person's sleeping patterns. In some people with dementia, the sleep–wake center of the brain has been damaged, which can lead to mixing up days and nights. In addition, there are the challenges of not understanding the usual environmental cues that it is nighttime and becoming unable to continue with lifelong habits independently (e.g., preparing for bed). Fear and disorientation likely disrupt sleep as well if the person wakes up in the night and cannot get his or her bearings.

As you know only too well, helping the person to get a lot of rest is important not only for his or her well-being but also for your own. If the person is restless and upset at night, your much-needed sleep is also disturbed. The following suggestions are guidelines for helping the person get rest.

Maintain Bedtime Routines

Over the years, most people develop a unique routine to prepare for bed. For example, one person may tidy up the kitchen, let the cat out, and wash his or her hands and face; another may have a warm drink and go to bed with a favorite book. Moreover, some people are night owls; others prefer to go to bed early. As dementia progresses, the person will have difficulty keeping up these routines independently. It then becomes essential for the caregiver to learn and help support these routines. These activities are important triggers that indicate it is bedtime, time to wind down and relax. It is also important to maintain a regular time for going to bed. It is important to avoid having the person go to bed too early, because this can lead to the person waking up in the middle of the night.

Help the Person Fall Asleep

Help the person fall asleep by offering abundant opportunities for physical exercise earlier in the day. In the last 3–4 hours before bedtime, however, avoid stimulating activities such as exercise, as well as rich or sugary snacks and products containing caffeine (e.g., coffee, tea, chocolate, certain soft drinks). Instead, offer warm milk or other dairy products at bedtime. Dairy products contain tryptophan, which raises body levels of serotonin (a neurochemical that helps induce sleep). Chamomile and some other herbal teas also help with sleep. Furthermore, it might be helpful to play soothing music that the person enjoys. If the person has trouble falling asleep because he or she is used to sleeping with a partner who is no longer there, try providing a comforting presence by lining up a row of pillows on the partner's side of the bed.

Many older people naturally develop a pattern of shorter sleep times during the night. As a result, they take daytime naps. This is fine, but discourage lengthy daytime naps that can disrupt the nighttime sleep cycle.

Take Safety Precautions

For safety purposes, push the bed against the wall or put a bureau across the end of the bed. This arrangement will give the person fewer ways to get out of bed. The safest response to concerns about the person falling out of bed is to put the mattress on the floor. Another safety concern is wandering at night. For persons who tend to do this, it can be safer to leave their shoes on. If they get up, they will at least have secure footing. You may want to know that the person is out of bed, however. In this case, it may be helpful to use a room monitor or to place a musical welcome mat (i.e., a mat that plays music when stepped on) beside the bed.

Limit Confusion

Avoid laying clothes out for the next day. This can be confusing, causing the person to think it is time to dress and get ready for the day, not time to go to sleep. Also avoid confusion by reserving the bedroom for rest, relaxation, and sleep. Sometimes people who have poor sleep habits use their bed or bedroom as an office or a living room. This can lead to associating the bed and bedroom with activity, making it even harder to fall asleep. For persons with dementia, try to keep things related to daytime activities (e.g., playing cards, craft materials) out of sight at bedtime.

If the person has gone to bed but wakes up in the night, provide comfort and reassurance. We can all be temporarily disoriented when we awake in the night, especially if we are not at home. It takes us a while to get our bearings. Persons with dementia will likely have even more difficulty getting their bearings and may need help. Make sure the person is comfortable and has neither too many nor too few blankets. If the person prefers, let him or her sit up in an easy chair or on the sofa, and cover the person with a blanket. Provide reassurance that you will always be available if anything is needed. Offer a back rub or a massage to help the person relax. If the person has wandered from bed, take him or her to the bathroom and then suggest a calming distraction, such as listening to music or eating a light snack.

A Word Regarding Paid Caregivers

Paid caregivers need to understand and support each person's lifelong routines and habits about bedtime and sleep. These become all the more important if the person is no longer living in his or her own home. A person with dementia should not be disturbed by nighttime checks unless these are medically necessary (e.g., repositioning to avoid skin breakdown). If the person awakens, paid caregivers should consider why (see Chapter 9 for details on problem solving). Does the person just need to go to the bathroom and be reassured? Is getting up a longtime habit? For example, staff at a care facility were puzzled and challenged by one resident who was always awake and looking for somebody after bedtime. One night they understood this behavior when they saw him helping a female resident down the hall to the bathroom. This man had been his wife's caregiver for years before coming to a care facility himself, so helping a female to the bathroom during the night was routine.

Taking Medications

Most people who take numerous medications find it difficult to sort out what gets taken when and, furthermore, to remember to actually take them. Dementia makes this already complicated task even more challenging. The challenge increases if the person never had to take medication before he or she developed dementia, as there are no old patterns and habits to rely on.

Conversely, taking medication can be different from other personal care activities because it is rather more straightforward and not as likely to have detailed personal routines attached. In the early stages of dementia, however, it is vital to ensure that the person is taking his or her medication properly. Unfortunately, people commonly take too many or too few pills, and asking the person if he or she has taken the medication often doesn't provide accurate information. The number of pills left in a prescription needs to be checked off according to a calendar. If you do not feel comfortable or able to do this, it must be done by a nurse, doctor, or other health care professional. Taking medication improperly can cause major problems, including a worsening of dementia symptoms. Further suggestions for managing medication follow.

Arrange for the Person's Physician to Conduct a Medication Review

Take all of the person's current medications to the review meeting, and be sure to share any information that you have observed on possible effects (negative or positive) of current medication. Drug reactions, interactions, dosages, and suitability can be very different with older people, especially persons with dementia. Caregivers need to keep a watchful eye and report any possible medication side effects immediately; as dementia advances, the person is not likely to be able to give this information accurately. Arrange for the dosages to be put on as simple a schedule as possible. Also, ensure that the prescriptions are accurate and still necessary. I'm always amazed to discover how many people are taking prescriptions that were given by previous doctors for conditions that no longer exist or haven't been reviewed in years. Geriatricians or family physicians specializing in the care of older persons can be especially helpful.

Include over-the-counter medications in this medication review. These medications—such as remedies for nausea and diarrhea; antihistamines; or cough, cold, and flu medications—can cause the person with dementia to become confused and fall. Combinations of these with prescription medication can cause extra problems and side effects. Over-the-counter medications should only be taken on the doctor's advice. Although herbal supplements are popular, they can have side effects and also should be reviewed with the doctor and/or the pharmacist.

Organize the Pills in Separate Doses

There are numerous ways to organize pills. Many medications can be put into dated, dosage bubble packs at the pharmacy. Pill minder boxes are also available; these containers are partitioned into sections for each dose. Some pill minders now have electronic systems that buzz or beep when it is time to take a pill. The person may be able to learn to use this or a combination of a regular pill minder and a watch or clock that beeps when pills are to be taken. If pills are to be taken several times per day, it is important to have a pill minder that has separate spaces for each dose. Once pills have been organized by dose, be sure to put all medication bottles away very securely. If the person lives alone, this approach may not work because he or she may need cuing to take each dose and may not know what day it is. For some persons, telephoned reminders may work. Whichever system is selected, remember that it is not enough to provide it and assume that it will work. Regular checks are needed to see that the pills are being taken properly.

A homemade system was worked out for Alice. Because she was a registered nurse, a regular pill minder did not work; it just served as an invitation to do her job of pouring meds and to move pills around from one slot to another. In order to ensure that Alice did not do this, I covered the pills with plastic, taped them to stiff cardboard, and wrote the date above each piece of tape (e.g., Friday, November 5). I would call in the morning and remind her to remove the pills for that day and take them while we were on the telephone.

Use Positive and Pleasant Communication Techniques

Support the person, but also let him or her know that taking medication is not up for discussion. For example, you might say, "I have brought you a nice glass of orange juice so that you can take the pills the doctor wants you to take." (Of course, this would need to be altered if the person has not had good experiences with doctors.) See Chapter 4 for more information on communication.

Even when using positive communication techniques, managing medication can become a hot issue. If necessary, involve a respected health professional as an outside authority. Having a nurse prepare the medication or having a nurse or doctor as an external authority can take the heat off the caregiver.

LIFE CARE ACTIVITIES

This chapter follows a practice that is common in the caregiving and rehabilitation literature: separating daily life activities into the two categories of those that are personal (taking care of the self) and those that are less personal (taking care of the household). I call household activities *life care activities*, although these are sometimes referred to as *instrumental activities of daily living (IADL)*. The ensuing subsections discuss several types of life care activities: managing finances; transportation and driving; shopping; preparing meals; and household maintenance, laundry, and cleaning. Generally, household care activities are even more complex than personal care activities. This means that the person with dementia will usually have problems with life care activities before he or she will have problems with personal care activities. Fortunately, it is also usually easier for a family caregiver to get outside help for these less personal activities.

Managing Finances

Lila lived alone and had no immediate family or close contacts. Remarkably, she still lived in her own small apartment at the age of 92. She was active and had friendly, casual relationships with the people in her

neighborhood. One day while getting on the bus, Lila fell and hurt her arm. She was taken to the emergency room, where it was determined that she had broken her arm. Normally, this would be a matter of setting her arm in a cast and sending her home. However, because Lila seemed so befuddled and lived alone, she was admitted to a hospital.

Of course, being a patient in an acute care orthopedic ward didn't lessen her confusion, but it did start the process of determining the source of her confusion. Although her confusion had been made worse by her fall and by being in the hospital, a careful comprehensive assessment found that Lila was in fact in mid- to late-stage Alzheimer's disease. She agreed that she didn't want to live alone anymore, but she believed that she couldn't afford to live in a care facility; she had already looked at one in the past and was overwhelmed by the cost. Because she grew up with a "you pay your own way" philosophy, Lila persisted in believing that she couldn't move, even when we told her that she would get financial assistance.

In trying to help Lila, we finally tracked down a distant cousin and were able to get into Lila's apartment. It was sparse and neat as a pin. It was also stuffed full of uncashed checks, unused bank accounts, and large sums of cash totaling almost half a million dollars! Lila had worked as a stenographer for a local company that had offered its employees shares. The company had prospered, so these shares had done very well. Unfortunately, Lila had been unable to manage her finances for so long that she didn't realize she was no longer a poor retired stenographer but a very wealthy woman. Although she continued to worry that she couldn't afford it, Lila did move to the care facility that she had visited and was very happy there.

Managing finances is a complicated activity involving high levels of skill in areas such as decision making and planning. For instance, the many steps and decisions needed to pay a bill by check can become too much even in the early stages of dementia. However, this difficulty may be hidden by the good graces of helpful bank tellers or others. This was certainly the case with Alice. An honest teller at the neighborhood bank later told Alice's son and me that for several years, Alice had come on a regular basis with a collection of bills that the teller helped her sort through and pay. Sadly, not everyone who a person with dementia turns to for financial help is that honest. It is especially important for partners or family members to put a system in place for managing finances in the early stages of dementia. (See Chapter 10 for more on care planning issues.)

Ensure that the Person Always Has Money in His or Her Wallet or Purse

Having our own money is a very important part of being an independent adult. This is particularly important for people who have lived through the Great Depression and have no real understanding of the different social support systems now in place. In addition, persons with dementia often have difficulty understanding the value of money and the fact that they have money in the bank. These concepts are too abstract. Having cash is something that they can understand, however. It need not be a lot—and probably shouldn't be because of the very real concern that the person may be taken advantage of. A few small bills and some change will usually suffice. For some people, going to the bank to withdraw money is important and helps to ease money worries.

Simplify Bill Paying as Much as Possible

With bank machines, charge cards, extended answering systems, and all of the many changes to how companies do business, banking and paying bills may be very different from the way the person was used to doing things. In this case, old habits may not do the person much good. However, it may be possible to have most bill paying and banking set up on an automatic basis, through direct debit and direct deposit. If you opt to take care of the person's banking in this way, also think about how to manage the statements for these bills, which may come in the mail. It is unlikely that the person will be able to read the statement and determine that the bill has already been paid; as a result, the person may become concerned about how he or she is going to pay the bill. It may be necessary to have the bills sent to another address.

Appoint One Reliable and Sensitive Person to Take Care of the Finances

It is essential to have someone in charge of the person's finances and to have this done in a legally correct way with which (as far as possible) all family members agree. This may be an ideal task for an out-of-town family member. The person in charge can also be a trusted friend or a lawyer. This difficult area can be simplified if there is an early diagnosis and the person can be involved in making these decisions. See Chapter 10 for further discussion of this challenging topic.

Transportation and Driving

Alice was a woman ahead of her time. In the 1930s, she had a career as a nurse and drove a sporty car that she owned. When she married, she followed the custom of the time. She stopped working outside of the home and stopped driving. During more than 40 years of marriage, she showed no interest in driving. She was perfectly happy to have her husband drive her wherever she needed. When her husband died, she was not only coping with this loss but also with losses due to Alzheimer's disease. As the disease progressed, she became more fixed on the idea that she should never have stopped driving. She wanted to start driving again, even though she had shown no interest in driving for many years.

For Alice and most others, driving a car is a mark of independence, held dearly since adolescence. It is also a complicated activity requiring judgment, perceptual abilities, decision-making skills, and many other complex brain functions. It is important to remember that a diagnosis of dementia does not automatically mean that the person is no longer able to drive. However, the person with dementia eventually will be unable to drive safely. In cases of early diagnosis, when the person has been involved in planning for the future, he or she may realize independently when he or she should no longer drive. Unfortunately, this is not always the case. You are likely aware that there are safety risks not only for the person and any passengers but also for others on the road. You are probably also concerned with how to discuss this sensitive topic with the person who you are caring for. It can be even more complicated if you don't drive and rely on the person with dementia for your transportation and shopping. This is a burden you shouldn't have to carry alone. The following suggestions may help.

Consult the Person's Physician

Because driving is such a complex skill, difficulties can start long before other cognitive losses may be obvious during a brief office visit. If there is uncertainty about the person's ability to drive, you may need to consult other professionals, such as a neuropsychologist or an occupational therapist. Some cities have driving assessment programs, although many of these are geared to persons with physical disabilities.

Physicians are obligated to contact the department of motor vehicles with their concerns. Every state and province has different regulations, but in most places, the department of motor vehicles will contact the person in question to request a driving test. (The department of motor vehicles will not indicate who reported the concerns.) In some states, the license may be revoked without a retest.

If the physician agrees that driving is no longer safe, he or she should be the one to tell the person directly. It should be presented as a medical issue, due to concerns about health and safety. This removes the decision, and the anger that may follow, from the caregiver. It can be helpful to have a written order from the doctor for future reference.

If the physician does not agree with your concerns, I urge you to get a second opinion. Failing that, report your concern to the department of motor vehicles.

After Consulting with the Physician

Reinforce concern for the safety of others, and remind the person of the doctor's order to no longer drive. If no one else in the household drives, it is best to remove the car so the person is not reminded of the loss. Remove car keys and other reminders of driving as well.

Understand that some people get satisfaction from giving advice to others about car maintenance or from helping with others' cars (e.g., washing and waxing). However, others are frustrated by these reminders of driving. In all cases, ensure that the person has other opportunities to support self-esteem and independence. In addition, provide opportunities for outings and drives with others.

Shopping

Ramona had always run the household and shopped with ease. When she started to complain that she didn't want to be bothered with shopping for groceries, her husband Richard became impatient because he thought she was being lazy. He would drop her off at the store and would get even more impatient with her poorly selected purchases.

One day when Richard picked her up at the store, he was startled to find that she had been stopped by a store security guard because she had not paid for the groceries. Ramona had also forgotten how to organize paying for her groceries. Unfortunately, Richard thought that this was a further sign of her becoming stupid and lazy and used this incident to make fun of her.

Fortunately, Ramona and Richard's adult children knew that something was wrong and arranged for an assessment, which confirmed that their mother had Alzheimer's disease. They began to help out with activities such as shopping. They tried to help their father understand that Ramona wasn't lazy or stupid but that she had a brain disease and couldn't manage things like shopping on her own anymore.

Shopping means different things to different people. For some people, it is a chore and a taxing experience. For other people, it is a favorite, pleasurable activity. Regardless of the meaning, some things, such as food, have to be purchased. Eventually, making these purchases will become a challenge for persons with dementia. Shopping is the ultimate decision-making experience, especially in large, modern stores. Even in familiar settings, a person in the early stages of dementia can find making basic choices difficult.

Alice loved to go to the grocery store. In fact it had been almost a daily ritual in the years after she retired. She was an expert bargain hunter and kept track of all the weekly specials at various grocery stores. She let this go as her memory and planning problems increased, but she still liked to walk over to the neighborhood grocery store almost every day. When she got there, she usually got three standard items, a head of lettuce, a pound of hamburger, and some tomatoes. This saved on decision making, but it didn't solve the problem of getting proper groceries. She seemed to realize that something was wrong and one day called her grandson at work. She was in a great state of panic because she had no food in the house. He left work and took her to the store where she got—you guessed it—a head of lettuce, a pound of hamburger, and some tomatoes. Some suggestions follow for helping people like Alice with shopping.

Take Stock of the Cupboards and Help the Person Make a Shopping List

If the person has always made shopping lists, this should be a joint activity. Otherwise, you will have to make the list. Be sure to include items that the person likes, not just those that you think he or she ought to have.

Help the Person Get Food and Other Necessities

Consider the person's lifelong habits and values. For Alice, going to the store was an outing. Therefore, I made sure that she shared in this activity at least once a week. Others are perfectly happy to have someone else get their groceries and even items such as clothes and shoes. If this is the case, you may want to find a grocery store that delivers telephone orders. You may be able to recruit a relative, neighbor, or friend who has previously offered to help. Catalog shopping may be a good option for clothing and other items. It may also be a good idea if the person becomes overstimulated by going to a store. This way, he or she can still make choices and be involved, but the experience is much less stressful (be sure to choose companies that have a convenient return policy).

Keep Shopping Trips Manageable

It is much more efficient to double up on errands and to make bigger, less frequent trips to the grocery store. However, these situations become overwhelming early on for the person with dementia. Caregivers who wish to make complicated or major shopping trips should probably do so on their own.

When shopping with the person with dementia, go to one or two stores for a few items only. Stay with the person as necessary and help him or her to make manageable choices and to participate. Perhaps you can ask the person to choose a dozen oranges, or you may need to simplify decision making even further by saying things such as, "Do you think we should buy this head of broccoli or that head of broccoli?" When shopping for clothing, help to narrow down choices by finding one or two items that you think the person would like. It may be necessary to go into the fitting room to help the person with dressing and undressing.

Preparing Meals

Bea had always lived with many challenges, including money shortages. Through it all, her cooking was a great source of pride for Bea and her family. She was an excellent cook and was renowned not only for her baking but also for preparing economical and nutritious meals. Bea and her husband Frank, as well as their children, were happy when an inheritance assisted with financial issues. Unfortunately, not long after this was received, it became clear that Bea was having mem-ory and cognitive problems. She would forget family events and names and began to suspect that Frank was seeing other women whenever he went out. At the same time, she became more reclu-sive and less interested in doing things such as pursuing her life-long interest in music.

However, she continued to try her best to make meals. These efforts included serving undercooked food. Both Frank and her children tried to intervene, suggesting that they would do more cooking, but Bea would have none of it. In fact, she ordered Frank out of the kitchen on numerous occasions. Frank was actually quite a good cook, but he was a gentle man and didn't want to hurt his wife's feelings, so he ate the rather poor offer-ings she presented. The rest of the family was especially con-cerned about the possibility of Frank and Bea eating improp-erly prepared food, but Bea stoutly refused suggestions about Frank doing more cooking or receiving deliveries from a meal service. Family members helped as best they could by keeping healthy food in the kitchen and coming in when their mother was away to throw out any spoiled food. Their concern moved to the need to act on the day when they learned that their mother had tried to serve sandwiches made with spoiled left-over meat.

With the help of day program staff, Bea and Frank's children connected with a person in the community who prepared and delivered excellent home-cooked meals for a reasonable price. On the advice of staff members, the children told their mother—very lovingly and kindly but firmly—that the first meal was arriving that afternoon. Bea was hesitant, but there was no further dis-cussion. When the first meal arrived, she ate it with enthusiasm; from then on, she accepted the delivered meals as part of her reg-ular, daily routine. In fact, Bea seemed to be relieved. When Bea started to worry about what she was going to make for supper,

Frank gently reminded her that their children had arranged for it to be delivered, and Bea relaxed.

Meal preparation is a life care activity that is strongly affected by the person's lifelong habits and values. For some people, meal preparation is a chore. The object is to get something to eat as easily and quickly as possible. For others, it is a joy, and every part of the activity contains pleasure and meaning. For these individuals, cooking and meal preparation is a hobby, a way to express themselves creatively, a way to give things to others. In addition, for many women who have been full-time homemakers, meal preparation has been a very important part of their life work. So, before you can understand how to help when meal preparation becomes difficult, it is important to know the meaning that cooking and preparing meals has held for that person. There is an extra challenge involved when the person lives alone. Although he or she may struggle to prepare meals, there is often reason to be concerned that the person is not eating properly. Suggestions about meal preparation activities follow.

Consider the Person's Habits and Values

Although nutrition is important, this is not the time to expect major changes in eating and cooking habits. Carefully weigh the importance of any change against the big picture. For instance, if the person only eats sweets and never eats a proper meal, action should be taken. Conversely, if the person insists on continuing with a lifelong diet of meat, potatoes, and canned vegetables, it is probably not worth making an issue about his or her diet unless there are serious health concerns. (In the latter case, any necessary changes should be introduced gradually.) Similarly, a person who has never eaten breakfast should not be expected to start now.

Respect the Person's Need
to Make Choices and Decisions

Regarding meal preparation, the need for choice and involvement applies at several different levels. At the most basic level, everyone needs to make choices about the type of food, the way it is prepared, and where and how it is eaten. Offering these choices to a person with dementia can make a huge difference in his or her enjoyment and eating habits. Persons with dementia who attend one day program where I once worked really seem to enjoy "make your own sandwich for lunch" day. The simple activity of choosing what to put on the sandwich and preparing it (with help as needed) is satisfying. It is essential to involve the person in decisions about meals and foods, making sure to offer choices that he or she can manage. For example, try asking questions such as, "Would you like to have peas or corn for supper?" and "Would you like to have lunch here in the kitchen or outside at the picnic table?" Note that the questions are not about whether to have a vegetable or whether there is going to be lunch; these are assumed.

Making choices about meals is complicated with regard to the big question: "Who is in charge of the kitchen?" This issue needs to be considered when the person starts to have difficulty with safely preparing nutritious meals. Individuals for whom cooking has been a chore will probably happily hand this duty over to someone else, provided the topic is approached with dignity and respect.

For individuals who have considered the kitchen their kingdom, offering help can be tricky. All positive communication skills must be used to offer choice and control and protect dignity. The person needs to be given the impression that he or she is still running the kitchen and that you are the helper. It is best not to hint that the person is no longer capable of doing something that has been a source of pride and self-esteem. Often, it is possible to call on this pride by suggesting that you would really enjoy eating the person's specialty dish and that you would like his or her help in learning how to make it. The person is probably no longer able to make this recipe, at least from start to finish, but he or she should be given the chance to participate in all of the steps and to feel like the chef in charge. (Refer to Chapter 6 for suggestions about breaking down activities into steps.) When the complicated activity of planning and preparing a meal becomes too much, the person can still do parts of it, such as preparing vegetables, mixing and stirring ingredients, or giving an opinion about seasoning. He or she can also probably manage a simpler and more routine meal, such as breakfast or lunch. If the person can't do simpler meal preparation independently, he or she may still be able to participate if things are laid out (e.g., bread, meat, and mustard for a sandwich) or hints are given for the various steps.

Address Safety Concerns

Kitchen utensils and appliances such as the stove can present safety risks for the person with dementia. Due to memory problems, the person may forget to turn off the stove, be unable to use appliances or knives safely, or be unable to exercise good judgment about things such as touching hot pots. (These issues are detailed in Chapter 5.) Ensuring that the person who values being in the kitchen still has the chance to do so safely can prevent accidents.

For some reason, Alice became worried about the noise the refrigerator was making and unplugged it. She also took food out of the freezer, put it in the refrigerator, and then put it back in the freezer. Because we did the grocery shopping together, it was relatively easy for me to date and label food as it was put away. This way, I could track things that had been moved around and were no longer safe to eat.

Poor judgment can also put the person at risk for eating spoiled food or using items inappropriately. People with dementia often have a damaged sense of smell, which can further increase the risk of food poisoning. Caregivers need to keep a careful check on food in the refrigerator and freezer and to remove any items (e.g., certain condiments) that may make the person sick if eaten in large quantities.

Use Lifelong Patterns to Guide Kitchen Organization and Ease of Use

Frequently used items should be easy to find or even left out on the counter. For instance, the person may still be able to make him- or herself a cup of tea or coffee if an electric kettle, spoon, cup, and so forth are organized in one spot on the counter. At the same time, it is important to avoid clutter, as this can make it more difficult for the person to function. Labeling cupboards and drawers may help. This may offend some individuals, however, so be sure to do it sensitively. Involving the person in the activity of creating the labels can help. Labels can then become something that the person can point to with pride.

Write Out the Steps for Frequent Kitchen Activities

Writing out steps may help a person who is still able to follow written directions. Make sure that the steps are separate (e.g., even making a cup of instant coffee involves several steps), and follow the person's usual routine. Favorite recipes can also be simplified and written out this way, as can the order of steps to prepare a meal.

Help the Person to Organize Simpler Meals

Again, lifestyle patterns and values are important. Some people may be happy with nutritious premade meals (commercial or homemade). Others may leave these sitting in the freezer. The best approach may be a respectful but firm "this is how it is going to be," as used with Bea in the section's opening vignette.

 Monica had raised a big family and had been an excellent cook. As her dementia progressed, she seemed to lose all interest in making meals. She said that she had done more than enough of it, which was certainly true. Whenever she went to the grocery store, she stocked up on pizzas. Her family found these hidden all over the house. Arnold, her husband, was angry that Monica had "stopped doing her duty," so he started cooking. Monica refused to eat what Arnold prepared and went in search of her cache of pizzas. When their children left prepared meals in the freezer, Monica forgot they were there and Arnold refused to eat them.

Obviously, there was a long history of difficulties in this relationship, and these difficulties were still being played out over meals. There were also issues of control and independence, as Arnold refused to have outside help with housework or anything else. He feared that doing so would mean that Monica would be put in a nursing facility because he couldn't manage.

Monica and Arnold's children spent a lot of time with health care providers trying to work out a solution. This was very difficult because Arnold also had a violent temper and there was real potential for abuse. In the end, it was decided that the only solution was to keep a careful eye on the situation and intervene in a dramatic way if necessary (i.e., move Monica out of the house).

As this challenging situation illustrates, there is unfortunately no "one size fits all" solution in so many aspects of dementia care.

A Word Regarding Persons Who Live Alone

Despite the preceding suggestions, helping with meals may be especially challenging with a person who lives alone. This was true with Alice. We were in daily contact with her, kept her kitchen well stocked with groceries, had her over at least twice per week for dinner, and had arranged for a housekeeper to help out three times per week. Even with all of this help, I was never sure that Alice had an adequate diet. This was confirmed when we cleaned out her apartment after she moved to a long-term care facility. Neatly stored in her cupboard was a 3-foot stack of foil plates from store-bought pies! Nonetheless, she was physically healthy during this time, and for the first time in her life, she wasn't overweight. All of those pies couldn't have done her too much harm, and she certainly deserved to enjoy them.

Caregivers can explore several options, such as premade frozen meals, delivered hot meals, or housekeeping services. The best choice depends on the situation; sometimes, unfortunately, there is no best choice. Issues of care planning and competency can arise in the most challenging of these situations. As Chapter 10 discusses, the most important thing is to start planning during the early stages of dementia.

Continuing Household Maintenance, Laundry, and Cleaning

The best way to help with cleaning tasks depends on lifelong values. For many people, these activities truly are chores. Handing them over to someone else is not too difficult. However, many people enjoy housework (hard as it is for me to understand). It is a valued and pleasurable activity for them. Making small repairs and doing other household maintenance jobs may be especially important for some men. It may be their work after retirement. Helping these people to continue doing these jobs is really important.

Whatever the value given to these activities, two concerns are likely to come up. If outside help is needed, the person is likely to worry about how to pay for it, even if he or she actually has the money to do so. Also, many people find it difficult to have someone else in their home doing things that they used to do. Some suggestions follow for helping with these types of challenges.

Support Lifelong Routines

"Support lifelong routines" may sound like a broken record at this point, but it bears repeating. Familiar routines remind the person how to do things and encourage him or her to participate. Help may be more easily accepted from others if the small details of life care activities are supported. For example, if the person has always swept the kitchen floor after finishing with the dishes, this routine should be continued. Supporting these lifelong habits may sometimes require a "grin and bear it" attitude on the caregiver's part, as you may have a faster or preferred way of doing things. The caregiver may find the person's sweeping the kitchen floor frustrating because it would be easier to run the vacuum through the kitchen. Yet, fitting in with the person's routine is easier in the long run, as the person is more content and less likely to be distressed.

These daily routines fit into a much larger picture of lifestyle and housekeeping standards. Beyond certain basic standards of cleanliness that affect health, there is an unlimited number of personal standards about cleanliness and tidiness. Imposing your standards on someone else is especially inappropriate when that person has dementia. If you are a spouse caregiver, you have probably long since worked out a mutually agreeable standard of housekeeping. If not, this is not the time to start. If the person is unable to keep the house clean enough for health purposes, however, action needs to be taken. This is a necessity that differs from imposing your standard.

Alice seemed to do a very good job of keeping her house neat and orderly, despite having Alzheimer's disease. However, on closer inspection, it was clear that she wasn't able to do basic necessities (e.g., keeping the toilet clean). Her struggle to keep tidy often led to some unusual combinations in drawers and cupboards. The bed was always made, but the sheets underneath didn't get laundered. As long as things looked tidy, she felt that her housework was done. We helped to keep the tidy look that she valued so much and filled in with some more difficult tasks that she couldn't manage, such as doing the laundry and cleaning the bathroom.

Introduce Necessary Changes Gradually and with Sensitivity

Early in my experience of caring for Alice, I learned the importance of introducing changes gradually and sensitively. As noted, Alice needed help with cleaning and laundry. I had just arranged for a cleaning service to care for my home—a huge treat for me because I worked outside the home. I thought Alice also would be thrilled to receive this service. However, she was understandably insulted and insisted that she could keep her house clean, just as she always had done. She angrily and suspiciously followed the cleaning staff around. Things worked much better when we arranged to have the cleaners come while Alice was out. However, the best solution was hiring a caring housekeeper who understood Alice's need to run her household. She worked with Alice to get the house tidy and clean.

The effects of dementia may necessitate some changes to household organization. The person who has always lived with clutter may no longer be able to cope with it because memory loss, perceptual problems, and so forth interfere with the ability to find things. Clutter may also be a safety risk, especially if it litters common walking paths. It is tempting to come in and restore order in one fell swoop. However, the person may well react to this loss of control with anger, and it is likely that more stuff will simply take its place. The best approach is to subtly remove a few things at a time, starting with the biggest hazards. Valued possessions need to remain in full view. Furniture in pathways may have been used as a support when walking. If so, it should be replaced with grab bars or sturdier pieces of furniture. (See Chapter 5 for more on home safety.)

Ensure that the Person Still Feels Like the Master of the House

Emma was having memory problems, but she was managing pretty well in her own home until she had a slight stroke, which affected her balance. Even with a walker, she was still unsteady. Her son, Stuart, was concerned and insisted that she move in with him and his wife. Stuart was acting with the best of intentions, but there was trouble from the start. Emma and her daughter-in-law, Francis, had never seen eye to eye. Francis let Emma know in no uncertain terms that she was no longer in her own home. Francis was absolutely in charge of the household. While Stuart was at work, a constant turf war raged inside the house.

Emma was still quite capable and wanted to help. Francis found this a nuisance. She always wanted things done in her way and according to her time frame. There was no room for give and take. If Emma was getting carrots ready for supper, they had to be cut up the way that Francis always did it, and they had to be done in a hurry. Understandably, Emma felt powerless. Sometimes when Francis went out, Emma would do things to help—or perhaps to get revenge—such as adding extra salt to the stew simmering on the stove.

Staff listened empathetically as Francis vented her frustration. Gentle attempts were made to help Francis understand Emma's feelings and to suggest ways in which Francis could give Emma some control. Francis continued to feel that Emma was ungrateful and spiteful. Unfortunately, the bitter history between the two women made change virtually impossible. The pleasant, good-humored, and helpful Emma that staff at the program knew just couldn't be supported in her daughter-in-law's house. Eventually, Emma agreed to move to a nursing facility, saying that she made too much work for Francis.

Having a sense of control about household tasks is especially important for persons who have valued being homemakers. Housekeeping is their job, their life work. Whether you are a spouse, other family member, or a paid caregiver, it is still the person's house. Even if the person doesn't own the building, as in a long-term care facility, it is his or her home. Do everything possible to give the person the sense that you are working with him or her as a helper. Consult on things big and small (e.g., ask, "Do you think we should hang the wash outside or put it in the dryer?"). Give compliments for past skills and accomplishments.

Finding ways to give the person a sense of control over household tasks can be challenging at the best of times. These challenges are even greater when the previous relationship was difficult, as in the case of Emma and Francis. When these challenges of control arise, it may help to step back and look at the big picture. In the overall scheme of things, is it better to have a happy relationship or to have the carrots cut the way you would like them cut?

Encourage the Person to Do Part of an Activity

Although doing the laundry from start to finish may no longer be possible, the person can help in various ways, such as hanging the clothes on the line or folding dry clothes. Drying dishes, dusting, sweeping, and raking leaves are a few of the many household tasks that the person can still help with if the task is broken down into steps or adapted as needed. For instance, if the person can no longer stand up to dry dishes, a tray of dishes can be put on the table so the person can sit down while drying them.

Focus on the Enjoyment of Doing the Activity, Not on Getting the Job Done

You are a busy caregiver, and there are many things that you have to get done as efficiently as possible. Out of all these many tasks, try to find things that the person can help with, that the person can enjoy and do at his or her own pace while you bustle around. Could the person sit at the table and slowly dry dishes while you clean up the rest of the kitchen and get things organized for the next meal? Could you vacuum while the person sorts and folds the laundry? Remind yourself that the point of the activity is not efficiency but an opportunity for the person to be active and feel needed.

CONCLUSION

The closing guideline for the preceding subsection—focus on the enjoyment of the activity in the moment, not getting the job done—is one of the most important and most challenging guidelines to enabling engagement in daily and other activities. For busy caregivers, who have so many things to do and probably have a lifelong focus on the end product (finishing various tasks and activities) instead of the process of doing, it can be very challenging to change gears, to appreciate the pleasure that persons with dementia can derive from the process of doing an activity. I am reminded of the story of a retired farmer who was invited to use his skill in building split-rail fences at a community heritage farm. He arrived with his ax and handsaw and went right to work. However, the museum director was astonished a few hours later to hear the sound of a chain saw. When he went to investigate he found the farmer happily cutting rails with his chain saw. By way of explanation the farmer said, "Well, that way of building fences was all right at the time, but now we have chain saws and there's no need to spend weeks building a fence."

The farmer was completely focused on the practical product (a fence) and had missed the importance of the process in creating an authentic, period, rail fence. I hope that the guidelines in this chapter, and those in Chapter 8 regarding recreational activities, will help caregivers to appreciate the great importance of the process of "building the fence" for authentic and life-enriching experience.

8

Using Leisure Activities for the Person's "Re-Creation"

I believe that the desire and the need to be creative lies within all of us, and that we all want to be expressive in some special way. This is done through creating items that give us pleasure to see, touch, hear, and even smell. It also gives us pleasure to offer these items of our inner expressions as gifts to our loved ones and friends. Creativity and self-expression are, I believe, very basic to enjoyment of life. From my own experience I believe we can enjoy the process of doing an activity as much as or even more than completing it and having the finished result in our hands. (Truscott, 2004, p. 93)

I hope I will always continue to look for new methods of creativity and self-expression, even should my current abilities decline. I hope the people around me, my family and friends, will help me find new adaptations. (Truscott, 2004, p. 97)

When I was in my mid-thirties, I was a mother, a wife, a family caregiver, a community volunteer, and a student occupational therapist. It was an interesting and challenging life, busy to the extreme. When first-year exams were finished, my classmates, who were a decade or more younger, were off to party downtown. I looked forward to a quiet meal with my family and to the pleasure of getting up early the next morning to immerse my hands, and my spirit, into fragrant bread dough. Then, I looked forward to—oh, luxury of luxuries—a few quiet moments poking about in my awakening and neglected garden.

Activities that bring meaning and value, those that make us feel good about ourselves and serve as a source of "re-creation" and renewal, are unique and personal. Furthermore, the same activity often has a different meaning for different people. For example, a dear friend of mine loves to iron. She finds pleasure in smoothing out the wrinkles and bringing order out of a rumpled mess. My personal view is that I am better off not owning anything that needs ironing! For my friend, ironing is pleasurable activity; for me, it is a detested duty.

Chapter 1 asked, "What do you do to take care of yourself?" I hope that you are also making time to take care of your self, to celebrate you. This is essential. As Marilyn Truscott's words outline at the start of the chapter, it is just as essential for persons with dementia, but perhaps it is no longer possible for them to do so independently. I would like you to consider what the person you are caring for did or does to re-create. To start the process, I will share a little bit of what I did today to take care of me, to re-create.

Today is a Sunday, a day that in my experience has meant time for a break, for restoration. I have a very long list of things that I ought to do—paying bills, washing windows, winterizing my house, and editing. I have done none of them. Today I have done a lot of things that are indulgences for me, activities that bring me pleasure, that take care of the self, that are "re-creation."

Because today marks the end of daylight-saving time, it is good for a type-A person like me. I got that whole extra hour that I have been waiting for since April. This meant that I could get up at 5:00 A.M., but it was really only 4:00 A.M. Getting up early is a pleasure for me, just like sleeping in is for others. I had tea and read part of the newspaper. (I enjoyed these activities so much that I did them again a few hours later.) I added a new color and crocheted a few rows on the afghan I am making for my daughter. I took a long, indulgent shower and dressed in my silk lounge pajamas, which I intend to wear all day. I made "real" (i.e., drip) coffee for the first time in a week and drank it in a Minton china cup that had belonged to my aunt. After this start, I felt so good that I managed to work productively on a paper for a conference that I have been struggling with for days. Then, more time for me—I had a long and fun talk with a special friend, ate a toasted bagel with apricot jam, and took a delicious nap. Right at this moment, it really does fill me with pleasure to be sitting here at my desk, writing about these things. Even sitting at the desk brings me pleasure. I am looking out a second-story patio door, which is framed by lace curtains at the top and red geraniums at the bottom, through silver maples dancing in the breeze, over to a shimmery blue lake. Because my silk pajamas are a tad cool on this October day, I am snuggled under a blanket knit by my mother. I am a lucky person, and today it feels good to celebrate it, to take time to celebrate and take care of me.

A person with dementia has a wonderful capacity to celebrate the moment, to find pleasure in the simple things of daily life. You can enrich this ability by providing opportunities for the person to do special things, things that have particular meaning to him or her. Lifelong interests and habits are the first place to turn when searching for these re-creation activities. You may also find that the person is interested in new activities. In some ways, dementia can be liberating. If novel activities are offered in appealing ways, old inhibitions (e.g., real men don't cook, woodworking is not for women) may be cast aside.

I know that you are busy trying to help the person continue with things that he or she needs to do, such as eating or getting dressed. These activities may be pleasurable for some people but not for others. In either case, everyone's day needs to be filled with duty and challenges as well as with activities that bring pleasure and help the person to maintain a familiar rhythm of activity. Doing so encourages engagement in life.

This chapter is not an exhaustive list of leisure activities, but I hope that it will trigger ideas about ways to help the person do things that bring pleasure in the moment, that re-create. It is not necessary to spend hours planning complicated activities. The best activities are connected with lifelong valued activities—those that fit in with the flow of everyday life. In fact, many older people may not have had time in their busy lives for leisure activities. As a result, the best activities are often connected with work.

Think about simple activities that are related to a favorite pastime. It can be helpful to have videotapes or magazines about such pastimes. Sometimes, just having the opportunity to touch and handle the things associated with a favorite activity can bring pleasure. For example, a person who enjoyed playing golf may find pleasure in using an indoor putter or hitting practice balls outside. Encourage him or her to watch a golf tournament on television, to clean his or her golf clubs or golf bag, or to sort through a collection of golf balls and tees. Another example of a simple, pastime-related activity comes from a friend who owns a yarn shop. This person reported that an older lady came into the store one day and said, "My dear, I can't knit anymore because I have Alzheimer's, but could I just smell the yarn and touch it?"

The challenge is to think of ways that help the person be involved in and gain pleasure from these activities. Usually, it is no longer enough to suggest that the person do something; you will need to organize the activity and get him or her started. As dementia progresses, you may play an increasing role, perhaps actually doing an activity with the person (e.g., looking at a book or magazine). See Chapter 6 for further suggestions on engaging the person in an activity or adapting it so the person can participate.

GENERAL ACTIVITY CHARACTERISTICS

Regardless of which leisure activities are chosen, those that help the person with dementia re-create share certain characteristics. The following list will help you remember these important qualities. The most rewarding activities are those that

Are familiar and overlearned—shaking hands, brushing hair, adding milk and sugar to tea or coffee, drying dishes

Are simple and repetitive but adult—putting flowers in a vase, winding yarn, looking at the newspaper or a magazine, sweeping the floor

Are failure free—offering an opinion; humming along with a song; looking out the window; sorting through items in a purse, briefcase, or junk drawer

Provide rich sensory experiences—feeling a fur muff or a felt hat; lifting, commenting on, cutting, and tasting a watermelon; looking at colorful photographs of familiar local sights; petting the dog; smelling a flower; rubbing on hand cream

Emphasize social skills—greeting others, gathering around a table to share a snack and a drink, sitting together to watch television or listen to music

Make use of movement—dancing or moving to music, walking, doing simple exercises, digging in the garden, filling the birdfeeder

Provide opportunities for reminiscence—looking at, trying on, or using vintage objects such as cameras, crank telephones, kitchen equipment, clothing, or school books; looking at family photos

Provide opportunities for making manageable choices—choosing which flower to wear for a boutonniere, which cookie to take from a plate, or what color background to use for a homemade greeting card

Provide opportunities for active participation—watering plants; grooming pets; signing a greeting card; singing, humming, or clapping with music (these contrast to passive activities such as looking at pets or just listening to music)

Are simple and repetitive—polishing shoes, wiping the table, dusting, mixing dough, stirring potting mix for plants

Have an obvious purpose—creating things for others (making Christmas ornaments, baking for visitors, sanding blocks for the grandchildren) or doing practical, everyday activities (folding clean towels, peeling vegetables, washing windows, getting dressed)

Emphasize nonverbal skills—listening to music; stuffing envelopes; cuddling children; sorting coins, buttons, socks, or coupons; raking leaves

Can be broken down into several steps—potting plants, baking, doing small woodworking projects (e.g., a birdhouse, a trivet)

Provide immediate positive feedback—baking, arranging flowers, tasting foods

Do not require immediate memory skills, verbal skills, or fine motor skills—singing familiar songs, misting plants, polishing silver

Do not confront the individual with his or her disability—asking questions that seek an opinion instead of a right or wrong answer, not prodding a person with advanced dementia to do something at which he or she used to be skilled (e.g., playing the piano)

Are related to seasons and familiar holidays—putting up Christmas decorations, preparing for Hanukkah, painting Easter eggs, setting the table for a special meal, raking leaves

Are meaningful—making a birthday card for a loved one, planting a garden, fixing a cup of coffee, getting dressed

Are rhythmic—moving or clapping to music, playing catch, shuffling cards, sanding wood

Are related to work—preparing meals, doing woodworking projects, gardening, engaging in self-care activities

SPECIFIC ACTIVITY CATEGORIES

The following subsections group activities according to types that may have had meaning for the person and include opportunities for independent participation. I hope that the ideas presented here trigger thoughts about activities that will bring pleasure and re-creation for the person you are caring for.

Self-Directed Activities

Some activities have a familiarity, rhythm, sensory appeal, and theme that entice the person to continue. Once started on such activities, the person may be able to do them independently. The person feels satisfied and occupied, and caregivers may be able to take a break. Some specific self-directed activities are listed next. By thinking about simple, repetitive activities that are connected with the person's interests, caregivers may be able to come up with many more.

- Shuffle or sort playing cards.
- Sort and look at greeting cards.
- Rearrange items in a purse, wallet, or briefcase.
- Manipulate beads on an abacus.
- Write or draw on paper (taped over the person's wheelchair tray as necessary).
- Feel or fold cloth book pages.
- Sand or polish a cutting board or other wooden item.
- Rock in a rocking chair (a great activity because it stimulates balance responses and provides comfort and pleasure).
- Ride an exercise bike.
- Stir or mix ingredients for a recipe.
- Look at a personal, labeled photo album.
- Mist plants.
- Tear old newspapers into shreds that can be used as litter at an animal shelter.
- Do repetitive cleaning activities such as sweeping, dusting, and wiping tables.
- Unravel and wind the yarn from an old hand-knit sweater.
- Use a stimulating apron. These often provide comfort in the later stages of dementia. They are available commercially (see Appendix B for resources), but you can also make one by stitching interesting objects of different

textures (e.g., zippers, snap fasteners, buttons, different fabrics) onto an apron that the person wears.

- Create a safe junk drawer for the person to sort and organize. Many people with dementia find pleasure in sorting through pens, coins, paper clips, rubber bands, spools of thread, buttons, coupons, twist ties, pieces of paper, string, and so forth. Up to a certain stage of dementia, this activity can be done repeatedly. However, this is not a safe activity for the later stages of dementia, during which some people put things in their mouth.

- Use respite videotapes if the person has enjoyed watching television. Respite videotapes, in which a person talks in a caring way directly to the viewer, may bring pleasure in the later stages of dementia. A commercial respite videotape is available (see Appendix B), but the person may be insulted by the content (i.e., it might be too basic or simple), so you should preview it first. You may also make your own respite videotape. In addition, short home videotapes of family members and activities may be appealing. Short videotapes of favorite programs or sports events also may be of interest.

- Create a work station providing repetitive activities that are connected to the person's past work. Desk activities are useful for a person who had an office job. A small table or desk is fine; if it is the person's own desk, all the better. Items of interest can include papers, envelopes, files, notebooks, and order books, as well as a desk organizer (in a disorganized state) with pens, paper clips, erasers, and so forth. For a homemaker, try setting up a bureau with interesting fabric remnants, socks to sort and roll, and clothes to fold. For someone who worked with his or her hands, have a workbench with safe locks, fasteners, plastic pipe fittings, handles to turn, and so forth. If you have a friend or relative who is handy, these materials can be securely mounted on a plywood background and put on the wall at eye level as interactive artwork. Such items kindle interest, provide an activity for the hands, and may be especially good for persons who like to work.

Quick, On-the-Spot Activities

Consider encouraging activity whenever the person seems responsive. This can include things that require little or no time and planning, such as the following:

- Listen to or sing a favorite song.
- Look at a favorite picture.
- Look out the window.
- Eat a simple snack or have a drink.
- Call a friend or relative for a quick chat.
- Sign a greeting card.
- Bring in the mail or the newspaper.
- Rub on hand cream.
- Brush hair.
- Pet the cat or dog.
- Water or mist a plant.
- Give a hug. We can never have too many hugs! A hug can provide quick reassurance for the person that you are there and you care. If the person doesn't respond well to hugs, a gentle touch on the arm or the shoulder, a warm handshake, a cheery smile, or a wave hello also conveys affection and caring.
- Play a game of catch. The automatic response to reach out to catch a ball seems to be preserved for some time through dementia. Of course, this shouldn't be done

without warning, and it should be presented in an adult way, suggesting that it is exercise for the person's hands. Playing catch with small beanbags in various colors and textures brings great satisfaction, especially during the later stages of dementia. Nerf balls can also be good.

Carpentry and Fix-It Work

At some point, working with power tools and even hand tools will become not only difficult but also dangerous for the person with dementia. If carpentry or fixing things has been an activity with great meaning for the person, it is important to find safe ways to continue with related activities.

- Offer simple sanding projects from precut wood pieces (e.g., bread boards cut in interesting shapes, birdhouses, trivets, blocks for grandchildren, magazine racks).

- Hand rub a wax finish on wooden items.

- Look at woodworking books and magazines.

- Help with or consult on fix-it jobs around the house.

- Sort and organize screws, nails, nuts, and bolts. Ordering these items in a multidrawer parts organizer can help the person to feel productive and happy for a long time. As memory loss increases, this is something that can be repeated every day. Remember that the object is not to actually have things sorted (although this may happen) but for the person to enjoy the process. This activity should be discontinued if the person begins to put things in his or her mouth.

- Clean up the workshop by organizing tools, organizing drill bits, and sweeping. Be aware of the person's limitations, and remove power tools and sharp objects as necessary.

Cooking

Long after Alice could no longer plan a meal or follow a recipe, she loved to be in the kitchen and to help prepare meals. While I was busy getting the rest of a meal ready, she did things such as breaking up lettuce for a salad or folding napkins. These activities were failure free and repetitive, and Alice became very involved in them. With her lifelong attention to detail, it took her quite a long time to do such activities. The key was for her to do things with no particular time frame (i.e., things that didn't require a long cooking time or were not needed at the start of the meal). One day Alice and my mother were making butter tarts. Alice's job was to put the raisins in each pastry shell. While Alice painstakingly put raisins in the tart shells, one at time, my mom prepared the rest of the dinner. Alice commented that it was good to be able to help.

A person who has always valued cooking and being in the kitchen will undoubtedly continue to enjoy these activities and should be involved. Yet, having the person involved in every stage of meal preparation may well take more time than you have. If you can find parts of the activity that the person can enjoy doing, it brings satisfaction to the person and gives you the chance to concentrate on other things. Examples include the following:

- Clip recipes out of magazines.
- Copy down recipes.
- Organize a recipe file.
- Prepare vegetables and fruits. Even when the person can no longer safely use a knife, he or she may still be able to help prepare foods in other ways (e.g., shelling peas, snapping beans, hulling strawberries, breaking up lettuce, washing fruits and vegetables).

- Mix, stir, and do other repetitive activities. These often can be continued by the person independently once habitual memory is triggered. Although fine cakes and pastries can be ruined by overstirring, there are many things that the person can work at without concern (e.g., separately mixing the dry or liquid ingredients for baking, cutting shortening into biscuit dough, shaking salad dressing, mixing salad greens). Remember that if it brings the person pleasure, just stirring flour in a bowl can be a good repetitive activity. Alice enjoyed using a rolling pin to make bread crumbs out of leftover bread bits.
- Clean up (e.g., wiping counters, drying dishes, sweeping the floor).
- Look at cookbooks and magazines with food and recipes. Ones with illustrations are the best.
- Serve as the head chef while someone else learns to make the person's specialty dish.
- Enjoy the rich sensory and memory experiences associated with food preparation. Use these experiences to stimulate the senses and trigger discussion about favorites foods, memories (e.g., what the person's mother used to make), and so forth.

Desk Work, Reading, and Writing

As noted previously, if the person has worked in an office or at a desk, continuing with related activities can have particular meaning. Keeping up with personal correspondence and doing things such as paying bills may have been an important part of another person's life. Opportunities to continue these activities can take the form of real work. Sometimes charitable or church organizations need help stuffing envelopes or affixing address labels or stamps for mass mailings. Some organizations may also need people to sort labels or coupons or roll cash register receipts that have been collected for redemption. Many persons with dementia enjoy doing these activities if the task is set up so that they can succeed. This may mean doing the activity at home.

Dementia makes it more difficult to concentrate on reading or to understand what is read. Abilities vary, so some people are still able to read during the later stages of dementia. Although they may not understand what they are reading, the activity itself will still have meaning. Some individuals may enjoy the opportunity to sit in a favorite chair with a book, newspaper, or magazine, as they have always done; whether they are able to read is no longer the point. It is important to keep book lovers in close connection with favorite books, just for the pleasure of touching them and turning the pages. (The caregiver may need to organize this activity.) Other people may find their interest held by adult books with pictures, such as travel books or other coffee-table books. This might be an activity that can be shared with others. Some may enjoy listening to audiobooks, and others may enjoy being read to—being read to by a child can be especially satisfying.

Other suggested activities follow for desk work and related themes.

- Sit at a desk or table to fold "letters" and put them in envelopes (this can be a perfect use for junk mail).
- Reorganize papers and file folders in a small portable file holder.
- Sort pens, paper clips, pencils, and so forth in a desk organizer.
- Copy addresses onto envelopes.

- Organize materials in a briefcase.
- Sort and roll coins.
- Look through old greeting cards and letters. These can be put into a scrapbook as well.
- Sign a card for a family member or friend. If such writing has been a familiar activity, the person may still be able to write (and the person's written skills may even exceed his or her verbal expression abilities). Another person may be able to tell the caregiver what to write down for him or her.
- Select a greeting card for someone special. If going to the store would be too overwhelming, you can provide two cards for the person to select from at home.

Games

For many older people, card games or board games (e.g., Crokinole, Scrabble, checkers, Chinese checkers, Monopoly) occupied many long winter evenings. These activities (or variations of them) may still bring pleasure. When I was girl growing up in rural Ontario, my parents' social life centered around an evening of playing the card game euchre, interspersed with lots of conversation and laughter, and followed by a substantial "lunch"—actually, an evening snack of sandwiches and sweets. Because babysitters were unheard of in that place at that time, we kids were part of this social event. We would sit at the table learning the game, sleep on the sofa, and join the grown-ups for the treats. Although I don't really enjoy playing cards and board games as such, I do still enjoy the re-creation of this experience. If such evenings have been part of the past for the person you are caring for, he or she may also enjoy a re-creation of the experience.

Lorna had always been an exceptional Crokinole player. The board game Crokinole involves shooting flat wooden disks across a polished wooden board toward a hole in the center. If a player shoots a disk into the hole, he or she earns 20 points. The further away from the center the disk stops, the fewer points the player earns. As Lorna's dementia progressed, she lost self-feeding and self-care skills and could no longer remember the rules of Crokinole, but she could still sink a 20 with dead accuracy. She needed guidance about things such as whose turn it was, but when a piece was placed in front of her finger, she was amazing. She got great satisfaction not only from participating but also from succeeding at a favorite pastime.

This is still another illustration of the importance of finding out what the person can still do, as skills are preserved in interesting ways through the course of dementia. The fact that Lorna could still accurately shoot Crokinole pieces, given her other losses, really stands in the face of logic. In fact, research has found that persons who have played games such as bridge maintain reasoning and logic skills longer through the course of dementia (Bowlby, 1993).

Think about any games or activities that the person you are caring for enjoys or used to enjoy. On the one hand, certain people find watching others play a satisfying activity. On the other hand, just watching may frustrate individuals who can no longer play. Suggestions follow for involving a person with dementia in games.

- Remember that simple card or board games can be good activities to do with grandchildren.
- Emphasize the social and fun aspects of games, and de-emphasize the competitive part. This way, the person is not so worried about failing and can enjoy the activity.
- Choose a task connected to a favorite game, such as shuffling cards or sorting the pieces of board games.

- Adapt the game or play simpler games so that the person can still participate. For example, the person may no longer be able to play a complicated game such as chess, but with some hints and cuing, he or she may enjoy playing checkers. Similarly, bridge or cribbage may be too difficult, but perhaps simpler card games will be of interest. You may be surprised that a person who played solitaire still remembers how to play; this game may also be adapted to be played together. Other games may be adapted to be played with a partner, so that the person with dementia has an understanding partner who is coach.

- Help the person maintain the social part of a group activity in which he or she once took part (e.g., a bridge or dart club). Attending for the whole time may be overwhelming for the person, but he or she may be able to attend for part of the activity.

- Help the person continue to play bingo, if this was an interest. Skills in maintaining numerous bingo cards and attending to the caller may persist; however, other aspects of bingo can be problematic, such as overstimulation from the noise and crowds of a public bingo hall. Find a way to continue playing bingo at home, perhaps as a few short games with a few understanding friends or family members. Consider using adapted, simpler versions of bingo (e.g., those with pictures), yet realize that this change could be difficult or upsetting if the person has been a great fan of traditional bingo.

Gardening

In Chapter 1, readers met John Angus, a man with advanced dementia who had a deep connection with the land. As described there, after months of living in various nursing facilities where he had not had an opportu-

nity to connect with the land or growing things, he had a power-
ful reaction when this opportunity was presented to him. As I
guided his hands to the potting soil, tears began to run down his
smiling cheeks. With hands immersed in his beloved soil, John
Angus said, "This is just heaven, just heaven, and I had no idea
that heaven was so handy to home."

With hand-over-hand guidance, John Angus potted several
begonias. On subsequent visits to the occupational therapy
department, he watered, fertilized, and pruned the plants, also
with assistance. By Christmas time, the begonias were in full
bloom. There are hardly words to describe the pleasure and satis-
faction it gave John Angus to present them to his family members
as Christmas gifts or the pleasure that they had in receiving the
plants.

Gardening is especially important for someone who has
always been involved with plants, but it can also be a valuable
new activity. Working with plants provides rich opportunities
for stimulating the senses. The very simple activity of touching and smelling a flower or the leaves of a plant can bring a
world of pleasure. Scented geraniums and herbs are especially wonderful for the senses. The mimosa, a simple to grow
and interesting plant, responds physically by curling up its
leaves when touched. The rich sensory experiences can also
stimulate long-term memories—for example, the smell of
sage or summer savory can trigger memories about turkey
dinners during holidays or other celebrations. Working with
plants provides an opportunity for nurturing living things,
and the therapeutic benefits of horticulture are well known
(Bowlby Sifton, 1998; Hewson, 1994). The following suggested activities relate to plants and gardening.

- Look at seed catalogs, gardening magazines, or photos of
  gardens.

- Turn over the soil in a garden.

- Repot a plant.

- Touch, feel, smell, and look at flowers or herbs.

- Mist or water houseplants. Note that the person may have difficulty knowing how much water to give a plant; however, misting is failure free—it is hard to do much harm, and indoor plants cannot have too much moisture for their leaves.

- Pick dead leaves or flowers off indoor or outdoor plants. A person who has always been involved with plants may be able to do this independently.

- Pick produce or flowers from an outdoor garden.

- Water an outdoor garden.

- Dig soil.

- Help plant the outdoor garden. This is a complicated activity, requiring many decisions. As dementia progresses, it will be necessary to break the activity into steps so the person can participate. For instance, when setting out transplants, if the transplant holes are all prepared, the person can be guided to put in each plant. The person may have difficulty planting fine seeds such as those for carrots, even if the planting space is prepared, but he or she may be able to manage larger seeds such as those for beans. A lifelong gardener may be happy to coach from the sidelines.

- Rake leaves or grass.

- Put flowers between the pages of a book to press them.

- Prepare herbs or flowers for drying.

- Crumble dried herbs and put them in containers.

Household Tasks

For a busy caregiver, completing the numerous daily house-hold tasks can be a challenge. It is easy to forget that doing these basic tasks repeatedly can bring pleasure to the person with dementia, especially if he or she has enjoyed housework. It is also an opportunity for the person to feel helpful and productive. Try to remember that the pleasure and the feel-ing that the person gets from the activity is what counts. It doesn't really matter if the dusting takes all afternoon (or doesn't need to be done anyway). Suggested household activ-ities follow.

- Fold laundry.
- Hang up clothes.
- Sweep.
- Dust.
- Pair socks.
- Sort and reorganize things in a dresser drawer (keep some drawers just for this purpose).
- Dry dishes.
- Sort cutlery into a cutlery tray.
- Wash windows.
- Polish silver or brass.
- Set the table.
- Take out the garbage.
- Bring in wood for the fireplace or wood stove. One rural caregiver who heated her home with wood found that although her husband could no longer safely tend the stove, he got great pleasure from constantly reorganizing the outdoor woodpile or the indoor wood box. If this used to be a valued activity for the person who you are

caring for, consider creating a wood box, even if you no longer use it for a fireplace or wood stove.

- Sort materials for recycling. Depending on the person's skill level, he or she can wash out jars or milk and juice cartons, remove labels from cans and bottles, remove caps from bottles, put newspapers into bags, or remove staples from printed material (if required).

Music Activities

In one form or another, music is a part of almost everyone's life. Experiences range from listening to the radio or stereo to playing an instrument or singing. Persons with dementia retain the ability to respond to and appreciate music, even when verbal and other abilities fail. Music can provide a way to continue expressing feelings and to return to past life experiences. It can also transport the person mentally to a richer, more comforting, and more engaged experience. Music can take the person beyond the limitations of dementia. For instance, close your eyes and recall a favorite song. Most likely, you won't just experience the song; you will also be reexperiencing a particular place with particular people. This activity in itself can provide great comfort for persons with dementia.

Music is a very personal experience. It is especially important to know the person's favorite types of music—that is, favorite songs and favorite performers. (Add these to the All About Me form in Appendix A.) Generally, the music that was popular between the ages of 15 and 25 is recalled most vividly. Music cannot work its magic all on its own, however. The effects of dementia can make it difficult for the person to initiate or even to respond to music that is played. Yet if the caregiver provides a bridge, a connection with the music, the effect can be amazing. For example, while making eye and touch contact with the person, sing or hum along with the tunes and encourage tapping toes, clapping in time with the music, or (if appropriate) dancing. Playing music all the time may not be helpful, as it can become unnoticed as part of the background. Continually playing music can also cause too much stimulation and distress the person.

For persons who were once skilled musicians, it will take understanding and sensitivity to involve them in music activities. These can be a reminder of what has been lost and a source of frustration if a person is no longer able to play an instrument. Nonetheless, some people remember how to play an instrument long into the course of dementia. One person, who was nonverbal and in the advanced stages of dementia, could still play the piano when he was cued by sitting at the piano and having his fingers put on the keys. The following activities are suggestions for using music.

- Play favorite pieces, remembering to help connect the person with the music. It is better to use audiotapes, records, or CDs than the radio, as you can select the person's favorites.

- Use different types of music according to needs. For example, calming music can be used at bedtime or if the person is distressed; more lively music can be used to cheer the person up or to encourage movement. It is important to start with music that has a rhythm close to the person's mood and then gradually move to the desired rhythm. For example, if the person is distressed and unable to settle down to sleep, start with some moderately lively music (e.g., "Home on the Range," "You Are My Sunshine"). As the person relaxes, play a calmer, quieter, instrumental piece.

- Play sing-along videotapes or videotapes of favorite musical programs (e.g., *The Lawrence Welk Show*) that may be enjoyed. Videotapes of favorite musicals (e.g., *The Sound of Music*) may also be good. As the person's ability to pay attention decreases, however, you may have to play longer videotapes in parts.
- Look at old songbooks and recall favorite tunes.
- Organize sheet music or look at and touch musical instruments. This activity may bring pleasure to someone with a musical past. However, it is important to know the person, as this activity may also cause distress over lost abilities.

Involvement with Pets

We gave Alice a canary, which she named Naomi. Alice found Naomi to be a wonderful companion. She chattered away to the bird, sharing opinions and thoughts, and Naomi responded to whatever was said with her cheerful song. Although bird books say that canaries won't sing if they are pestered or their cage is disturbed, Naomi obviously hadn't read these books! Every time Alice walked by, she would affectionately tap at Naomi's cage and Naomi would sing her heart out. She only stopped singing when Alice went into a nursing facility and wasn't there to tap at her cage anymore.

Spending time with pets can be a successful activity for persons with dementia. Animals respond to nonverbal communication and are not troubled by speech and memory difficulties. Spending time with a pet provides opportunities for nurturing, rich sensory experiences, and connection with a living being. These experiences are especially valued by a person who has always had a pet, but they may become important for a person like Alice, who had been previously indifferent to pets.

Remember that not everyone is fond of animals and that this should be respected. Some people may have had a negative experience, such as being attacked by a dog, which may *seem* to have faded over the years. However, it is possible that with losses in recent memory and reasoning skills, the presence of an animal can rekindle these old, traumatic memories. If the animal is a visitor, take precautions to ensure that it is calm, good natured, and healthy. Keeping these cautions in mind, here are suggested activities connected with pets.

- Pet, hold, and cuddle animals.
- Take the dog for a walk.
- Groom and comb the animal's coat.
- Feed the animal.
- Look at picture books of animals.
- Do home volunteer work for an animal shelter, such as tearing up newspapers to be used as litter.
- Provide a good-quality stuffed animal. I make this suggestion with extreme caution. Although many young adults have stuffed animals, they are not so common with older people. Stuffed animals may bring comfort, but they can also lead to distress if they cause others not to think of the person as a dignified adult.
- Watch short videotapes or television programs about animals.

Arts and Crafts

For many older women, sewing, knitting, hooking rugs, and quilting were creative outlets, but they were also real work done to clothe the family. As dementia progresses, the many complicated steps involved in following new patterns or even recalling old patterns becomes difficult. Alice had made hundreds of pairs of socks and was so familiar with the basic process that she could knit without looking. One of the first signs of her memory difficulty was trouble with turning the heel of a sock. Because she had been such a skilled knitter, she wasn't interested in knitting simpler items, such as scarves. However, she still got great pleasure out of sorting through her collection of yarns, patterns, and needles. She also enjoyed darning holes in socks.

A crafter might continue to enjoy the following activities. These suggestions may also bring pleasure to others who have never done these sorts of activities.

- Sort through and organize sewing or craft materials. Just touching the objects can bring pleasure and stimulation. This is an activity that can be repeated over and over, as the process of sorting (not the end product) is enjoyable. A sewing basket, box, or parts organizer can make the activity more interesting, and you can encourage involvement by asking the person to sort the sewing basket as a favor to you.

- Wind yarn. Winding yarn from a skein to a ball may be too complicated, but unraveling a hand-knit sweater may be easier. This activity usually provides pleasure and stimulation, but one lady refused to do it, horrified at the waste of taking apart a perfectly good sweater! This example serves as a reminder that there are no guarantees and that explanations must be offered for any activity.

- Cut simple, predrawn fabric patterns for quilts or pot holders.

- Do simpler versions of previous favorite activities. For example, knit scarves or afghan squares instead of sweaters, or quilt a sampler that is already pieced.

- Make a simple craft project from a homemade or purchased kit. These allow the steps to be laid out in advance. Usually, the person will need help with each step. These projects can be particularly meaningful if the completed results are intended as gifts for others.

Spiritual Activities

Going to church and church activities had always been very important to Alice. These activities continued to be highly valued as her dementia progressed. Although she had difficulty paying attention to the sermon and finding hymns in the hymnal, she seemed to find great comfort in being at church and responded enthusiastically to the music. When Alice moved to a Catholic nursing home, she began going to Mass for the first time in her life. She started this completely on her own and went every day. Despite the unfamiliar service, Mass brought great comfort to her.

Like Alice, many persons with dementia find spiritual activities uplifting and comforting. Perhaps the person's enhanced intuitive and emotional ability supports a deep internal connection, which overrides the problems that he or she may have with memory and thinking. I witnessed this during a Christmas Eve service. One member of the congregation was in the later stages of dementia. Throughout the service, she made various sounds that could not be understood. At the close of the service, the minister took Communion to this lady's seat. After receiving Communion, she proclaimed in a joyous voice, "That was just beautiful." Although she may not have grasped the spoken parts of the service, the sacrament of Communion obviously spoke to her at a deep, personal level. Here are some suggested ways to help others to have these experiences. It may be helpful to share these ideas (and information about dementia and the person who you are caring for) with leaders and other members of the person's spiritual community.

- Help the person continue to attend his or her preferred religious services for as long as possible. If the typical service is too long or taxing, try attending only part or see if another house of worship offers a similar but shorter service. Some individuals may appreciate a videotape of a service, allowing them to watch it in shorter, more manageable bits.

- Provide opportunities to listen to and sing music that is part of the person's spiritual tradition.

- Remember that favorite and familiar readings from religious texts can continue to have great meaning for the person. The person may be able to read these independently, and reading to children can give the person an opportunity to pass on traditions. If the person can no longer read, he or she may enjoy being read to by others.

- Encourage the person to continue with religious traditions that have been a part of daily life. For example, the person can participate in the Jewish tradition of the Sabbath meal or in the Christian tradition of saying grace at mealtimes. You may be surprised at what the person is still able to do from these lifelong traditions. One lady with dementia could say little about her family or other life events, but when she was called upon to say grace, she did so wonderfully. She didn't simply recite a memorized verse but shared insightful and moving prayers.

- Provide opportunities for the person to touch and handle sacred books and other objects that are part of the person's religious tradition (e.g., a menorah, a rosary, a prayer wheel).

Sports Activities

Many people have a passionate interest in particular sports. Fortunately, even after the person is no longer able to play the game itself, there are ready-made opportunities for armchair players. The person can continue to enjoy sports in the following ways.

- Do part of the activity that he or she can still manage. The chapter introduction gave suggestions about activities that a golfer might still enjoy. If the person loves baseball and is no longer able to play the game, he or she may still enjoy a game of catch. This can be further adapted to a simple tossing of a ball while the person is seated. If you are concerned about using an actual baseball, there are many excellent balls that allow a safe and satisfying game of catch (e.g., foam Nerf balls). Games of catch that involve foam balls or beanbags and are presented in an adult fashion (as a form of exercise) may be enjoyed by many. The automatic response to reach out and catch a tossed object persists into the later stages of dementia and can be a valuable activity, even for a person who has never been involved with sports.

- Do simple physical activities. Research shows that exercise is especially important for persons with dementia (Bowlby Sifton, 2000f). Exercise not only maintains good physical health but also stimulates thinking and mental function and helps the person to feel less frustrated and agitated. Exercise is also important for caregivers. Walking or swimming are two of the best exercises and may be something that you and the person with dementia can do together. There are many excellent exercise videotapes meant for older adults or ones that can be done while seated, which you may enjoy doing together. Some individuals may enjoy using an exercise bike. If the person has used equipment such as a treadmill, he or she may be able to continue doing so, with encouragement, for some time.

- Recall the social aspects that go with certain sporting events, such as eating hot dogs at a baseball game, going to a tailgate party before a football game, or going to "the 19th hole" after a game of golf. Although the person may no longer be able to fully participate in these activities, having short get-togethers with understanding friends can be very meaningful. If the person should avoid alcohol, serve nonalcoholic beer or other nonalcoholic drinks.

- Watch a game on television. This may be difficult as the person's attention span fades, but taping games and playing them in short bits can bring pleasure. Championship or playoff games may be enjoyed repeatedly.

- Listen to the sports news on radio or television.

- Look at a sports magazine or the sports section of the newspaper. It may be necessary to read to the person and make explanatory comments.

- Reminisce about past sports accomplishments. Joking about the fish that got away and recalling other types of sports accomplishments (by the person or by someone else) can bring pleasure.

- Look at photographs of the person's past sporting activities. The person also may enjoy looking at a coffee-table book containing photos of great moments in sports.

- Handle, clean, or sort the gear associated with favorite sports. Suggestions include oiling a baseball glove, waxing skis, cleaning golf clubs, or sorting through a tackle box.

Travel and Photography

Even when with a companion, traveling and being in unfamiliar places eventually becomes too challenging for persons with dementia. Fortunately, most people who loved to travel are used to reliving their experiences by recalling their adventures. This should be encouraged and supported by the following activities.

- Look at photographs and memorabilia from trips.
- Encourage the person to tell favorite travel stories.
- Watch travelogue videotapes.
- Look at travel books and brochures.
- Eat foods and listen to music associated with favorite places to which the person has traveled.
- Take a small trip, such as a drive to get ice cream or have a picnic.

CONCLUSION

This chapter has focused on the importance of having opportunities to re-create, to engage in leisure activities for pleasure and renewal. The chapter has offered guidelines for engaging persons with dementia in only a few of the hundreds of possible leisure activities. The chapter's last suggested area of interest touches on photography, which leads me to recall a valuable piece of folk wisdom: "The human mind does not take photographs; it paints pictures." This an excellent reminder that the preferred activities *and* the memories and experiences of being involved in those activities are uniquely personal. Caregivers who are able to step into the picture with persons who have dementia and enable engagement in meaningful leisure activities offer opportunities for increased pleasure and decreased distress. Unfortunately, however, it is impossible to eliminate all sources of distress for persons with dementia. Chapter 9 discusses ways to understand, prevent, and respond to distress that leads to challenging behavioral symptoms.

9

Understanding, Preventing, and Responding to Behavioral Symptoms

I tax my family's patience so many times, because how I behave in just so many situations triggers in them quite normal emotional responses to someone else's 'bad behavior'. Even I wonder at times why I can't be more 'normal'. But my behavior comes from a disease process in my brain—I can't help it, however much I try. (Boden, 1998, p. 63)

Very often I wander around looking for something which I know is very pertinent, then after a while I forget all about what it was I was looking for. When I am wandering around, I'm trying to touch base with—anything, actually. If anything appeared I'd probably look at it, or look at it or examine it and wonder how it got there. I feel very foolish when I am wandering around not knowing what I'm doing and I'm not always quite sure how to do any better. It's not easy to figure out what the heck I'm looking for. (Henderson & Andrews, 1998, p. 24)

THE BASICS ON
CHALLENGING BEHAVIORAL SYMPTOMS

Mrs. Chisholm was in the advanced stage of dementia and lived in a long-term care facility. She retained many social skills and thoroughly enjoyed social and entertainment activities. She was usually the life of the party, so it was surprising one day when she stayed in her room and refused to join the staff, students, and residents who were preparing food for a party. As I approached her room, I realized that she was very distressed. She was crying and constantly repeating, "It is just too embarrassing, all of those other ladies, with their beautiful dresses, and here I am with absolutely nothing on at all." I tried all of the usual approaches, telling her what a lovely dress she was wearing and gently running her hands over her dress so she could feel the fabric. None of these approaches were successful in relieving her distress. I thought that perhaps she was uncomfortable in her chair, so I shifted her seating position and then I saw the source of the problem. Mrs. Chisholm was wearing a wrap-around dress, and the back was entirely open. As a result, she was sitting with her bare skin next to the chair upholstery. As far as she was concerned, she was wearing absolutely nothing.

The preceding story illustrates several points about behaviors that challenge caregivers.

The Behavior, Not the Person, Is Challenging

Before starting any discussion about care challenges, it is important to remember that the behavior, not the person, is challenging. Mrs. Chisholm and other persons with dementia are trying their best to manage with day-to-day life. They are first and foremost people—whole people with a wide range of abilities and needs. Whatever distress the symptoms of dementia are causing a person at the moment, he or she is not the distress, the behavior, the challenge. Nobody likes to be summed up by some particular negative characteristic. Remember the pain inflicted by schoolyard nicknames such as "fatty," "dummy," or "clumsy"? It is important to avoid referring to the person with dementia as a particular behavior—for example, calling him or her a wanderer, a hoarder, difficult, aggressive, and so forth. These labels box caregivers and the person into a corner, making it difficult to see the strengths and needs of the whole person and to use these strengths to respond to the challenge.

For this reason, I was reluctant to name the challenges in this chapter. However, to ease understanding, it seems best to use the names that are commonly used to describe such challenges. Please remember, though, that these terms are used to describe the behavior, not the person.

All Behavior Has Meaning

As puzzling as certain behaviors may be, they represent the person's best attempt to communicate. These behaviors are often the expression of an unmet need. As caregivers, we are challenged to step inside the person's world, to stand in his or her shoes to understand what he or she is trying to tell us. In the preceding vignette, Mrs. Chisholm was understandably distressed at the seeming violation of long-standing social values—that is, she felt as if she was naked. Mrs. Chisholm needed to have her dignity protected, and she was unable to do anything about this herself.

Behaviors that Challenge Caregivers Are Symptoms of a Physical Brain Condition

Challenging behaviors are not under the person's conscious control, nor are they deliberate attempts to be difficult or aggravating. Persons with dementia are struggling to cope with deteriorating skills in a world that is becoming increasingly difficult to understand. Just as we would not expect the person with arthritis to stop having painful, restricted joints, we cannot expect the person with dementia to stop having symptoms such as misinterpretation, memory loss, or repetitive questioning. It is essential to recall that by the time the first symptoms of dementia are evident, 80% of the damage to the brain has already been done.

Arguing with the Person About Firmly Held Beliefs Only Causes Distress

People with dementia tend to use the most powerful sensory information available to them to understand a situation. Deteriorating sensory and perceptual abilities, combined with impaired reasoning and other cognitive deficits, led Mrs. Chisholm to believe that she was not dressed. In this case, the sensation of her bare skin against the chair's fabric was overwhelming and led Mrs. Chisholm to conclude that she was naked. Although this perception was inaccurate, it was her firmly held understanding of the situation. No amount of verbal reasoning would persuade her otherwise. (In fact, the more that staff members tried to tell her that she was dressed, the more upset and distressed she became.) Caregivers are advised to enter into the person's world, not to deny its existence. If we try to understand where the person is coming from, we can often get to the source of the distress.

Caregivers Must Find Creative Ways to Meet the Needs Expressed Through Behavior

As caregivers, we cannot expect the person with dementia to try any harder. Instead, we must try harder to understand what the person is attempting to communicate, why a symptom is occurring, and what we can do about it. The onus is not on the person with dementia to change his or her behavior; rather, it's on caregivers to reframe responses in order to relieve the person's distress.

Although neither chemical nor physical restraints were suggested in Mrs. Chisholm's case, this method is unfortunately a frequent response. There is no evidence in research or in practice to suggest that using chemical or physical restraints has a significant long-term effect in treating the behavioral symptoms of dementia. In many cases, the use of restraints just makes things worse (Cohen-Mansfield, 2000; Richards, Lambert, & Beck, 2000; Talerico & Evans, 2000). It is startling to realize that all medications currently given for behavior management for persons with dementia are used on an off-label basis (Cummings, 2000). That is, behavior management is not one of the uses recognized by manufacturers.

While caring for Alice, I found it frustrating that even though she loved to go in the car, she always refused to put on her seat belt. Explaining and arguing every time wore my patience thin, and I had to insist on her buckling up before we could go anywhere. At the time, I thought that this was an issue of control. Now, too late, I think Alice was trying to let me know that the seat belt was uncomfortable. She was very short, so a seat belt would cut across her neck. If I had been thinking about what she was trying to tell me, I could have provided a soft fabric cover for the belt so it wasn't uncomfortable.

Alzheimer's Disease and Related Dementias Are Neurologically Based and Have Primarily Behavioral Symptoms

Even if the perfect caregiver and the perfect care situation existed, the person with dementia would still have challenging behaviors. These are the complex symptoms of a brain condition. No one can possibly anticipate every situation that may cause distress for the person. The goal is to provide care in such a way that these challenges are less frequent and less distressing to all involved. When a challenge does occur, try to take a problem-solving approach. In addition, try not to feel that either you have failed as a caregiver or that the person is being difficult on purpose. These challenges are the symptoms of a brain condition; no one is to blame or at fault.

PREVENTING CHALLENGES

An ounce of prevention is worth a pound of cure.

I hope that all of the information presented in the previous chapters has been helpful in understanding and preventing challenges. These ideas are reviewed next, and some new suggestions for prevention are introduced.

Help Maintain Long-Established Habits and a Familiar Lifestyle

As a toddler, my niece Erin had a particular fondness for bananas. She was very excited when her mother said that she could have half a banana. A helpful visitor peeled back the skin and passed the top half of the banana to Erin. You can imagine this person's surprise when Erin began to sob and wouldn't eat the banana. The problem was solved when Erin's mother suggested trading and giving Erin the half with the peel!

Parents know their children's habits and preferences and share this information with baby sitters. These routines are the small rhythms of daily life that ensure the child that there is order in the world, that provide comfort. As adults, we continue to rely on routines for reassurance and comfort. We are all creatures of habit, down to the tiniest detail. When others don't know these habits or we are unable to carry them out ourselves, we feel out of sorts.

Think about your own personal routines and how you feel if you can't continue with them—for example, someone is sitting in your favorite chair just when you need to relax, you can't watch your favorite television program because the playoffs are on, you are sick and need a cup of tea but you've run out of tea bags, or the dog destroyed your favorite pillow. Now think about how you might respond to these situations if you had dementia and couldn't understand or talk about what's wrong. You would be upset, so you might shout, swear, throw things, or become agitated.

For example, I prefer very hot coffee with a really small amount of cream. My family and friends are now used to seeing me go to the sink and dump out a half a cup of coffee because it has become too cold for me to enjoy. Suppose that I develop dementia and my caregiver lovingly brings a cup of lukewarm coffee loaded with cream and sugar. I respond by taking one sip, making a dreadful face, and dumping the rest of the coffee down the drain (or maybe even throwing the coffee). What is the caregiver, who doesn't know me and my habits, to think except that I am a cantankerous, ungrateful person who is difficult to take care of?

Now, take this a few stages further and think about when you are unwell or upset. For most of us, personal routines and the comfort and reassurance that they provide become even more important. The same must certainly be true of persons with dementia. As the brain deteriorates, it becomes harder to make sense of the world and to do the things needed to follow familiar habits. Just when these old habits are most needed to provide comfort, the person finds it difficult either to do these things independently or to tell others what they would like.

This is where family members, close friends, and partners play such a vital role. You know the person better than anyone else. Even if you aren't providing care directly, sharing this information with hands-on caregivers can make all the difference in meeting the person's needs and preventing the person from becoming upset and distressed, from presenting challenging behaviors. Please take the time to fill out the All About Me form in Appendix A. Add to this form as you discover things that work or that cause distress. Share it with all of the person's caregivers.

Support Involvement in Meaningful Activity

This point cannot be overemphasized: Anyone who is deprived of being able to do things that have personal meaning can become cranky and upset. A person with dementia is likely to become even more distressed because of the losses that he or she is already experiencing. It is understandable that one of the first concerns of caregivers is how to deal with challenging behavioral symptoms (negative behavior). However, I suggest that we try to turn this question around and instead ask, "How can we support involvement in meaningful activity (positive behavior)?" If the person has things to do that bring meaning to his or her days, it is less likely that the person will have an unmet need that is expressed as a behavioral symptom. Please see Chapters 6, 7, and 8 for more examples about and information on supporting involvement in meaningful activity.

Support Success

Undoubtedly, persons with dementia are very aware of their slipping abilities and are probably more sensitive than usual to failure. The experience of repeated failures can cause anyone to be frustrated and distressed. Whatever you do with the person, strive for success, supporting the person's sense of self. Supporting success also supports dignity and self-esteem.

Explain Everything, Assume Nothing

Often, persons with dementia have such well-preserved social skills that it is easy to forget that brain damage affects their ability to understand the people and events around them. For instance, persons with dementia may not recognize that the meal in front of them is there for them to eat. Rather than assuming that these persons are unable to feed themselves, we need to explain—using a lot of ways besides words (e.g., appealing to the senses, using gestures, helping them to start)—that this is their meal and it is time to eat. Explaining and asking permission becomes especially important when invading personal space for care activities such as bathing, toileting, and dressing.

Support the Need to Feel in Control

Physical illness had required Fred to live in a long-term care facility for years. He had a happy, positive relationship with the staff members; they cared for and about each other, much like a family. This positive relationship continued after Fred developed Alzheimer's disease, right through to the later stages. However, when Fred was no longer able to do his own personal care, his caregivers were surprised that he became angry and resistive when they tried to help. They explained what they were doing and were very gentle and caring, but no amount of explanation seemed to help. A routine was developed in which one person would hold Fred's hands while the other washed his private areas. It should be no surprise that Fred reacted with physical and verbal anger to this loss of control and

seeming invasion of his privacy. Although he was sweet and coop-
erative at other times, bathing Fred became a dreaded chore. The
situation changed entirely when Fred was given some control and
reassurance. His hands were freed and he was given a washcloth.
Sometimes he used this to try to wash himself; other times, he
used it to wipe the sink. After his upper body was washed, he was
helped to put on a warm and comfortable robe, which added to
his sense of security. While staff members washed his private
areas, Fred often enjoyed looking at and talking about a pleasant
poster of dogs, which was put up on the bathroom wall. Fred had
regained a sense of control and dignity, and bathing him was no
longer such a challenge.

Having a sense of control is a basic adult need. When this
is violated, it leads to distress. In every activity and situation,
there is opportunity for the person to have some control, to
feel that his or her personhood has been honored and
respected. We need to search for and provide these opportunities to prevent distress.

Encourage and Acknowledge
the Expression of Emotions and Feelings

Changes in the ability for verbal expression can lead to bot-
tled-up feelings and cause great frustration. Even if we can't
understand what the person is saying, it is important to listen
and acknowledge the feeling behind it. Comments such as,
"John, you sound sad; I am sorry," are calming and reassuring. If we are unable to understand the source of the person's
feelings, just letting him or her know that we are aware is
calming. It is critical to support the emotional message of
what may appear to be confused speech. It is also important
to offer numerous nonverbal ways to express feelings (e.g.,
listening to music, engaging in physical activity). See Chapter
4 for more suggestions.

Establish a Calm, Reassuring, Supportive, and Safe Environment

A living environment that provides comfort and security and says "you belong here" supports contentment. In turn, this environment helps to overcome anxiety and distress. For details and suggestions, see Chapter 5.

Avoid Arguing and Confrontation

Alice had always disliked the cold, and as her dementia progressed, she developed an even greater need to be really warm. For instance, she turned up the thermostat and then complained about it being too warm. When I checked the thermostat setting, Alice was surprised that it had been turned up so high. She said that the tenant upstairs must have come in when she was out and turned it up. My first (unstated) reaction was to say, "That's ridiculous and impossible." However, I bit my tongue, turned the thermostat down, and opened a window for a bit. As a long-term solution, we got an automatic thermostat that couldn't be tampered with and set it at a comfortably warm temperature.

A person with dementia is able to reason and often reaches a conclusion that seems correct to him or her. It is his or her best attempt to explain what is happening. Reasoning or arguing does little good. It is better to offer a distraction and change the topic than to get into a heated discussion.

Try New Solutions and Approaches

Our history of communicating with others—and the person we are caring for—is based on logic and reasoning. For example, when someone asks us where the bathroom is, we tell them, they go there, end of story. When someone with dementia asks us a similar question, he or she may wander down the hall in the correct direction but turn around and wander back, asking the same question and perhaps showing signs of incontinence. The natural response is to repeat the directions while feeling exasperated.

This is just one illustration of how easy it is to forget that the person who looks so normal has a damaged brain. It is also an illustration of how easy it is to get into a rut—of giving the same response over and over and thinking that if we repeat it often enough, the person will understand. In Chapter 2, I shared how I had become stuck in a rut, believing that if I just worked at it long enough, Alice would learn her new address. Of course she couldn't, and I was just causing us both distress by insisting that she try. It is difficult to make the leap—to realize that the way we are trying isn't working, that the person does not have the brain capacity to follow this method and we need to try something else. In the preceding example, rather than concluding that the person cannot learn to find the bathroom, we could try walking with the person to the bathroom every time he or she asks (so that the motor pattern can be learned) or placing artwork, an awning, or another three-dimensional object near the bathroom door so that the person can see it when he or she looks down the hall.

It is vital to appreciate that persons with dementia can learn if we set up learning for success. Being flexible and adaptable in our responses is an art form that is well worth learning. However, this flexibility needs to be balanced with the reassurance of a consistent, daily routine. Avoid introducing too many changes at once.

Learn from Past Experiences

It is important to avoid situations that have caused distress in the past (e.g., overstimulating visits or outings). Remember that although persons with dementia continue to need stimulation, they have a decreased threshold for coping with it. Also watch for signs that the person is becoming distressed (e.g., facial expressions, changes in physical activity).

Avoid Demanding Explanations
or Asking too Many Questions

The cognitive losses associated with dementia make it increasingly difficult for the person to answer questions that have right and wrong answers or to provide explanations. Caregivers need to learn to fill in the blanks based on other forms of communication. Asking too many questions can trigger challenging behaviors.

GETTING UNSTUCK: CREATIVE PROBLEM SOLVING

By making use of the guidelines in the previous chapters, you can help the person you are caring for to maintain a familiar lifestyle, to be involved. Unfortunately, despite our best efforts, there will continue to be challenging and frustrating caregiving situations when none of the previous suggestions seem to help. The unique ways in which dementia affects each person call for unique solutions. This may be especially true regarding required activities such as bathing.

While in the midst of trying to solve a complicated problem, especially one related to caregiving, it is easy to become so overwhelmed that you can't see the forest for the trees. It is also easy to become like a stuck record, hoping that the person will finally get it if you repeat solutions that worked when the person was well or that work for you. When I was a family caregiver, I found myself in this situation many times. After we moved Alice from another province to live in an apartment near us, she couldn't recite her address. I was concerned for her safety but focused on the problem instead of the person and her present abilities. When I finally realized that Alice could not learn her address, I was able to move out of the groove that I was stuck in and come up with other solutions. Because she loved jewelry, we gave Alice a necklace engraved with her name and address and emergency contact numbers. She always carried a purse with her, so we made sure it contained plenty of identification. Emergency numbers were placed by the telephone, and we practiced how to use them.

It is indeed wonderful that in so many ways, a person with dementia looks and acts like the same person that we have always known. Although social skills and other continuing abilities are great strengths to use during care, we also need to remember that these can camouflage the damage to the person's brain. It bears repeating that by the time we see the first signs of memory loss, 80% of the brain damage has already happened (Cummings, 1993).

The only window on the changes in the person's brain are the changes in the person's behavior. Outside, the person may appear the same; inside the brain, the changes are huge. This means that we caregivers have to change our way of doing things, to come up with different approaches that don't require persons with dementia to use the damaged part of their brain. Most important, we need to drop approaches that assume the person can still reason, think, and remember in the same way. Just as we don't expect a person who had a stroke to stop having symptoms (paralysis on one side), we cannot expect persons with dementia to stop having their symptoms (memory loss, disorientation).

Problem-Solving Steps

 When Cora began to wet her clothes, her caregiver, Eleanor, realized that Cora didn't understand when she needed to go to the bathroom. Using an approach that focused on the problem (rather than the person), Eleanor began to regularly ask Cora if she had to go to the bathroom. Because of the damage to her brain, Cora couldn't understand this question and always said no; thus, the accidents continued. Next, Eleanor began to regularly tell Cora to go to the bathroom. Cora was insulted, became angry, and refused to go to the bathroom; the problem continued.

Caregivers at Cora's day center suggested a person-centered approach, which respected Cora's dignity as an adult but also compensated for her difficulty in realizing when she needed to use the bathroom. Every couple of hours and after meals, the caregiver gently took Cora's arm and said, "Cora, I will help you to the bathroom." Cora felt better to be recognized as a person but also got the cues she needed, and the accidents happened much less often.

Problem solving is a very important caregiver skill, but remember to focus on the person, not on the problem. Combining an understanding of the person—his or her life story, values, and needs—with general care guidelines can provide direction (but not recipes) for solving some caregiving problems. In the preceding example, gently directing Cora to the bathroom was the most successful approach because it took into account both brain limitations and Cora's dignity.

A better understanding of the source of these challenging behaviors can trigger creative ideas to solve care challenges and get unstuck from unsuccessful care patterns. It is important to realize that there is no one right answer. By trying different ideas, you can often find a solution. Some may work; some may not. Whatever works this week might not work next week. You are invited to take a risk and try a different way; the payoff could be tremendous. There is not much to lose and much to be gained.

Because you as a caregiver are so close to the person and the problem, it may help to have a wise friend, a family member, or a professional work through the 11 problem-solving steps with you. The process is reviewed here and applied to the ensuing example of difficulty with bathing.

Step 1: Identify one challenge.

Although asking the question "What is the problem?" may sound ridiculous, it is an important place to start. Simple, pointed questions often untangle the complicated challenges of caregiving. Caregivers are understandably overwhelmed with a desire for the person to be the way that he or she used to be. This is a natural but impossible wish. Because of brain damage, the person simply cannot be the way that he or she was. This means that we need to change our behavior as caregivers. In addition, this approach ameliorates the feeling that everything is a problem, that everything needs to be changed. We are only human and can only deal with one thing at a time.

First, list all of your concerns. This helps to break caregiving challenges down into manageable pieces, so they can be dealt with one at a time. Sometimes just doing this exercise alone is helpful, as airing all of your concerns can release feelings and frustrations. Try to make these concerns very specific, such as repetitive questioning, wandering at night, not sitting to eat, restless pacing, and so forth.

Next, pick the one challenge or problem that is the most difficult for you and your loved one. Wandering at night is potentially the biggest concern, but only you can decide. After you have chosen one challenge, it is a good idea to keep notes about what time of day the problem occurs, what happens before and after, who is there, and so forth. These notes may be kept on a calendar and can help you organize your thoughts at a time when you may feel upset and distressed. If a certain behavior is really troubling, you may think that it is happening more often than it really is. This record also helps at the solution stage, when you're trying to determine whether something works.

 The main problem that Angela identified was Sam's restlessness at night. After recording details on the calendar for 2 weeks, she realized that Sam had a restless night on occasions when there was too much activity, such as when he visited his friend Al, attended his card club, waited in the car during shopping outings, or had long visits from grandchildren. Although Sam seemed to enjoy most of these activities for a while, he eventually became overstimulated and tired. With the help of the staff at Sam's day center, Angela was able to plan enjoyable activities that didn't cause Sam so much stress. For example, grandchildren visited only one or two at a time, and during these visits, Sam read their favorite stories to them. Then Angela took the grandchildren outside for more active play, which Sam could enjoy watching from inside. Playing cards had become difficult for Sam, so Angela found that it worked better if Sam attended the card club only for the socialization, which he could manage very well. Because Sam enjoyed going to church, he and Angela went together but skipped the fellowship coffee time after-

ward, which seemed to be too much for Sam. Angela also found ways to encourage Sam to help with chores at home. All of these changes helped Sam have fewer restless nights.

Step 2: Identify the owner of the problem.

Before trying to understand and respond creatively to the problem, asking the following question invites us to step back from the issue at hand: Is this a problem for the person or for the caregiver? Activities such as eating with a spoon instead of a fork, wearing mismatched clothing, telling the same story repeatedly, pacing, or constantly dusting the furniture may be frustrating and sometimes embarrassing for caregivers. But when you stop and think about it, do these things really cause any harm to the person or to you? For instance, having a safe area in which to pace, not the pacing itself, is the problem.

Conversely, I do understand just how difficult it can be to step back and look at a problem this way. As noted, Alice had two favorite outfits that she liked to wear all of the time. We shopped for clothes and Alice was delighted with the new outfits, but no amount of persuasion could convince her to wear them. Finally, I realized that it didn't matter all that much. Alice obviously felt most comfortable in her favorite dresses and that was what really counted.

Understanding the reasons behind challenging behaviors can reduce frustration and help us to step back from a problem. Working through Steps 3, 4, and 5, which follow, can aid your understanding. Asking yourself the question, "Whose problem is this?" involves considering how you feel about the problem. It can be that even when you understand the reasons behind a behavior, such as why the person constantly hums the same tune, it nonetheless drives you batty. This is perfectly natural.

If you can claim ownership of the problem, then it is important to ask yourself, "Is this behavior so troubling that it is impossible to ignore?" For instance, one caregiver reported that her husband constantly whistled through his teeth and asked what she could do to get him to stop. Just as I was about to ask, "Why does he need to stop?" she said, with gritted teeth, "It drives me crazy." Then I knew why we needed to work on a way to redirect this behavior (e.g., by distracting him with another repetitive activity such as chewing gum).

**Step 3: Identify what is going on
with the person that may explain the problem.**

Thinking about this concept is crucial. We need to stand in the person's shoes, to think about how he or she experiences the situation. We need to use an understanding of lifelong habits and values to get inside the behavior from the person's point of view. Having an intimate knowledge of the person is critical. It is especially important that paid caregivers learn as much as possible about the person from family and significant others.

By considering this concept and the one that follows in Step 4 (aspects of dementia's progress that may explain the problem), we are trying to get to the meaning, the feeling behind the behavior. Persons with dementia often have difficulty expressing their needs and feelings in words. When words fail, behaving in a certain manner can be the only way to express needs and feelings. As mentioned at the start of this chapter, challenging behaviors can best be understood as an expression of unmet needs.

All behavior has meaning; sometimes, we just can't figure out what the meaning is. Knowing the details of the person's habits and past life experiences is a tremendous help in understanding behavior. These details can be big, such as the name we use to refer to the person, or even seemingly minor, such as the type of toothpaste the person prefers. For example, one person understandably changed from being pleasant and helpful to agitated and physically aggressive when care facility staff members called him "Johnnie" instead of "John" or "Reverend Smith." Another illustration is the story about the man who had worked in a mill and wouldn't eat lunch unless his caregiver blew the noon lunch whistle.

Step 4: Identify aspects of dementia's progress that may explain the problem.

Now it is time to shift our attention to the symptoms of dementia and how they may be contributing to the problem. Although behavioral changes are themselves symptoms, at this point we are thinking about how changes in communication, memory, cognition, and perception contribute to the problem. For example, a common behavioral symptom is sundowning, which often includes searching for home at the end of the day. Among the many causes that have been suggested are certain dementia-related factors:

- Perceptual deficits—the way the brain understands what is seen is probably made much worse with the light changes as the sun goes down, and the person may not recognize that he or she is in fact at home
- Increased sensitivity to stimulation—caregivers often engage in a higher level of activity at this time of day (e.g., preparing for dinner)
- Difficulty communicating concerns and fears

Home caregivers are understandably upset when their loved one talks about wanting to go home at this time of day. This must feel like the ultimate insult, given all of your efforts to keep the person at home. It helps if you understand that the person has perceptual problems, which may make it difficult to recognize where he or she is or who you are. Wishing to go home may also be related to communication difficulties. Perhaps the person is really trying to say that he or she is feeling frightened and insecure and is seeking the comfort or emotional shelter that is associated with the concept of *home*. See Chapter 5 for more details on this challenge.

Step 5: Ask yourself how you would *feel* if this were you.

It is essential to take a moment and put yourself in the shoes of the person that you are caring for and try to imagine how you would feel if you were in similar circumstances. This gives not only more empathy and compassion for the person but also often provides solutions to the challenges. For instance, how stressful would it be if you *knew* that you had to be at work or at home caring for your children but you could not get there because you were in a place that you did not recognize and nobody would let you leave?

When we appreciate how stressful and real these feelings are, we can find ways to reassure the person that his or her work was valued in the past (i.e., by talking to him or her about the work) and now (i.e., by finding ways that he or she can help you).

Step 6: Decide whether a change is needed or the behavior can be accepted.

This step is connected with Step 2, regarding whose problem this challenging behavior is. After having worked through Steps 3 and 4, do you feel more able to accept, for example, that the person can't help asking the same questions or telling the same story repeatedly? Chapter 1 suggested strategies for expressing your feelings as a caregiver and managing stress; these may be useful in helping you accept the situation.

If the problem continues to cause frustration, ask yourself, "Is the goal to eliminate the behavior or to have it happen less often?" Some challenging behaviors, such as wandering into the street, are so dangerous that we need to work toward eliminating them altogether. However, for many challenges, such as rummaging in drawers, it is unrealistic to expect that the behavior will disappear completely. If we expect to reach this goal, we often set ourselves up for failure. It may help to think about this behavior as the person's way of telling us something. For instance, a person who rummages in drawers may be expressing a need to continue with lifelong activities. From this point of view, perhaps the behavior can be thought of as shopping, sorting, or organizing. It would be more realistic to aim for preventing rummaging in certain drawers (i.e., those containing important, dangerous, or fragile items). This goal might be accomplished by providing drawers of safe things that can be sorted and rearranged and locking up other drawers.

Some behavioral symptoms, though frustrating, are simply inevitable; there isn't much that can be done except to try to change our response as caregivers. For example, there is little hope that persons with profound memory loss can learn not to repeatedly ask about the same concerns. Caregivers who learn to accept this as fact usually experience less frustration. Previous chapters suggested ways to provide reassurance and structure, which may help to reduce the frequency of repeated questions.

**Step 7: Determine what happens
just before and just after the challenging behavior.**

Thinking about the people and places that surround a challenging behavior can help with understanding and finding solutions. Does the difficulty occur at a certain time of day, with a particular caregiver, or when the person is tired? Keeping a record is helpful.

It is also important to think about the usual response to the challenging behavior. As discussed previously, a person with dementia, like anyone else, has an ongoing need to experience pleasure and to get attention from others. If these needs are not met, it is only natural that the person will seek to have his or her needs met in any way possible. For example, if the person is ignored when he or she is quiet and gets a lot of attention when he or she shouts, it is likely that the person will continue to shout. It doesn't really matter if the attention is positive or negative; negative attention (e.g., scolding) is better than no attention at all. It could be that the person is starved for attention. This is a worst-case example, but, unfortunately, it does happen.

Step 8: Generate a list of possible solutions that use persisting strengths.

At last, we're getting to the main point. Because the challenges of care can be so overwhelming, it is understandable that you may be tempted to jump in with solutions. However, the point of the preceding steps is to foster understanding so that you can come up with workable solutions. Throw every possible idea onto the table. This creative process is important because one solution rarely works every time. There is no right answer. Remember to include the person's continuing strengths in your list (as discussed in Chapter 3).

Step 9: Evaluate the solutions and pick the best one(s).

Use your intimate experience with and understanding of the person to organize ideas according to what is likely to work and what is easiest to put in place. It is important to appreciate that probably no single solution will work every time due to the variability of dementia. The goal is to come up with a range of possible solutions, so if Plan A doesn't work, you always have a Plan B, C, or D. However, only try one solution at a time.

Because you know the person best and know what you have tried in the past, you are the best judge of what might work. The word *might* is really important here—you never know if something will work until you try it.

Step 10: Implement the selected solution.

When trying possible solutions, it's particularly important to be patient and to remember the reasons why the challenging behavior may be occurring. Unless the trial is a total disaster, you may need to give it several tries before deciding that it does not work. For example, Chapter 7 suggested changes that make the bathroom a more welcoming place. The person needs time to adjust to these changes, so the bathroom also becomes a more familiar place, before it's determined whether the changes have made a difference. Sometimes, we need to change more than one thing; it may be that a combination of several things will work. We also need to give ourselves time as caregivers to become comfortable with this different way of doing things.

Step 11: Evaluate the effectiveness of
the solution; if it was unsuccessful, try another.

Never let a good failure go to waste! Try not to invest too much in one particular solution. As you know, nothing in dementia care is a guaranteed success. If something doesn't work well, back up and try again. Remember that it is not your caregiving that failed; it is this particular solution that failed. Again, sometimes a combination of several solutions finally works. Remember that trying and failing is not a problem, as you never know until you try.

Problem Solving Applied to Challenges with Bathing

For most adults bathing is a pleasant, relaxing activity. We may have a shower or a bath to relax at the end of a busy day or to wake up in the morning. As noted in Rader and Barrick (2000), if it wasn't pleasant, we would all find other ways to keep clean! Unfortunately, as dementia progresses, the complicated activity of bathing becomes so difficult that the person needs help from others. When this happens, the person has to give up control of this previously personal, adult activity. Unfortunately, bathing can then become a dreaded task rather than a pleasure. I hope that considering this particular challenge will help caregivers to give the person control and to find pleasure in bathing.

Step 1: Identify one challenge.

The main challenge is not washing properly.

Step 2: Identify the owner of the problem.

Carefully consider this question to be sure that you are not imposing your standards for type or frequency of bathing. If the person is happy with a sponge bath but doesn't like to get in the tub, there really is no problem. Caregivers from a younger generation, who may be used to daily showers, can be especially challenged by caring for someone who grew up in the era of the "Saturday night bath." (This was even my experience growing up in rural Ontario just 50 years ago!) If the person is continent, there is no need for the person to bathe more than once per week. As a nursing colleague, Geri Hall, remarked, "No one ever died because they didn't have a bath!"

**Step 3: Identify what is going on
with the person that may explain the problem.**

- Embarrassment and frustration that he or she can't bathe independently

- Frustration and anger at the loss of personal control and the invasion of personal space by the caregiver who is assisting
- Embarrassment at being undressed in front of others (many older adults were never even naked in front of their spouses)
- Confusion due to an unfamiliar method of bathing (perhaps the use of a bath bench or other equipment makes the task unfamiliar)
- Discomfort regarding temperature (age-related changes in temperature regulation mean that the room temperature may have to be as much as 10 degrees Fahrenheit warmer to feel comfortable)
- Fear of getting sick (some people hold firmly to the myth that bathing in the winter is unhealthy and causes pneumonia)
- Different standards of hygiene

Step 4: Identify aspects of dementia's progress that may explain the problem.

The following dementia-related issues may contribute to difficulty with bathing:

- Inability to organize the many complicated steps involved in bathing
- Lack of awareness that he or she needs a bath (due to memory loss)
- Difficulty getting in and out of the tub (due to motor and coordination problems)
- Inability to see the bottom of the bathtub (due to perceptual problems, the person becomes frightened about getting in)

- Fear of being drawn down the drain with the water (due to faulty reasoning)
- Fear of drowning or suffocating from the water rushing over his or her face during a shower or hair washing (due to faulty reasoning)
- Unable to understand what is expected (due to communication problems)
- Inability to recognize the caregiver; thus, the person resists the stranger who is undressing him or her
- A collapse of intervening years and events (due to memory loss)—the person may be transported back to a past traumatic experience and become very frightened

Step 5: Ask yourself how you would *feel* if this were you.

Take a moment and stand in the person's shoes. How would you feel if you had to have someone else, either someone close to you (e.g., your spouse, your daughter) or a stranger (or someone who seems like a stranger to you), help you bathe? Really experiencing these feelings can help us all to be more empathetic and supportive. In training new long-term care staff, Joanne Rader actually asks people to pair up and meet her at the showers with their towels and shampoo, prepared to bathe each other. Although she does not actually have the staff take showers, she finds that this exercise evokes dismay and other sentiments that effectively give staff insight into what persons with dementia may be feeling and why they may resist help with bathing (Rader & Barrick, 2000).

Step 6: Decide whether a change is needed or the behavior can be accepted.

This is a highly individualized decision. How often is it really necessary to bathe? Modern standards of a daily bath or

shower need not be the standard for the person you are caring for. Of course when there is a need for a bath, for the sake
of the person and ourselves, we would like it to be a positive
and pleasant experience. We would like to reduce the level of
distress for all involved.

Step 7: Determine what happens just before and just after the challenging behavior.

Unfortunately, bathing has become so stressful and upsetting
for some people with dementia and their caregivers that the
very mention of a bath sets up a negative and fearful tone. In
these cases, hard work is needed to develop more positive
associations with bath time. It may be necessary to include
soft towels or robes in a favorite color, music, or pretty bathroom decorations.

Step 8: Generate a list of possible solutions that use persisting strengths.

Consider every possible idea at this step. Some possible solutions follow:

- Approach bathing in ways that respect adult dignity, yet
  expect a positive response. Bathing is a very sensitive and
  personal activity; care must be taken not to offend the
  person. It is also important to reassure the person that
  you will be there to help. You might say, "I have a nice
  warm bath all ready for you; I will go with you to the
  bathroom." Gently take the person's arm and start walking toward the bathroom. Always give step-by-step
  explanations of everything that is happening. This is
  especially important regarding the invasion of personal
  space, such as helping the person to undress. It may be
  helpful to avoid using the word "bath" and to use less
  threatening expressions such as "getting cleaned up" or
  "freshening up."

- Provide pleasant experiences by using favorite towels, soft robes, scented soaps and powders, candles, or music. Use the techniques of sensory stimulation described in Chapter 6. Drawing attention to the smell of the soap or the pretty color of the towel not only provides pleasure but also encourages the person to participate. Baby washcloths and soaps are gentler. Pleasant conversation is reassuring and can help make bathing a more social occasion that is less embarrassing for both of you. As discussed in Chapter 7, the bathroom itself should be a pleasant and inviting place.

- Explore the many ways to get clean besides taking a tub bath. Examples include a sponge bath, a shower, a bed bath, or cleansing with rinseless soap.

- Provide personal control by encouraging the person to do as much as possible independently. Even persons with advanced dementia can hold a washcloth, which helps them to feel like they are participating. The caregiver should always try to give the impression that the person is bathing and the caregiver is just helping. (Some individuals may be used to having others help wash their back, so this may be a comfortable way to start.) Provide choices about towels, clothing, and so forth; also offer a choice about timing (e.g., ask "Would you like your bath now or after breakfast?").

- Protect the person's privacy. Never let the person be totally naked (e.g., use a bath blanket, drape a robe around the person's shoulders). If sponge bathing, the person doesn't need to be completely undressed at once. The person's upper body can be washed and dressed before his or her lower body is undressed and washed. As noted, one caregiver reported that when her mother agreed to help with her bath, she came to the bathroom wearing her bathing suit. In another situation, the person got into the bathtub fully dressed and removed her own clothing as it got wet.

- Give the person a positive reason to have a bath (e.g., for going to church, for receiving a visitor the next day).

- Separate hair washing and bathing. Sometimes, hair washing is actually more frightening than bathing. Some women may be happy and comfortable to continue with having their hair done by a hairdresser. One creative caregiver created a weekly contest for a free hairdo. The person who had been reluctant to have her hair washed was thrilled with the prize she had won!

- Start with a more neutral activity if the person is upset by the whole idea of assistance with bathing. For instance, suggest something that is relaxing and comforting (e.g., a foot soak, a massage).

- Get the room as warm as possible, and warm towels and clothes by putting them in the dryer briefly.

- Consider assistance from a paid caregiver for this activity. Bathing can be one of the most difficult activities for family caregivers to be involved in because it is such a departure from their usual role.

- Have the person's doctor write a prescription for bathing if the person respects the advice of his or her physician.

- Let the water drain before the person gets out to reduce the risk of falling. Ensure that this action will not cause fear that he or she will be pulled down the drain.

- Put a colored bath mat in the bottom of the bathtub so the person can clearly see the bottom.

- Install sturdy grab bars to help the person feel more secure when getting in and out of the tub.

Step 9: Evaluate the solutions and pick the best one(s).

You know the person best and know what you have tried in the past, so you are the best judge of what might work. The word *might* is really important here. You will never know if something will work until you try it, as shown in the following illustration.

Suppose that Priscilla is a very private person who has always been concerned about being properly groomed and dressed. As Priscilla's dementia progresses, however, Priscilla's daughter and caregiver, Joan, notices that her mother is not bathing properly. Joan offers to help, but Priscilla insists she is doing fine and does not need any help. Joan then tries the following plan. Because she knows that her mother has always bathed on Sundays before church, she chooses this as a logical bath time. She also takes her mother shopping to purchase a new outfit to wear to church. In addition, Joan decides to offer Priscilla a surprise "home spa" treatment. She buys a lovely new robe in her mother's favorite color and a special selection of soaps and shampoos to arrange attractively in a basket.

Step 10: Implement the selected solution.

It is unlikely that you will happen upon the perfect solution with your first attempt. Try to be patient and realize that all plans will need some fine tuning. Unless the solution attempted was a total disaster, it may require several tries and giving everyone time to get comfortable before turning to another plan. Here is how things worked out for Joan and Priscilla:

At bath time, Joan told her mother that to celebrate the new outfit they had bought for Priscilla, Joan had a big surprise. She gently took her mother's arm and walked with enthusiasm to the bathroom. She had the bathroom all set up to look like a spa, with some new plants, Priscilla's favorite music, and things arranged just to Priscilla's liking. Joan also had a nice warm bath ready. Her mother was delighted with the surprise and responded positively to Joan's suggestion to get in before the water got too cool. Joan held out the new robe and offered to help her mother get undressed. However, Priscilla said that she would rather undress on her own. Joan accepted this need for privacy and said that she would be nearby if her mother needed help washing her back.

Step 11: Evaluate the effectiveness of the solution; if it was unsuccessful, try another.

Problem solving involves coming up with a range of possible solutions, so backtrack and try again if something doesn't work. Sometimes a combination of several solutions may finally work, but remember that nothing is going to work 100% every time, as shown in the continuing story of Joan and Priscilla.

Joan's solution worked well at getting Priscilla into the tub on Sunday morning. Priscilla was pleased with Joan's attention and looked forward to this time, which established a positive association with bathing and a good rapport between mother and daughter about this issue. Unfortunately, although Priscilla got in the tub and got wet, Joan knew, by body odor, that Priscilla was not actually washing. Joan now needs to find some other solutions for offering her mother help with the actual washing. These might inclhude Joan's suggesting that she will come in the bathroom at a certain time to help her mother wash her back (leaving a towel on the edge of the tub for Pricilla to use to protect her privacy) or Joan's knocking before entering with her mother's church clothes and saying, "While I am here, I will just wash your back." If these and other solutions prove unsuccessful, Joan may need to involve a paid caregiver to help with her mother's bath.

Responding to Challenging Behavioral Symptoms

Despite the best prevention efforts, there will be times the person will become upset or distressed. You will need to respond in ways that will help restore calm. General guidelines for on-the-spot responses follow:

- Provide emotional support, reassurance, and caring attention. Be mindful of the basic human need for caring and quiet attention by using every opportunity to speak with, touch, and acknowledge the person. This can help to avoid situations in which the person may get so desperate that he or she calls out for attention by shouting or other means. People tend to continue with behavior that gets rewarded (i.e., meets their needs). If the person's need for caring attention is not being met in positive ways, negative behaviors will often result. As noted previously, for a person who is not getting any attention, negative attention is better than no attention at all. These negative ways of getting attention should be neither rewarded nor dismissed. Instead, they should prompt caregivers into immediate action to address the person's unmet need. For example, one gentleman in a long-term care facility was regularly falling because he kept trying to get out of his wheelchair, even though he knew that he was unable to walk. This situation and the person's need were dismissed by staff as "attention seeking"—end of story! When a person is so desperate for attention that he undergoes pain from falling and the anger of staff members, it is really just the beginning of the story.

- Listen to the emotional message of the behavior and the communication and respond accordingly. (See Chapter 5 for more details.)

- Distract the person rather than confront him or her.
- Redirect the person with meaningful activities. Gross motor activities—such as walking, vacuuming, and sweeping—are especially good.
- Think about what the person used to do when he or she was stressed (e.g., walking, cleaning, listening to music), and try to involve him or her in these activities.
- Use gentle humor.
- Find ways for the person to maintain control; help the person to save face.
- Avoid power struggles.
- Avoid shouting or displaying anger.

ADDRESSING SPECIFIC BEHAVIORAL SYMPTOMS

Walking About (Wandering, Pacing, and Restlessness)

Because wandering is commonly a high concern, it is addressed again in this chapter. Walking about is not, in itself, a problem. In fact, it is a way to relieve stress and can be good exercise. Persons with dementia who walk about are often more physically healthy than those who don't. This behavior becomes a problem only when the person walks into areas that are unsafe, tries to leave the care environment (and risks getting lost), or becomes exhausted (and risks falling). The challenge is to find ways that the person can walk about safely. In addition, keep in mind that this exercise can burn a lot of calories, so the person may need extra high-energy snacks (e.g., pieces of cheese, high-protein milk shakes).

What Might the Person Need?

- Regular exercise
- Access to the outdoors

- Involvement in meaningful activities
- A safe place to walk about
- Reassurance that he or she will be taken care of
- Assistance meeting a personal need
- Distraction from the repetitive activity of walking, if he or she is becoming tired

How Can These Needs Be Met?

- Safety proof an area of the home and/or outdoors for safe walking. A circular path with points of interest is usually best. See Chapter 5 for more details.
- Involve the person in meaningful activity.
- Disguise exits. Use a curtain, removable cloth strips, or a mural; paint the handle and door frame the same color as the door; or try a two-dimensional grid in front of the door. For further information, see Chapter 5.
- Attend to personal needs. The person may be unable to verbalize that this restlessness is caused by needing to go to the bathroom, being hungry or thirsty, feeling uncomfortable because of his or her footwear or clothing, or being too hot or too cold.
- Remember that at least a part of the wandering behavior is related to searching for the familiar, for reassurance. Constant reassurance provides a message that the person is safe and cared for.
- Provide a safe outlet for the energy used in pacing (e.g., using a rocking chair or exercise bicycle, taking walks with caregivers, engaging in meaningful activity). Plan a physical activity at least once during the day. If the person is unsteady on his or her feet, an adult walker can provide a safe way to move about independently. See

Appendix B for resources, and consult a physical therapist or an occupational therapist for help in choosing a walking aid.

- Don't tell the person about planned activities too far in advance. Doing so may increase restlessness because of difficulty with memory or concern about how he or she will cope.
- Ensure that the circumstances are not over- or under-stimulating. If the restlessness is relatively new or has a sudden onset, have a medical professional check for an infection or illness.
- Address the perserveration (uncontrollable, repetitive activity) that is caused by brain damage. The person may become stuck in the repetitive activity of pacing and may continue to do so even when he or she is obviously tired and at risk of falling. Sometimes, simply offering a pleasant distraction (e.g., sitting down with the person to enjoy a snack) helps the person rest and "get unstuck."

What Are Some Possible Responses?

- Provide a positive distraction (e.g., listening to music, chatting).
- Walk with the person if he or she wanders outside. Begin a nonconfrontational conversation that addresses present emotional concerns or distracts by focusing on a favorite topic. Gradually change the direction in which you and the person are walking and return to home. Orders, commands, or expressions of anger should be avoided at all costs, as these may make the person even more determined to leave.

Nighttime Restlessness

This topic is discussed in Chapter 7 in the section titled "Sleeping."

Sundowning

Sundowning describes the extra restlessness that some persons with dementia experience at the end of the day (i.e., as the sun goes down). The many possible explanations for this behavior are undoubtedly related. Examples include increased difficulty understanding the environment as natural daylight fades, increased stimulation from caregivers' extra activity at this time of day (e.g., family members coming home and preparing for dinner, staff members changing shifts at a care facility), fatigue and reduced ability to cope, and the natural tendency to want to go home at the end of the day (e.g., to go home after a long day at the office). Perceptual deficits and other dementia-related problems often contribute as well.

What Might the Person Need?

- A calm reassuring environment that says, "Stay here with me"
- A quiet place that avoids the overstimulation caused by increased caregiver activities at this time of day
- Knowledge that someone is going to take care of him or her
- Extra clues about the time of day
- Adequate exercise and activity earlier in the day
- Support for personal routines that occur during this time of day

How Can These Needs Be Met?

- Keep the levels of noise and stimulation to a minimum.
- Provide constant reassurance that someone is there to care for the person.
- Identify with the emotional need for home—that is, emotional shelter (see Chapter 5).

- Close the blinds or curtains and turn on plenty of lights.
- Provide an outlet for the person's energy by giving opportunities for exercise and activity earlier in the day.
- Ask the person to help with the evening meal preparation.

Repetitive Questioning

Try to learn to accept repeated questioning. Because of severe memory loss, a person with dementia really doesn't recall that he or she just asked the same question. Be patient and reassuring. If the question has to do with finding a loved one (e.g., a parent, a spouse, a child), tell the person that you are there and will care for him or her. Identify with the person's need to recall this loved one, and assist him or her to reminisce.

What Might the Person Need?

- Reassurance
- Regular routines
- Manageable stimulation

How Can These Needs Be Met?

- Support the emotional need and meaning behind repeated questions (see Chapter 4).
- Offer a variety of experiences and activities.
- Offer an interesting and distracting activity or item to redirect a person who perseverates (gets stuck on one phrase). Motor activities, such as going for a walk or folding towels, are particularly good.
- Provide a large card printed with the answers to frequently asked questions. Incorporating movement into

the use of the card can help the person learn how to use it. For example, place the card on the refrigerator or in another familiar location. Then, every time the person asks the question, walk with him or her to the card. The person will probably never learn not to ask the question, but he or she often can learn to walk to the card to find the answer independently.

- Provide ample orienting cues in the environment, such as calendars and clocks, and reality reassurance during conversation (see Chapter 5).
- Try to maintain a consistent and predictable daily routine.

Shadowing

Due to the many cognitive and perceptual problems associated with dementia, the person is prone to becoming anxious and fearful. This anxiety may be especially heightened if the caregiver—the person's lifeline and solace—leaves the room. To compensate for the fear of being abandoned, the person may shadow the caregiver, following the caregiver everywhere. This can be very frustrating because the caregiver never seems to have a moment alone. As discussed in Chapter 1, it is important for caregivers to find a way to have a regular break from caregiving, whether in the home or outside of the home (i.e., using respite care).

What Might the Person Need?

- Reassurance and consistency

How Can This Need Be Met?

- Provide a consistent daily routine.
- Frequently reassure the person that you will always be there to take care of him or her.

- Avoid talking about planned activities too far in advance.
- Tell the person where you are going and what you are doing. If the person can still read, leave a note saying where you have gone and when you will be back.
- Try to set up your daily chores, such as meal preparation, so that the person can see you as you work.
- Plan activities that can be done together.

Saving and Shopping (Hoarding and Hiding)

For some persons with dementia, the combination of shopping and saving can become a favorite self-created activity. This is very inventive but can be troublesome for caregivers because it becomes hard to keep track of things. In addition, the person may gather and hide food, which can create an odor problem and the risk of food poisoning (if the person finds and eats spoiled food).

Grace had mid-stage Alzheimer's disease and lived happily at home with her husband. The only difficulty was Grace's concern about losing her money and her purse.

Several times per month, Grace called her daughter Elizabeth to say that her purse was missing. After a few times, Elizabeth learned where to look. Grace felt the need to secure her purse; therefore, she wrapped it in several layers of paper and string and tucked it into a suitcase at the back of a closet. Elizabeth was able to decrease Grace's anxiety (and the resulting telephone calls) by buying a second purse, exactly the same, and placing some money and a bank book inside. Elizabeth also helped her father understand that Grace, who had always done the family finances, still needed to be involved with the finances by going on trips to the bank, signing checks, and being kept up to date on the bank balance.

What Might the Person Need?

- Extra reassurance that food will always be available
- Participation in meaningful activities
- Opportunities for control
- Help organizing personal possessions so they don't get lost

How Can These Needs Be Met?

- Put healthy snacks (e.g., fruit or vegetable pieces) in accessible areas so the person can get them independently.
- Provide a cupboard and/or a bureau containing safe and interesting things that the person can sort through and reorganize. Be sure to prevent access to other areas by using childproof locks or the other suggestions found in Chapter 5.
- Safety proof favorite but dangerous hiding places such as the oven, stove burner elements, drains, or the garbage disposal.
- Provide adequate opportunities for the person to make choices and have control, as suggested in Chapters 6 and 7.
- Always put important personal possessions (e.g., photos, purse) in the same place.
- Get duplicates of important items (e.g., glasses) if necessary.
- Learn the person's favorite hiding places.

Repetitive Behaviors

In the later stages of dementia, repetitive hand clapping, banging, or shouting can be a problem. These behaviors often are the result of boredom—lacking stimulation, persons provide their own. This behavior may be complicated by the tendency to perseverate on a particular activity or phrase and by the attention that such behavior receives, even if it is negative.

What Might the Person Need?

- Stimulation
- Attention

How Can These Needs Be Met?

- Provide stimulation that the person can manage. The best approach is to provide a self-directed, repetitive activity that is not disruptive—for example, looking at a book or magazine, feeling or holding onto a various-textured quilt, or sanding wood. For more suggestions, see the "Self-Directed Activities" section in Chapter 8.

- Remember to provide caring attention. Keep in mind the basic human need for caring and quiet attention by using every chance to speak with, touch, and acknowledge the person. Doing so can help avoid situations in which the person becomes desperate for attention and resorts to shouting or other means to get it.

Suspiciousness

Due to cognitive losses, especially difficulties in remembering and understanding what's going on around them, persons with dementia may become suspicious that family members, home helpers, or others are taking their things, trying to harm them, and so forth. Such suspicious ideas are a person's best attempt at making sense of the increasingly confusing world around him or her. Despite memory loss, these ideas can become remarkably fixed. It is, of course, extremely upsetting for a struggling caregiver to be accused of taking the person's money or of having an affair with the neighbor.

Visual or auditory hallucinations may contribute to suspicion in some persons with dementia. A physician who has expertise in the care of persons with dementia should be consulted to determine whether medication may be of assistance.

What Might the Person Need?

- Help in keeping track of personal possessions
- Help interpreting the world around him or her
- An environment that is easy to manage

How Can These Needs Be Met?

- Keep the environment and personal possessions organized so there is less chance that things will get lost.
- Have duplicates of favorite or important items (e.g., purse, glasses, photos).
- Learn the person's favorite hiding places.
- Provide safe, secure, accessible places for prized personal possessions. Mount family photos on the wall near the person's bed, attach a pouch or carry bag to the person's favorite chairs, or provide a fanny pack to hold personal possessions. Such carry bags and fanny packs can be made in materials of various textures so that they also provide sensory stimulation.
- Ensure that the person's vision and hearing are checked regularly and that his or her glasses or hearing aids are properly cleaned and used.
- Avoid ambiguous or confusing designs and pictures.

- Explain sounds or events that may cause alarm or confusion. For example, let the person know that the noise outside is a truck picking up the garbage.

What Are Some Possible Responses?

- Provide reassurance, and respond to the emotion of the concern. For example, if a person says, "That housekeeper is stealing all of my money," respond to the person's concern about having enough money. Offer reassurance about personal finances in ways that the person can understand, such as showing him or her the bank account balance, making sure that the person always has some money in his or her wallet, or giving general verbal reassurance. If you are concerned about the person losing money, providing a few small bills may be enough to offer reassurance. Often, persons with dementia no longer understand the actual value of particular bills, so they may be just as happy having a few dollars as they would be having a $20 bill.
- Never lie or deceive. The person may not remember the content of what was said, but he or she will remember the feeling of being deceived.
- Neither play into a misconception or hallucination nor attempt to argue or reason the person out of it. Such misconceptions are not reasonable to us, but they are firmly fixed in the person's mind and represent his or her best attempt to explain what's happening to him or her.

Extreme Distress (Agitation)

Because it is never possible to anticipate and meet all care needs, there will be situations when the person becomes distressed or upset. With patience and experience, you can keep these times to a minimum. The person will usually become happier and less distressed as you work to meet his or her needs.

Nonetheless, extreme agitation or aggression is not to be expected. This behavior is rare and means that the person's needs are not being met. If the person suddenly becomes agitated and aggressive, a physical problem (e.g., an infection) is highly possible. Consult a physician immediately.

If extreme distress or agitation is a regular pattern, it is necessary to make a thoughtful and careful study of the person's needs and how they are being met in the care situation. Outside professional help from experts in the care of persons with dementia is recommended. The local Alzheimer's Association or Alzheimer Society chapter may be able to direct you to such services in your area.

All of the preceding ideas are suggestions for preventing the escalation of distress, which may lead the person to strike others. It should be stressed again that a calming, reassuring environment and approach is of utmost importance in preventing these incidents. If a person is becoming agitated or upset, intervene at once, either moving him or her to a quieter setting or trying some of the procedures already suggested. Other pointers follow.

- Remain calm.
- Offer a distraction, such as eating a snack, taking a walk, or doing another favorite activity. Motor activities are especially good for venting frustration.
- Never approach or move the person unexpectedly. Persons with dementia may have a return of the startle response, a reflexive reaction to a sudden noise, touch, or change of position.
- Avoid confrontation except in cases of safety risks. Even in these cases, it is often better to leave the situation and get immediate help.

- Speak calmly and quietly, responding to the person's emotional concerns.

- Call for help if you are at all concerned for your safety or the safety of others. You should have a preorganized plan of action for such emergencies (e.g., a neighbor or family member who can be called).

- Keep your distance and give the upset individual personal space.

- Reduce stimulation in the area (e.g., turn off the radio).

- Remove any potentially harmful objects from the environment.

Catastrophic Reactions

A *catastrophic reaction* is an expression of extreme distress (e.g., anger, agitation, crying) to what may appear to be a simple or unimportant occurrence. These reactions occur when the person with dementia feels overwhelmed, perhaps by something as apparently simple as dropping a sandwich or being unable to recall a particular word. Again, these reactions are best avoided by following the preventive actions already discussed and by watching for signs of increasing distress and concern.

What Might the Person Need?

- Successful experiences
- Nurturing and understanding
- A less demanding environment

How Can These Needs Be Met?

- Avoid challenging the person beyond his or her capacity to act and respond.
- Avoid overstimulating environments.

- Analyze the circumstances surrounding the reaction and try to avoid them in future.
- Evaluate the action taken and determine its effectiveness.

What Are Some Possible Responses?

- Speak calmly and reassuringly.
- Move slowly.
- Don't restrain the person, but use reassuring physical touch as appropriate.
- Move the person to a calmer environment.
- Call for assistance, if necessary.
- Use gradual distraction.

Inappropriate Sexual Behavior

Dementia rarely causes sexual disinhibition. However, when this behavior occurs, it is extremely embarrassing and distressing for the caregiver; as a result, it may appear to be more common than it actually is. When problem solving, it is especially important to consider the role of misinterpretation or misunderstanding. Sometimes a person's confused actions—such as fiddling with buttons or zippers or attempting to remove clothing—may be incorrectly interpreted as sexual behavior. In reality, the person may have to go to the bathroom and be unaware that he or she is in a public place or may be unable to find the toilet. In addition, a person may masturbate without being aware that he or she is in a public place. Furthermore, removing clothing or undoing buttons and zippers can be a form of self-stimulation or self-directed activity.

Sometimes, however, a person with dementia may misinterpret a caregiver's touch as a sexual gesture. This is an extremely sensitive and difficult subject for all caregivers, but it is especially so for family members, who will be upset at their relative's seeming loss of social control. For spouse care-givers, the issue is even more complicated. Some guidelines follow; see Chapter 7 for more details.

- Be aware that the individual with dementia has continu-ing needs for caring attention and affection, and these needs may be unmet. Provide appropriate caring personal touch to meet those needs: touching the person on the arm, shoulder, or hand; giving a hug around the person's shoulders; taking a person's arm or hand as you walk together; rubbing on hand cream; or, if appropriate for the person, offering a shoulder or neck massage. Make sure actions cannot be misunderstood; for example, avoid sitting close to the person on the bed.

- Protect individual dignity. Never make a game or a joke of sexual overtures. (This is particularly applicable to care facility environments.)

- Provide and respect the need for privacy.

- Provide ample opportunity for bolstering self-esteem and receiving important positive attention.

CONCLUSION

Understanding and responding to what appears to be inap-propriate sexual behavior by persons with dementia is perhaps one of the most challenging aspects of dementia care. Although there are no easy solutions, caregivers who can appreciate that these and other challenging behaviors are in fact symptoms of Alzheimer's disease and other dementias are more likely to find solutions. Like all other symptoms, these behaviors cannot be consciously controlled by the person. Understanding challenging behaviors as expressions of unmet needs and approaching them from a creative problem-solving perspective often enables caregivers to find solutions.

Chapter 10 offers caregivers guidelines for solutions to care planning issues.

10

Care Planning

The best advice we received was from a physician who told my mother, my brother, and me to "get a plan." Don't wait until a crisis comes. If, for instance, the caregiver becomes ill or dies, what will you do? This advice made all the difference in the world compared to the difficulties we faced without a plan when my father was diagnosed 20 years earlier. (Anne Hallisey, caregiver to both of her parents, who were diagnosed 20 years apart with Alzheimer's disease)

Planning for the future should be a priority from the very beginning of the caregiving journey. This strong position comes from years of experience in dementia care in my own family and in community, acute, and long-term care settings. I have agonized with persons who have dementia and their families as they struggled with the pain and difficulty of moving through the stages of different care requirements (e.g., needing help and supervision at home, moving to a long-term care facility).

These transitions and decisions are never easy, even with the most careful planning. The path of caregiving often takes a steep uphill turn; the way ahead is a narrow, twisting path strewn with loose rock and scrubby brush. Fortunately, a few have climbed this way before and there are some markers and handholds to help you scale the cliff. Because you have been preparing for this climb, you find the strength in your limbs and in the rope and sturdy shoes in your pack that will somehow help you reach the top. It is tough going, but you know you can make it.

Without planning, challenges multiply and can become overwhelming. This is more like falling over the cliff, like a hazard in the path ahead that you didn't see coming and weren't prepared for. Tragically, I have often been part of the rescue crew at the bottom of the cliff, trying to help persons with dementia and their caregivers make emergency care plans. The trauma and stress of such situations leaves shattered relationships and broken spirits that may take longer to heal than the time available.

What can you as a caregiver do to keep from falling over the cliff? Prepare for the journey ahead by learning as much as you can about what the journey is going to be like. Use this information to plan with the person who has dementia how you will take care of each other on the journey and how you will manage the "stuff" needed for the road ahead.

When I stress the importance of care planning, I don't mean to suggest that caregivers need a concrete, step-by-step plan. Caregiving is not a place or a destination; it is a path or a journey. Likewise, care planning is not a one-time-only event; it is a process that takes place over time. As dementia progresses, needs change and plans must also change. Instead of making a fixed plan, you need to gather information and consider preferences and various options (e.g., resources for extra help at home, respite care). This type of preparation helps you to make the best decision possible when the need arises. In this way, you and the person you are caring for can reach a decision, having had time to discuss and reflect on various options. Your decision will also be informed by the present circumstances rather than by how you imagined it weeks, months, or years before.

Certainly one of the most challenging decisions you will face is deciding when it is time for care outside of the home. Many times I have suffered with family members who promised that they would never put their loved one in a nursing facility. This promise was made when the person was well or in the early stages of dementia. At that time, there was no way to know what the care needs would become. The promise was also often made without knowing the range of helpful and positive care options available. This promise, made with neither enough experience nor information, can cause tremendous heartache and guilt if the realities of care do lead to placement in a long-term care facility. I urge you to avoid making such promises and decisions in advance. Hindsight is 20/20.

Please also remind yourself that all you can do is give difficult decisions your best possible effort, based on the information and understanding available. Often, there is no right decision, just the best option out of the available alternatives. Try to avoid second-guessing yourself and regretting past decisions. You did the best that you could at that time.

This chapter is only a brief introduction to areas that need to be considered in planning care. Other books and resources, such as those listed in Appendix B, will provide the detailed information that you need. Your local Alzheimer's Association and Alzheimer Society chapter is a key resource in care planning. In addition to providing information, many have staff members who can give advice about daily care needs and long-range planning. If staff help is not available, they may be able to refer you to a community agency or professional to help with the important but challenging task of planning for future care.

Brief guidelines on three areas of care planning follow: learning about dementia, taking care of people, and taking care of practical matters.

LEARNING ABOUT DEMENTIA

Knowledge is power.

Some caregivers need to leap right in and read and learn everything possible about dementia; others can't cope with even thinking about it. Like most circumstances, neither extreme is very helpful. There is so much information—and so much of it is focused on losses—that it is easy to become overwhelmed, both by what there is to be learned and by what lies ahead. The following suggestions are provided to guide your learning.

Celebrate Your Successes

Take some time to look back. Where was your understanding a few weeks or even a few days ago? I think you will be surprised at how you have already grown and how much you have learned. Give yourself a well-deserved pat on the back.

Remember that No Two People with Dementia or Care Situations Are Alike

If you have seen one person with Alzheimer's disease, you have seen one person with Alzheimer's disease.

As emphasized throughout this book, and as you have no doubt learned from your own caregiving experience, the changes that come with dementia differ from person to person and even for the same person daily and hourly. Any learning material can only offer general suggestions on how dementia progresses. We do know that the person will gradually lose many cognitive abilities that will make independent daily living increasingly difficult. Although these losses follow a roughly similar pattern, it is simply not possible to say that at this stage the person can do A, B, and C but not E, F, or G. Nor can anyone say for sure what particular changes may mean about care needs.

Although it is understandable that family and professional caregivers would like markers to indicate exactly when changes are needed in care arrangements, this is not possible. Two very difficult times of transition are determining when the person can no longer be left on his or her own and when it is time to consider a move out of the home. However, by learning as much as you can in advance, you can be better prepared to make these decisions.

Each care situation and each person is unique; many factors need to be considered. Be wary of information that suggests otherwise. Dementia care is complex; no one has all the answers, and there is no one-size-fits-all solution. The advice of an experienced health care practitioner may be helpful in customizing information and planning for your particular situation.

Break Learning into Manageable Pieces

The only way to eat an elephant is one bite at a time.

Although you need to make general plans for the future, try to focus on what you need to know now to help on a daily basis. It is probably best to start with a brief overview of the general progression of dementia but not to get bogged down in the details of what may lie ahead. It is easy to become overwhelmed worrying about how you will cope with some future change, such as when the person is no longer able to eat independently. Focusing on future worries distracts from the ability both to cope with and appreciate what is happening right now (e.g., the person is having difficulty preparing meals but takes great pleasure in eating and currently is able to feed him- or herself). Remind yourself to take one day at time, to celebrate the moment, and not to borrow trouble.

Seek Information that Balances Losses with Continuing Strengths

Because dementia causes progressive losses, much of the available information focuses on these losses. Although this is important, it is even more important to remember that the inner self, the person, is not lost and that each person with dementia has many continuing strengths. The wise learner and caregiver seeks ways to use these strengths to compensate for losses. The preceding chapters of this book offer information on strengths and abilities and on compensating for losses.

Learn from the Person with Dementia

This suggestion applies on two levels. In the big picture, we can learn from the person with dementia to capture the joy of the moment, to live more fully in the now (see Chapter 2). On a smaller scale—that is, in day-to-day life and activities—the person with dementia is our best teacher about preferences and successful approaches. Sometimes we just need to fine-tune our listening and looking skills to understand what the person is teaching us.

Learn from Mistakes

As noted previously, never let a good failure go to waste. Nobody is perfect. There are bound to be mistakes and things that don't go well. Remember that the caregiving journey does not have a precise route plan, only a trail guide. The real tragedy is missing the opportunity to learn from mistakes.

Share Learning with the Person You Are Caring For

For yourself, learning needs to be a gentle process. Trying to absorb too much information or information at the wrong time is overwhelming. If the person has been diagnosed in the early stages of dementia, he or she may have an active interest and a need to learn as much as possible. Conversely, the person may need more time to adjust, to grieve, and to process such a major piece of information.

It may be helpful to think of the ways in which we teach children about sex. We probably all have a story about the child who asks where babies come from. Some overzealous parents take this as a signal to overwhelm a 6-year-old with all of the details of intercourse. This is more information than the child can handle and more than he or she asked for. Other parents may give the stock reply, "You'll find out when you are older." This is equally unsatisfactory and doesn't answer the child's need to know. Fortunately, there is a middle way, by which the child will get an answer that meets her or his need to know without providing overwhelming details. Although talking about sex may make the parents uncomfortable, the children learn that sex is a natural part of life, not a dirty word.

In the same way, we need to understand that dementia is a brain condition, not a dirty word. Not talking about it with the person doesn't take it away, nor does it take away the person's need to know. The topic may make us uncomfortable and sad, but a head-in-the-sand approach doesn't serve the caregiver or the person with dementia. Christine Boden shared her feelings on her diagnosis:

Even once a diagnosis is made, families are still left to cope with very difficult behavior, and are often ashamed, pretending nothing is wrong. We would not be ashamed of our relative or friend with cancer, heart attack or stroke, so why are we so ashamed of a disease that attacks us just as physically, but in the brain? (1998, p. 53)

Saying that persons with dementia can only cope with so much information at once is not to say that it is appropriate to keep the diagnosis from them. It is their life, their future; they have a right to know. Of course, getting the news is painful, but it is even more painful for people with dementia to feel their abilities sliding and not know why. Deep inside, all persons with dementia know something is wrong. Without a name for this something, they may blame themselves and believe they are stupid, or they may blame others, leading to strife with family members, co-workers, or friends. It is much kinder for persons with dementia to know that they have a brain condition and that their difficulties are not their fault.

I can speak about this so frankly because we made this mistake with Alice. I would do things very differently if I knew then what I know now. It was 1985 when we realized that there was a very real problem, that the memory loss and difficulty with managing daily activities was more than grief at losing her husband of 44 years. Alice was living 1,200 miles away from us, and as far as her doctor and family and friends there could tell, she was getting along quite well. With every visit, we knew differently.

Although this book stresses the importance of early diagnosis and assessment, that is not what we did. It took several months before we could even admit out loud that there was a problem and then take action to address the problem. In all of these stages, which included moving Alice to a home near us, we were never up-front with her about the real reason for the move. When Alice moved, we arranged for her to see our family doctor, with whom I shared the details of her challenges. Based only on the information that I provided (something else that I would do differently), Alice was diagnosed with probable Alzheimer's disease. Neither the doctor nor Alice's family ever told her this.

Alice was happy to be wanted and to be near her only child and her grandchildren, but in her heart of hearts, she knew there was more to it than this. Often she would say things such as "I am in a terrible mess," "I don't know why I can't remember anything," and "I am just getting so stupid." These were really questions, calls for information, which to my regret now, I never answered. I did offer reassurance that she wasn't stupid, that she was managing very well with the upheaval of the move and that she need not worry because we would always be there to take care of her. This was all important information, but it was not the same as letting her know that the real cause of her difficulties was a brain condition.

As the saying goes, that was then and this is now. I can only urge you not to make this same mistake. Take cues about what the person needs to know and how much he or she can handle from the comments the person makes or the questions he or she asks. Timing is everything; we can only hear things when we are ready to hear them. Rather than planning a careful talk, caregivers should be prepared to seize the moment when they hear comments such as "I can't understand why I can't remember things." This is especially important if the person is diagnosed in the later stages of dementia, when he or she may be unable to ask direct questions. Although the person may react with anger and sorrow, knowing that there is a reason for the problems experienced is more comforting than not knowing. Some persons with dementia learn to short-cut their own frustrations by saying things such as

"Well, I have Alzheimer's disease; I can't help forgetting."
Conversely, direct confrontations when the person is embarrassed, challenged, or frustrated are seldom helpful.

It is helpful to emphasize that the diagnosis came from a
doctor, not from yourself. Whenever possible, involve the
person's doctor or other health professionals in giving information about the disease and its effects. This takes you off the
hook and helps to preserve your relationship with the person.
Unfortunately, however, one cannot assume that all health
care professionals will give this information in a caring and
sensitive way. If at all possible, shop around for an understanding clinician. Good sources for such referrals include
other caregivers and your local Alzheimer's Association or
Alzheimer Society chapter.

Sharing Information with Family Members, Friends, and Other Caregivers

Sharing information with others is important but complex.
We all have our own timing and needs regarding how much
and what sort of information we can handle. No one takes
well to "should's" (i.e., "You should read this"; "You have to
know this"). Yet, I have worked with many families in which
one or more members are reluctant to even admit that their
relative has a problem. This places a great burden on other
family members, who must not only struggle with the responsibility for care needs and decisions but also with the responsibility of sharing information with others. From her years of
experience working with families, Lisa Gwyther commented
as follows: "Few incentives (money, religious or motivational)
will make an unwilling family assume care for someone with
Alzheimer's. Few disincentives (stress, lost opportunity, physical risk) will keep a determined family from honoring a commitment to care" (1995, p. 17).

In my experience, the preceding advice applies not only to care but also to each family member's willingness to learn. Inevitably, reluctance to know gets mixed in with existing family beliefs and feuds, as shown in the following example.

Susan was thought to be bossy and interfering. She was also the first person to notice that her mother-in-law was having serious problems with memory, cooking, shopping, and maintaining her household. Other family members dismissed these observations, putting them down to normal aging, and became furious when the "interfering" daughter-in-law tried to insist on getting a specialist appointment. Existing family dynamics, the daughter-in-law's "you should do this" attitude, and the reluctance of other family members to admit to the problem all worked together to delay receiving a diagnosis of Alzheimer's disease and planning for care until there was a crisis (a hospital admission).

Despite different views, all family members were concerned about the mother's welfare. When the diagnosis was made, they did pull together to develop a family care plan, with the help of the care team. It was a large family, and meetings were challenging but productive. All of the children and their spouses agreed that their mother's well-being was the first priority. They also agreed that their father was domineering, stubborn, and potentially violent. From these two points of agreement, it was fascinating to watch the family members (with guidance from the health care team) take on different roles to develop a care plan. The plan was far from perfect, but it did keep their mother safe and at home for some time. Even the father, who refused to come to such meetings or openly acknowledge the problem, was trying to act in his wife's best interest. It became apparent that he really did care about his wife and that his reluctance to accept the diagnosis or outside help was based on his belief that she would be better off at home.

In this complex situation, some family members wanted to know everything about the disease and the future. They were the ones who, with the help of the care team, took over sharing information with others and making long-range plans. Some got along better with their father than others and were able to share pieces of information with him. Others were good at practical tasks and were able to help with housework, shopping, and transportation. At the request of her husband, the "interfering" daughter-in-law didn't come to the meetings. However, she was an efficient organizer and used this skill to take care of many practical details.

Like most family situations, this one was very complex. At times of crisis, negative relationship histories tend to become amplified. This is not the time when family members are likely to take on new roles; instead, they are likely to resume old ones. When under stress, we all tend to return to old patterns of coping and relating, as it is complicated to learn new ways. A family member who has always been distant and disinterested is likely to stay that way or become more so. It is unlikely that trying to force understanding or involvement is going to work. In fact, this approach is likely to drive the person further away. Likewise, the organizer and director will go into high gear. The member who has always been the caregiver will increasingly assume this role, and other family members will likely assume that the person will continue to fulfill this role, never thinking that there is a need to pitch in.

If you have been the traditional caregiver in your family, these are tough times. You are likely to become the principal caregiver, either directly or indirectly, for the person with dementia. This may have happened more by default than choice. Either way, it is likely that you not only have care responsibilities for the person with dementia but also that you feel responsible for sharing the information about the diagnosis.

Ideally, everyone who has a significant relationship with the person should be involved in a family meeting to hear about the diagnosis. In the real world, this seldom happens. In some cases, other family members may have been sharing your concern up to the time of diagnosis. These persons are also likely to share your interest in learning more about the condition and about planning for the future.

But what about others who either reject the diagnosis or don't want to learn anything more? As the old adage goes, "You can lead a horse to water but you can't make it drink." It is up to you to tell others when a diagnosis has been made. Beyond this, your responsibility ends. It is up to family members to take care of their own needs for learning and coping. Likewise, when other situations arise, such as needing to make decisions about living arrangements or a health crisis, other family members should be informed. You can *suggest* that others read certain materials or talk to the doctor or others. "Should's" or "have to's" are unlikely to have much effect.

Although it is difficult, try to limit what you feel responsible for; you have enough on your plate. As noted previously, if you have traditionally been the caregiver in your family, you may feel a strong responsibility to continue in this role—not only with the person with dementia but also with other family members who may be struggling with the news.

I had a struggle in this regard. Alice and her sister Eula had always been very close. This relationship remained vital, even though they were separated by distance and physical and cognitive conditions (Eula had severe arthritis; Alice had Alzheimer's disease). After we helped Alice to move near us (which was 1,200 miles away from Eula), I tried to help Alice to make at least weekly telephone calls to Eula. Although Alice couldn't make the telephone calls independently, she was highly skilled socially, and she and her sister would have happy conversations. Without seeing the challenges that Alice faced on a daily basis or the times that Alice turned to me for the details of what she was trying to say, it may have been easy for Eula to assume that Alice was just fine.

When we had to help Alice move to a long-term care facility for her own safety, Eula was surprised. A couple of months after the move, Eula visited. During face-to-face conversations, Eula came to understand that Alice could no longer live on her own. The sisters had a happy reunion, although Eula was saddened to see the progression of Alice's disease. Because Alice was a retired nurse, she believed that she worked at the nursing facility rather than lived there. Initially, Eula believed that she could talk Alice out of this notion. This didn't work, and Eula began to consider the causes of these changes in her sister. After each trip to the nursing facility, Eula asked questions to learn a little more about Alzheimer's. Gradually, she began to understand that Alice wasn't just being stubborn or difficult. When it was time for Eula to go home, she took a copy of a book on family caregiving for persons with Alzheimer's disease to learn more.

Eula's birthday was about a month after this visit. Unfortunately, in the busy whirl of working full-time, caring for my own teenage children, running a household, and maintaining daily contact with Alice, the birthday got overlooked. In a later telephone call, Eula's daughter told me that her mother was heartbroken: For the first time in 79 years, Alice didn't wish Eula a happy birthday. I felt absolutely terrible and still do. I felt that I had failed in my responsibility as caregiver, not only for Alice but also for Eula. A wise colleague pointed out that it wasn't my responsibility to take care of Eula's feelings or to protect Eula from the reality of Alice's disease. Although I know that this is true and that this event pushed Eula to a deeper and more personal understanding of Alice's situation, I still wish I could have saved Eula the pain.

I am sure that the conflicting feelings and challenges represented by this one small event are repeated a thousand times over in the lives of most caregivers. Caregivers, by nature, try to nurture, protect, and support not only the person with dementia but also many others. This is a virtue. However, one person has only so much nurturing to go around. I urge you to focus this energy on the person with dementia and yourself. Although maintaining healthy, balanced relationships with other family members and friends is vital, giving energy to meet the needs of other healthy adults is not a priority at this time.

In the experience that I just shared, I struggled to let go of feeling responsible for Eula. I am very fond of Eula so this was challenging. Conversely, Eula is an adult who is able to cope with life's joys and sorrows. She needed and deserved to be treated with sensitivity and respect; she did not need me to take care of or protect her.

Although family members and friends deserve to be treated with sensitivity and respect, they do not need you to take responsibility for their learning needs about dementia. As discussed in the previous section on sharing information with the person with dementia, take your cues from others about what they would like to know and are ready to know. Take opportunities when others ask questions, either directly or indirectly, to share pieces of information or point them toward learning materials. Gear your responses according to the person's need. There is no doubt that waiting for others to open up to information can be frustrating. However, it has been my experience that any other approach leads to resentment.

To maintain family relationships, make use of outside expertise. Involve your physician and other health care professionals in helping to share information and in making difficult decisions. Contact the Alzheimer's Association or the

Alzheimer Society for advice and information. Provide printed or videotaped learning materials, such as those suggested
in Appendix B.

If you are the principal caregiver, making opportunities for
other family members to spend time with the person with
dementia is not only of great value to the person, it also can
help others appreciate some of the changes and challenges
that you live with daily. This can, in turn, provide an excellent
stepping stone for sharing information.

Friends, Neighbors, and
Acquaintances Also Need to Be Informed

In the case of early diagnosis, the person may tell others. In
other cases, it is helpful if the caregiver sensitively tells others. Sharing this information can be a good time to suggest
that it is important for the person to keep up social contacts
and continue with familiar activities and routines. It is also
important to stress that the changes seen in the person are the
result of a brain condition.

If others are interested in reading materials or guides, refer
them to the resources listed in Appendix B in connection with
this chapter and Chapter 3. If a brief guide is needed, consider suggesting Lisa Gwyther's excellent book *You Are One of
Us*. Although it is written for clergy and church members, it
is a superb, easy-to-read guide for all friends and visitors. It
offers easily applied information about dementia as well as
talking to, visiting with, and doing things with the person
with dementia. It also reinforces the importance of continuing contact for caregivers.

Use a Variety of Ways of Learning

Appendix B lists videotapes, pamphlets, and newsletters—all
of which are excellent ways of learning. Many local
Alzheimer's Association or Alzheimer Society of Canada

chapters have resource centers from which these materials can be borrowed. They also provide a great deal of free materials, which can be mailed to family caregivers.

A growing amount of information is available on the Internet. A number of helpful web sites and on-line resources are listed in Appendix B. If you do not have access to the Internet at home, many public libraries offer access.

Talks and presentations are often organized by the local chapters of Alzheimer's groups, and many times these are also available on videotape or cassette. Talking with other caregivers, in support groups or through a telephone support connection, is also a good source of information.

Don't Believe Everything You Read or Hear

The explosion of information on Alzheimer's disease and other dementias is almost overwhelming. The increased interest and understanding is encouraging. In the early 1980s, when I first began this work, it was possible to read just about everything there was on dementia care in a couple of weekends. Now it is nearly impossible to keep up with the exciting array of high-quality information that is available. Nevertheless, there are also some questionable suggestions and ideas that may be reported as fact, especially in the popular press. Remember that day-to-day dementia care is not a hard science; one size does not fit all. Information that offers prescriptions or recipes, as opposed to guidelines, is open to question. Question things you disagree with, as you are also an expert in your own right, and consult with your local Alzheimer's Association or Alzheimer Society chapter to verify information.

Talk with Other Caregivers

Other caregivers can help you understand how suggestions for care have worked for them or have been adapted in their caregiving situations. Other caregivers can also help you apply problem-solving techniques and other information to your particular caregiving situation. Keep in mind, however, that although other caregivers are experts in their own caregiving situations, they may not be general experts on care or dementia.

TAKING CARE OF PEOPLE

Although long-range planning is essential, it is also crucial to keep a balance, to take one day at a time, and not to become overwhelmed by what the future may hold. Above all else, remember that while you are planning how to meet the future care needs of the person with dementia, you also must take good care of yourself. For more details, please see Chapter 1.

The following topics are offered only as the briefest of introductions to the complicated process and practicalities of care planning. For more details, I refer you to the resources for this chapter found in Appendix B. The comments in the previous sections on sharing information with the person with dementia and with others also apply here.

Planning Together

For many reasons, it is encouraging that dementia is being diagnosed earlier. This gives a person with dementia and his or her family members time to adjust and to enjoy life now as well as to make plans together for future care. As noted previously, these plans are not meant to be fixed in stone; rather, making them presents an opportunity to discuss wishes and options. It is also essential to assure the person that you will be there with him or her, that whatever the location or whoever is providing daily care, you will continue to care about the person and be involved in his or her life. Making plans for future care is looking out for the person's best interests. It is an act of care and concern, an assurance that he or she will continue to receive quality care if you should become unable to do so on a full-time basis yourself. It does not suggest that you will abandon the person as dementia progresses.

It is vital not to make promises now that you will regret or be unable to keep in the future. You can promise that you will always care about the person and be involved in his or her care, but it is unrealistic to promise anything about where this care may take place. Never say never as it is a long time indeed. The path of dementia care can be long; no one can see around the many twists and turns to what the future journey will look like. Although you may now feel that you would, for instance, never put your loved one in a nursing facility, there is simply not enough information to make this promise now. Such a promise is not only unwise, it is unfair to everyone for the following reasons:

- You may find yourself physically or emotionally unable to meet the increasing care needs of your family member with dementia.
- The person with dementia may benefit from a nursing facility environment, with its increased number of people available to provide care and special services.
- Many long-term care facilities have made great strides in improving the care available to persons with dementia.

One caregiver shared these thoughts on making absolute promises:

I swore with every fibre of my being that I would never put my husband in a nursing home. I had made him give me the same promise. I took care of him at home for 12 years. My doctor finally said to me, "You must put Jack in a nursing home or you'll die, then we'll put him in a nursing home." In my heart of hearts, I knew he was right. But now I have so many concerns about the care he's getting. There are nights I can't sleep. I feel I have abandoned him, though I visit him almost every day. I am not sure this is a better answer. (Ballard & Poer, 1999)

It is important to remind yourself that even when there has been an early diagnosis, people vary in the degree to which they are able and willing to be involved with making plans. Review the suggestions on sharing information and use these suggestions to involve the person with dementia in the planning process, as he or she is able.

Some people have had a lifelong tendency to avoid planning for the future and/or discussing difficult topics. In these cases, there is little point in trying to force the issue. All you can do is give the person the opportunity to talk about the future. People also vary greatly in their understanding or insight about what is happening to their brain and what this may mean for the future. Although a person's insight usually decreases as the dementia progresses, some people have limited insight even in the early stages. In this case, or when the person is at a more advanced stage of dementia, caregivers may be left to make plans and decisions on their own. Although this is stressful, I urge you to move forward with making plans for the future as best as you are able. In the end, this is for everyone's benefit. It is time for you take leadership. One of the signs of a good leader is someone who hears all of the opinions and options, then makes the best decision possible based on this information.

Although the person you are caring for may be unable or unwilling to express an opinion, you can still take the person's views into account by considering lifelong values and wishes. It may help both of you if plans also include trips or other fun things that you have always planned to do together.

Be Honest

 Nancy and Jake had shared more than 60 years of each other's lives. Although buffeted by the usual sorrows and uncertainties that life brings, theirs was a loving and sustaining relationship. The light of love shone from their eyes, much as it had when they were 18.

Unfortunately, health concerns began to cast shadows. Jake had leukemia and required increasingly frequent blood transfusions. In addition to the severe arthritis that had troubled her for years, Nancy began to have serious memory problems. Despite these challenges, Nancy and Jake were able to manage in their own home, with the help of family and friends. Unfortunately, this became more challenging as Jake's physical health and Nancy's cognitive abilities deteriorated. Their son Earle, who had moved back to the area, was concerned enough to call a family friend to stay with Nancy while Jake was in the hospital and to get the couple's finances in order; he was not concerned enough to visit or provide direct care on occasion or to try to stand in his parents' shoes.

Finally, during one of Jake's hospital stays, Earle decided that something had to be done. He persuaded Jake that it would be best to have Nancy admitted to a nursing facility. Tragically, he also persuaded his father that the best way to handle this was to not to tell Nancy what was taking place. With the assistance of the family doctor, Nancy was admitted to a hospital and then transferred to a nursing facility. She was told only that she required more medical care.

In spite of advanced dementia, Nancy was painfully aware that she had been tricked. She refused to talk to or eat with Jake, the man she had looked at with such wonder and love for more than 60 years. Until she died, she continued to remark about how terrible it was to be tricked by the person you love. No amount of reassurance from Jake, who died a few months later, could over-

come Nancy's anger and resentment and restore trust to their relationship.

This story is shared as a reminder that persons with memory loss not only have the absolute right to be treated with honesty and respect but also retain the capacity to understand when they are not treated this way. Although other care arrangements for Nancy may have been necessary, it was not necessary to make these arrangements deceitfully. The pain of living with dementia is enough in itself without adding the pain of relationships shattered by dishonesty. The details of care planning are unique to each care situation. The need for compassion and honesty is common to all.

Shared Caring

 Albert is the loving caregiver for his mother, who is physically frail and has mild cognitive problems. Through his sensitive and loving support, his mother has been able to remain in her own home, which is a 2-hour drive away. Albert is fond of saying that he just "helps out a little" with vacuuming, cleaning, doing laundry, and preparing meals. Over the last couple of years, however, the little bit of help has broadened to include activities such as helping to write letters and Christmas cards, shopping, and driving to medical appointments. Although Albert considers it a privilege to be able to care for his mother and she considers it a privilege to receive his care, the travel and the ever-increasing tasks have begun to take a physical and emotional toll.

Albert was really looking forward to sharing caregiving with his brother and sister-in-law, who had just retired and moved back to the area. However, when they offered no help, Albert became annoyed. He took various opportunities to suggest that he was finding the care overwhelming, but they simply replied by sug-

gesting that outside help be hired. And besides, they wondered, what else did Albert have to do with his time now that he was retired?

Naturally Albert was hurt and frustrated by these remarks. The lack of sensitivity to his and his mother's dignity and needs was painful. He gave up making comments and spent a long time carrying resentment and frustration. After a period of conversation with friends, prayer, reflection, and reading, he was able to free himself of much resentment and accept that the situation with his brother and sister-in-law was not going to change. They were not going to wake up one day and realize that they needed to pitch in. When he was able to let go of the resentment, he found that he had more energy and less distress. He realized that he was using a lot of emotional energy by feeling angry and resentful. He has dropped the hope that help will be volunteered and instead occasionally asks them to do specific tasks.

A sister who lives at a distance has a much better understanding; she offers emotional support through telephone calls and practical help when she visits. This sister also arranged for paid help with housekeeping tasks, giving Albert more time to do the personal things that he enjoys doing for his mother and that no one else can do in quite the same way.

From this experience, and that of other caregivers, I offer the following suggestions about sharing care with others:

- As noted, family members are likely to continue with their lifelong roles within the family. The person(s) who has been the caregiver will be the first to respond. If one member has always been distant and disinterested, he or she is likely to remain or become more so.

- Do not expect that others will automatically understand what needs to be done and volunteer to help. If they do, it is a bonus; unfortunately, this is a rarity.

- Holding unspoken expectations of help from others can lead to resentment and saps emotional energy

- Others cannot know what is needed unless you ask. It is usually best to ask for help with specific tasks, such as housework, shopping, or spending an afternoon with the person to give you a break.

- Consider the skills and interests of family members when asking them to help. For example, a person who likes to shop may be able to go grocery shopping or help the person get new shoes or clothes. Another who likes to garden may be able to help with yard work, and, with some guidance from you, share gardening activities with the person with dementia. The practical person may be able to take on paying bills and organizing business matters. A busy family with young children may bring the children to visit, giving you a break and the person a chance to read to or spend time with children. Family members who live at a distance can keep in touch by telephone (you may need to make the telephone call); they also may be able to manage practical things such as business planning.

It is essential to plan visits and activities so that the person is not overwhelmed. Consider the following suggestions and see Chapters 6, 7, and 8 for guidelines on these activities.

- Work on the All About Me form in Appendix A or a memory book as a family project.

- Involve experts to help with specific issues and make long-range plans. Involving other family members with the doctor and the health care team from the time of diagnosis is valuable. Doing so can avoid emergency meetings and making decisions in a crisis; it also begins the sharing of responsibilities right from the start.

Nevertheless, this isn't always possible. Your local Alzheimer's Association or Alzheimer Society chapter or other community agency may have a professional staff member who is skilled in helping families develop care plans. Making use of these services brings in an objective third party who is both aware of the community services and understands how to work within the dynamics of the family. Getting this assistance can take a great deal of pressure off of the primary caregiver. A lawyer can help with making decisions about power of attorney and other legal matters. An accountant may be helpful with financial planning.

- Contact neighbors, friends, and community organizations in which the person has been involved (e.g., church groups, hobby clubs, service organizations) with specific suggestions about how they can help. Like family members, these people can't understand what you and the person you are caring for may need unless you let them know. If you sit and wait for these people to reach out, you are likely to be disappointed. Although most of us are used to being independent and find it hard to ask for help, this is no time to let pride stand in your way. If you can't ask for yourself, perhaps you can ask for the sake of the person who you are caring for. It is my experience that most people will appreciate suggestions on how they can help. The worst thing that someone can say is no.

Taking Care of the Person

Most of this book's previous chapters have focused on ways to take care of the person with dementia. One further suggestion is to seek a support group for persons with dementia. There is a growing number of these groups in both large and small communities. Many persons with dementia have found that participation in such groups is pleasurable and helps them cope with their condition. This much-needed source of support takes some pressure off caregivers. The following thoughts of one person with dementia are often repeated by others who participate in support groups:

> It is important to have hope, though. What we're going to do in creating a support group will give us hope. It may not last long, or it may run out, but it's better than not doing it at all. The worst things in Alzheimer's is that people don't get out. And there have to be things to get them out. I don't want to vegetate. (Bill, cited in Snyder, 1999, p. 49)

Possible Barriers to Getting the Help You Need

I was standing in the grocery store, totally exhausted, trying to decide what I had come for. I looked down at my cart and all I had were diapers for my incontinent mother and for my two-year-old grandson. Diapers were the only thing I could remember. I had asked a neighbor to stay with my mother and Tim because we were out of everything and there I was. I couldn't remember what I had come for. It was this simple incident that forced me to consider getting help. For almost a year I had been walking around in a semi-trance trying to do everything myself. I had to face the fact that this situation was no longer safe for my mother, for Tim, or for me. (E. Wakefield, cited in Ballard & Poer, 1999)

Many people are reluctant to make use of paid in-home help or other services, such as adult day care or respite care. Getting extra help is one of the most challenging steps for primary caregivers. In fact, caregivers of persons with dementia use outside help and services much less often than caregivers of persons with physical disabilities, even though in the

Canadian Study on Health and Aging, persons with dementia faced considerably more disability than persons with physical problems: 6.1 problems in doing activities of daily living versus 0.9 problems in doing activities of daily living (Lindsay, 1994b). However, despite this high level of disability, outside help was used by caregivers one quarter as often.

The following subsections share thoughts I have collected from other caregivers on why getting help can be challenging. There are valid reasons for this reluctance; perhaps understanding these reasons can help you overcome barriers in getting the help you need.

Services Are Not Available or Do Not Meet Caregiver Needs

In far too many cases, services such as in-home care or respite care or day programs are not available. There are also cases in which these services are available but are underused by persons with dementia and their caregivers. Unfortunately, caregivers are sometimes faulted for this underuse. However, care planners and professional caregivers should ask more questions before reaching this conclusion. Do these services meet the real needs of the people that they are meant to serve? Adult day programs are a good example. Does the particular program have transportation? Does the program run at times that are convenient for caregivers? Does the programming meet the needs of the participants? Are the staff members skilled in working with persons with dementia? What is the community's level of awareness about the program?

It is important to validate reasons why caregivers may not use available services. Providers are called on to advocate for services to meet the identified needs of persons with dementia and their caregivers. Perhaps when you are not so busy with caregiving, you will join in this campaign.

Paid Care Providers May Not
Have the Skills to Offer Quality Services

To provide excellence in care, two skills must work hand in hand: 1) It is necessary to know about dementia and dementia caregiving in general and 2) it is necessary to know the detailed information about the person being cared for.

Although still far from ideal, there have been tremendous improvements in the dementia-specific training and skills of paid caregivers, both paraprofessional and professional. When selecting services, it is important to find out whether workers have dementia-specific training and, if so, what sort. Your local chapter of the Alzheimer's Association or the Alzheimer Society may be able to suggest providers with staff who are trained in dementia care. It is also possible that you may play a role, especially with in-home care workers. Many workers may not have formal training but have wonderful interpersonal and intuitive skills. You may be able to share some of your dementia-specific knowledge or resources such as booklets or videotapes.

Primary family caregivers have an intimate knowledge of the person who they are caring for. This is based on a shared life history and on experience with providing day-to-day care. Caregivers may be understandably reluctant to share care with paid caregivers who do not have this history and experience. An organized way of sharing this information with all caregivers is essential in overcoming this barrier. Try using the All About Me form in Appendix A or *A Personal Care Book* (Alzheimer Society, 1993).

Having In-Home Helpers or Going
to a Day Program Is Too Disruptive

This concern is closely connected with the previous points about lack of training and services that do not meet caregiving needs. Services provided by caregivers without skills in dementia care can indeed be disruptive. For some caregivers, there may be no choice, but I urge you to shop around for services and workers that can meet your needs.

Some caregivers may find satisfaction and strength from advocating for changes, big or small, in the services available. Others may find the prospect of taking on another challenge too overwhelming. Still others may have family members who can become advocates for both the caregiver and the person being cared for.

Some Myths Affect Decision Making About Getting Help

MYTH: Getting outside help is a sign of weakness.
REALITY: Knowing when you need help is a sign of great wisdom and strength.

Although it is understandable that you may feel like a failure when you ask for help, nothing could be further from the truth. As discussed in detail in Chapter 1, providing care for someone with dementia is rewarding yet extremely demanding. There is only so much of you to go around, and as dementia progresses, it will be impossible to do everything. Just as a car can only go so far on a tank of gas, you can only do so much with the energy available to you. Please also understand that your caregiving situation is unique. It is not reasonable to compare other caregiving situations with your own.

Chapter 1 discussed the importance of taking care of yourself—if not for your own sake, then for the sake of the person for whom you are providing care. These same principles apply to getting outside help. If you find it too difficult to do something just for yourself, stop and imagine how the person you are caring for will manage if you become too sick or exhausted to carry on. It is a fact that caregivers of persons with dementia have much higher levels of physical health problems. In the Canadian Study on Health and Aging, these caregivers had six times the level of health problems as compared with caregivers of persons without dementia. In addition, 75% of caregivers of persons with dementia are depressed at one time or another. The Canadian Study on Health and Aging found twice the levels of clinical depression for caregivers of persons with dementia compared with other caregivers (Lindsay, 1994b). Caregiving is a long journey. The end result of not taking care of yourself and getting help when it is needed may be that you will not be able to finish the journey.

MYTH: Only I can provide the care the person needs. REALITY: Although the care you provide is irreplaceable, others can make a different but equally valuable contribution, both in doing practical tasks and in developing their own unique relationships with the person.

There is no doubt that no other person can offer the kind of caring relationship that you do. However, others definitely can enrich the person's life by sharing in different sorts of relationships. Opening yourself to such opportunities has the potential to enrich your life and the life of the person you are caring for. Even with two healthy partners, no relationship can be expected to meet all of the needs of both partners. This point becomes even more important when one partner in a relationship has dementia. Many caregivers find that dementia caregiving can be a lonely journey, as friends and family sometimes find it difficult to cope and come around less often. Sharing care with others, paid and unpaid, enlarges your world and frees you from some tasks. Caregivers who have time to refuel find that they can bring more emotional and physical energy to their time with the person with dementia.

In some cases, it is easier to have a paid helper for personal care activities such as bathing. Both you and the person you are caring for may feel uncomfortable with stepping outside of the usual bounds of your relationship to do personal care activities. In addition, paid caregivers can help with practical tasks such as housework or shopping.

MYTH: The person with dementia can control his or her behavior if desired.
REALITY: Dementia is a physical condition of the brain. Many of the symptoms of dementia are changes in behavior.

Unfortunately, there is a long way to go in public understanding that the dementias are brain conditions. Lack of understanding leads to a continued stigma about Alzheimer's disease and other dementias. Some may wrongly believe that the person with dementia is behaving in an odd or difficult way on purpose. In turn, this may mean that caregivers are reluctant to get outside help because they are embarrassed by the person's behavior and by the fact that a family member has dementia.

Spreading the word about the realities of dementia is a slow process; however, the cause will not be furthered by hiding yourself and the person away from others. Furthermore, the well-being of both of you depends on continuing to be involved in the web of activities and contacts that make up daily living.

Money Is Not Available for These Services

Many caregivers simply do not have the financial resources to hire others to help. Although I wish that this was a myth, it isn't. I am truly sorry if this is your situation. I can only say that advocacy groups, such as the Alzheimer's Association and the Alzheimer Society organizations, are working hard to ensure that every person with dementia has access to the kind of care services that he or she needs.

It is hard to keep track of what may be available in your community. The local Alzheimer's Association or Alzheimer Society chapter, as well as other service organizations, can help you find community services and programs that are available at no charge or on a prorated basis. A social worker or health care professional from a community organization can be of great assistance in helping you to gain access to these services. In addition, in some communities or through some social service organizations, caregivers may have the option of receiving payment for at least some of the care that they provide.

Suggestions for Using Outside Help to Its Fullest

If you have decided to make use of outside help, here are some brief suggestions to guide you. Please refer to Appendix B for additional resources.

Get Professional Help to Assess
Which Services May Be Needed and Available

Services are available without charge from many Alzheimer's organizations or community social services agencies. The range of programs and agencies varies greatly from community to community. A professional skilled in dementia care can help you develop a plan that is customized to your caregiving situation. Like all aspects of dementia care, one size does not fit all and there is no perfect plan. For some caregivers, adult day programs are very helpful. For others, in-home help with certain tasks is the way to go; still others benefit from a prolonged break provided by respite care. Many find that a combination of these options helps. A skilled and sensitive professional can also assist with coordinating these services, as can family and friends.

Unfortunately, no plan can be fixed in stone; changes to the plan will be needed as care needs change. A skilled professional can be an objective third party to reassess care needs from time to time.

Be Selective

Some caregivers may not have a choice about the selection of workers or agencies. However, if you do have a choice, shop around for the agency and/or the person who is likely to best fit your caregiving situation. The local Alzheimer's Association or Alzheimer Society chapter or another community service agency may provide you with a list. Ask other caregivers about their experiences.

Unless a wonderful private care worker falls into your lap, it saves a lot of worry to use agency workers rather than hiring someone yourself. It may cost more, but there is a huge advantage to having someone else responsible for personnel and payment issues. In addition, if one worker doesn't pan out, the agency can provide others, and you are not back at square one again.

When selecting an agency, interview the agency. Ask if care workers have had training in dementia care. Find out the policy on scheduling and assigning workers. Does the agency try to have the same person come all the time? If a paid caregiver does not work out well with your loved one, will the agency send another? Are workers bonded?

Suggest that the Help Is for You
Rather than for the Person with Dementia

Although the person may resist the idea of personally needing help, he or she may be willing to accommodate a worker in the home to help you. If you are the primary caregiver for someone who lives alone, you may be able to use this same approach to encourage the person to get services such as an emergency help call system or delivered meals. Tell the person that you are worried about his or her safety or that he or she is not getting enough to eat and that these services will relieve you of the worry.

Introduce the Person to a Service Gradually

As discussed throughout this book, change is especially difficult for persons with dementia. It is important to introduce change gradually and sensitively, making use of the information in the preceding chapters to guide you. For example, Chapter 6 contains an example of an individualized introduction to a day program. Yet, it is probably best to assume control over big decisions, such as obtaining in-home help. You can then offer real choices about some other aspect. For example, you could say, "We have a housekeeper coming today, as I am finding the work too much for me. Which of these sheet sets would you like her to put on your bed?"

Help Paid Care Workers to Build a Relationship with the Person

Some care workers have a particular gift at developing a caring and collaborative relationship with persons with dementia. Most, however, will need your guidance in getting to know the person—his or her likes, dislikes, interests, and habits—to develop a therapeutic relationship. Family caregivers know more about the person than anyone else. Sharing the person's story, through conversation, family photos and memorabilia, and written information (e.g., the All About Me form in Appendix A) is essential for fostering a caring connection. As these relationships flourish, paid caregivers should be encouraged to share their own discoveries about the person and effective ways of providing care.

These suggestions are even more important in longer-term care arrangements, such as day programs or respite or long-term care. In fact, a good indicator of a quality service is one that seeks the person's story from family members. Likewise, positive relationships between paid and family caregivers encourage a two-way street in sharing information and ideas about the person. For example, some day programs share a diary of the person's day with family members.

Times with paid caregivers should have spaces for fun and joy as well as for tasks. In this way, both the person and the paid caregiver will look forward to the visit, and necessary tasks such as bathing or housework will be done with greater ease. Family caregivers should not only share information about tasks to be done but also let the paid caregiver know about activities the person enjoys (even something as simple as singing the person's favorite song) and ways the person likes to help. Involving the person in a brief pleasurable activity, such as sharing a snack or a short conversation, builds rapport and often transforms a task into a pleasant social time. Please see Chapters 6, 7, 8, and 9 for more information.

Suggest Both Tasks and Fun Activities

As suggested previously, even when care workers come only for brief periods to do specific tasks, such as bathing or housework, it is essential to incorporate elements of fun and relationship building. Care workers who spend longer periods of time in the home may need encouragement to involve the person in pleasurable activities such as baking, walking, gardening, and listening to music. If participation in such activities is seen as part of the person's job expectations, it relieves the paid caregiver of feeling he or she has to do tasks all the time or just sit with the person once the tasks are done.

Let Go of the Notion that
There Is Only One Way to Do Things

One of the challenges of involving others in caregiving is the need to let go, to some degree, of control over how tasks are done. This may be a particular challenge for tasks around your home. Try to focus on the big picture. For example, if the laundry is done—the clothes are clean and fresh—and you didn't have to do it, does it really matter how things were folded? There are numerous ways of doing things, and not all may be your way. Taking a "my way or the highway approach" to household tasks is not likely to help anyone.

As the primary caregiver, you need to decide what needs to be done and which details truly affect you or the person who you are caring for. Yet, for paid caregivers to feel satisfied with their work, they need to have some control over the process of the doing. Suppose that a paid caregiver is asked to prepare a pot of stew. Of course, the paid caregiver will need to know about any ingredients that cause allergies or are disliked. If the paid caregiver simply makes a wonderful pot of stew according to her family recipe and not yours, however, try to celebrate her skills and enjoy the meal rather than fretting that the stew wasn't made your way.

Give Feedback

Like you, paid caregivers have a difficult job. It is unlikely that they are in it for the money. In fact, research has found that the majority are involved for the satisfaction that the work brings (Pillemer, 1996). Offering praise when things have been well done is essential to the worker's well-being, helps to build a relationship between you and the worker, and—most of all—ensures that your loved one receives the best possible care.

At the same time, it is essential to inform a paid caregiver when you are not pleased or when things have not gone well. It does little good to complain to others; you need to speak to the person directly. I truly understand how difficult this can be for some people. Although I have been working on it for years, I would rather do just about anything than deal with a personal conflict. However, with practice and a few techniques, my confidence has improved and my frustrations have decreased. There are whole books written on this topic, so I will just offer a few suggestions.

The first rule of giving negative feedback is that it should be constructive rather than destructive. It is the person's actions, not the person, that is a problem. Launching a full-scale attack on the person is unlikely to result in improved care and it certainly is destructive for relationships. Keep your comments focused on the behavior, not the person.

The most effective feedback begins with positive comments. It is essential, first of all, to let the person know what he or she has done well. This can than lead into areas for improvement. Try to use questions and reflections, rather than orders or commands. Beginning these questions with phrases such as "Could you try . . ." and "How would it work if . . ." involves the person in solving the problem and makes it more likely that he or she will try to do things differently.

Constructive feedback seeks to build strengths and relationships, not to embarrass or humiliate the person. Such conversations should be conducted in private and at a time when both of you are as calm as possible. Nevertheless, a much stronger approach (or speaking to the supervisor) is

essential if the paid caregiver does something that is dangerous to the person's physical or emotional well-being.

Take Advantage of the Time
Made Available by Service Providers
to Do Something for You

Please refer to Chapter 1 to read about the extreme importance of care for the caregiver. You need to reserve at least
part of the time that the person is in someone else's care to
pamper yourself. Taking this time allows you to refuel and
recharge so that you return to full-time care with renewed
energy. There will always be many practical tasks that need to
be done; don't let precious time for yourself be entirely con-
sumed by doing these tasks.

TAKING CARE OF PRACTICAL MATTERS

Planning the Setting for Care

Undoubtedly, we all hope to live all of our days in our own
home. Unfortunately, circumstances in our own lives or in the
lives of family members caring for us may mean that this is
not possible. It is, however, possible to take steps now so that
your future home (wherever it is) includes the features of
home that you cherish most.

Similarly, caregivers can talk, share, and plan with the person with dementia so that if it becomes necessary for the person to receive out-of-home care, the setting feels as much like
home as possible. Persons with dementia and their caregivers
are advised to embark on a voyage of discovery; discovering
and sharing both the most treasured features of living at
home and exploring the types of care settings available. It is
unlikely that this voyage will lead to a perfect match (the ideal

setting), but the options discovered will probably be closer to ideal than waiting until a crisis forces a move from home.

For this to be truly a voyage of discovery, you are called on to let go of biases and unfounded beliefs, to bring an open mind to the process. Although it is still far from perfect, the long-term care sector has made tremendous strides in improving the quality of care offered to persons with dementia and their caregivers. This change has taken place on two different levels.

First and foremost, it is becoming increasingly understood that the best possible care is individualized, supporting the person to continue with a familiar lifestyle in a setting that is as homelike as possible. This major change in thinking has transformed many existing nursing and care facilities and has served as the founding philosophy for numerous others. Be sure to explore for yourself the kind of care that is provided in facilities in your community. There may have been many changes.

Second, there is a growing range of options for care. These options include freestanding dementia care homes or apartments, assisted living facilities, group homes, private board and care homes, retirement homes, nursing facilities, and facilities that combine many of these features and provide "life care" (i.e., the person moves within a residential complex to a different type of care as needed).

Considering the possibility of leaving the family home, of being cared for by someone other than family members is painful for everyone involved. However, I can assure you that not thinking about and planning for this possibility will increase everyone's pain if such a move becomes necessary.

Take a proactive response; find out which care options are available in your community. Talk with other caregivers, the local Alzheimer's Association or Alzheimer Society chapter, support group members, and social services agencies. Decide which places are of interest to you, and find out more about them through telephone calls. Visit facilities to gain firsthand knowledge.

Learn the Details of the Application Process and the Costs of Various Options

The cost of long-term care is overwhelming for most families and, unfortunately, may stop the planning process in its tracks. Please try not to let this happen to you. Clearly, the cost is enormous; however, help is available. Just as there is a growing range of care options, there is also a wide range of programs and plans, which differ from state to state and province to province, to assist families with these costs. As taxpayers and contributing members to your community, you have earned and deserve this assistance. In addition, be sure to explore the full range of long-term care options; there can be important differences between for-profit, not-for-profit, and government-funded facilities.

Sorting through the complexities of available programs is a big job. Before you take this on yourself, find out whether your local Alzheimer's Association or Alzheimer Society chapter has a staff member who helps families with this process. If not, ask about a community service organization that can help. Some areas have a coordinated application process for all long-term care services, whether in-home or facility based. In this case, only one application needs to be made. Another family member may be able to help with gathering this information.

Tour Facilities and Talk with Residents and Staff

When touring facilities, observe the following: Do staff treat the residents with dignity and respect? Does this facility feel welcoming and warm? In addition to noting these two crucial factors, observe things such as the availability of structured activity as well as the opportunity to make independent decisions, the design of the rooms, the opportunity to bring in personal possessions, the appearance of the dining room (institutional or homelike), the opportunity for residents to eat at their own pace, and the availability and appearance of bathrooms.

These observations indicate a sense of the quality of life that residents may experience. Observations about the physical design and decor are important. However, no amount of interior decoration can compensate for an uncaring atmosphere. There are facilities that look absolutely wonderful but provide distant and impersonal care. As folk wisdom tells us, beauty is only skin deep. Consider the following questions:

- Are direct care staff trained to work with persons with dementia?

- Is there opportunity for individualized daily routines and resident choice?

- Is there a special care unit? If so, what are the admission and discharge criteria (i.e., will the person have to move within the facility or go somewhere else at a certain stage of progression)?

- Are specialty services available (e.g., dietary, occupational therapy, physiotherapy)? If so, how often?

- Are there team meetings for developing resident care plans? How often do these occur, and who is involved?

- Can the resident maintain his or her own family physician if desired? Is there an examining room on site?

- What is the policy on restraints?

- Is there a safe path for residents who wander?

- What are the security measures for persons who wander?
- Is there a safe outdoor area for residents?
- What is the policy on palliative care?
- Are family members encouraged to be present and involved in care planning and care routines?

Submit Early Applications to One or More of the Facilities that You Like Best

Although the need for long-term care may seem a long way off, every possible step should be taken to avoid having to make a decision in a crisis situation. For instance, if either the primary caregiver or the person with dementia becomes ill, temporary or long-term placement may become an unexpected necessity. If the application process has begun, there is at least a possibility that the person may be able to go the facility of choice. If a space becomes available before there is a need for out-of-home care, the person's name can be moved down the list for later entry.

Financial and Legal Matters

The detailed information that you will need to deal with financial and legal matters is beyond the scope of this book. However, getting your financial and legal affairs in order as soon as a diagnosis is made is absolutely vital for you and the person with dementia. Make decisions about long-range financial and legal issues while the person is still capable of participating, both in a practical and legal sense. For couples, if the partner with dementia has always done the family finances, taking immediate action becomes even more vital. Although the topic must be approached with great sensitivity, the other partner will need to take over this job, or it will need to be passed on to another family member, trusted friend, or professional.

Whatever you decide to do, do it now and put it in writing. This can save endless heartache and distress down the road. Although you may think that such problems will never arise in your family, far too often I have witnessed how money issues can change people in unexpected ways. In addition, dementia complicates legal considerations tremendously. Once the person becomes legally incompetent, arrangements such as an enduring power of attorney can no longer be made. Caregivers are advised to seek expert advice about practicalities and legal implications. Both the law and the practical application of concepts such as competency and living wills vary widely from one jurisdiction to another. For example, in some jurisdictions, competency is divided into different areas, so that a person may be competent to make decisions about his or her personal care but not about financial matters.

I wish you well in this difficult undertaking and hope that the suggestions in previous chapters on communication and working with the person's strengths are of some assistance. Please see Appendix B for some suggested resources. You will also find information in Chapter 7 on working with the person with dementia to address finances.

CONCLUSION

I bring this chapter—and this book—to a close with good wishes for the journey ahead and a strong suggestion to think about and plan for the future. The appendices at the end of this book offer information to assist you in planning for the journey. In particular, I invite you and the person you are caring for to jointly complete the All About Me form in Appendix A, as this can provide an opportunity for both of you to celebrate the person with dementia, and, it is hoped, a chance to capture the joys of the precious present together, to live in the moment. By engaging in joint activities such as filling out this form, caregivers can be enabled to become care partners. In addition, other caregivers can be given the opportunity to know and celebrate the whole person cloaked by dementia. And this is truly the heart of dementia care.

References

Altman, H. (Ed.). (1987). *Alzheimer's disease: Problems, prospects and perspectives.* New York: Kluwer Academic/Plenum Publishers.

Alzheimer Society of Canada. (1993). *A personal care book.* Toronto: Author.

Ballard, E. (1993). *Managing grief and bereavement: A guide for families and professionals caring for memory-impaired adults and other chronically ill persons.* Durham, NC: Duke University Medical Center, Office of Communications.

Ballard, E., & Poer, C. (1999). *Lessons learned: Shared experiences in coping.* Durham, NC: Duke University Medical Center.

Boden, C. (1998). *Who will I be when I die?* East Melbourne: HarperCollins Publishers Australia.

Bourgeois, M., Schulz, R., & Burgio, L. (1996). Interventions for caregivers of patients with Alzheimer's disease: A review and analysis of content, process, and outcomes. *International Journal of Aging and Human Development, 43,* 35–92.

Bowlby, C. (1993). *Therapeutic activities with persons disabled by Alzheimer's disease and related disorders.* New York: Aspen Publishers.

Bowlby Sifton, C. (1998). *Living at home with Alzheimer's disease and related dementias.* Ottawa, Ontario: Canadian Association of Occupational Therapists.

Bowlby Sifton, C. (2000a). Caregiver focus: It's the little things that matter. *Alzheimer's Care Quarterly, 1*(1), 1–4.

Bowlby Sifton, C. (2000b). Caregiving challenges: Searching for home. *Alzheimer's Care Quarterly, 1*(1), 81–85.

Bowlby Sifton, C. (2000c). Caregiving challenges: Sexuality and persons with dementia. *Alzheimer's Care Quarterly, 1*(2), 87–90

Bowlby Sifton, C. (2000d). It is in the shelter of each other that people live. *Alzheimer's Care Quarterly, 1*(1), iv–v.

Bowlby Sifton, C. (2000e). Meeting needs. *Alzheimer's Care Quarterly*, *1*(4), iv–vi.

Bowlby Sifton, C. (2000f). Well-being and doing: Enabling occupation with persons with dementia. *Alzheimer's Care Quarterly*, *1*(2), 7–28.

Bowlby Sifton, C. (2001a). Life is what happens when we are making other plans. *Alzheimer's Care Quarterly*, *2*(2), iv–vii.

Bowlby Sifton, C. (2001b). Making dollars and sense: The cost-effectiveness of psychosocial therapeutic treatment. *Alzheimer's Care Quarterly*, *2*(4), 81–85.

Bowlby Sifton, C. (2002). Lessons on listening: The *art* of communication. *Alzheimer's Care Quarterly*, *3*(2), iv–vi.

Brawley, B. (1997). *Designing for Alzheimer's disease: Strategies for creating better care environments*. New York: John Wiley & Sons.

Buchanan, J. (1989). *Encounters: The experience of disease*. Charlottesville: The University of Virginia Press.

Burns, A., Jacoby, R., & Levy, R., (1991). Progression of cognitive impairment in Alzheimer's disease. *Journal of the American Geriatrics Society*, *39*, 39–45.

Calkins, M., & Marsden, J. (2000). Home is where the heart is: Designing to recreate home. *Alzheimer's Care Quarterly*, *1*(1), 8–16.

Callahan, S. (2000). *My mother's voice*. Forest Knolls, CA: Elder Books.

Canadian Study of Health and Aging (CSHA) Working Group. (1994). Canadian Study of Health and Aging: Study methods and prevalence of dementia. *Canadian Medical Association Journal*, *150*, 899–914.

Cohen, D., & Eisdorfer, C. (1986). *The loss of self*. New York: W.W. Norton.

Cohen-Mansfield, J. (2000). Nonpharmacological management of behavioral problems in persons with dementia: The TREA model. *Alzheimer's Care Quarterly*, *1*(4), 22–34.

Cohen-Mansfield, J., Werner, P., Marx, M., & Freedman, L. (1991). Two studies of pacing in the nursing home. *Journal of Gerontology*, *46*(3), 77–88.

Coleman, P. (Ed.). (2000). *Neurobiology of aging: Abstracts from the 7th International Conference on Alzheimer's Disease and Related Disorders*. New York: Elsevier.

Clarfield, M. (1991). Assessing dementia: The Canadian consensus. *Canadian Medical Association Journal*, *144*(7), 851–853.

Clarfield, M., & Foley, J. (1993). The American and Canadian consensus conferences on dementia: Is there consensus? *Journal of American Geriatric Society, 41*(8), 883–886.

Cousins, N. (1979). *Anatomy of an illness as perceived by the patient.* New York: W.W. Norton.

Cress, M., Buchner, D., Questad, K., Esselman, D., deLateur, B., & Schwartz, R. (1999). Exercise: Effects on physical functional performance in independent older adults. *Journal of Gerontology, 54,* M242–M245.

Csikszentmihalyi, M. (1988). *Beyond boredom and anxiety.* San Francisco: Jossey-Bass.

Cummings, J. (1993, September). *An overview of Alzheimer's disease.* Paper presented at the Alzheimer's International Conference, Toronto.

Cummings, J. (2000, July). Managing non-cognitive symptoms in AD. Paper presented at *Alzheimer's disease: A debate defining the value of treatment.* Preconference symposium of the World Alzheimer's Congress, Washington, DC.

Dartigues, J.F., Gagnon, M., Michel, P., Letenneur, L., Commenges, D., Barberger-Gateau, P., Auriacombe, S., Rigal, B., Bedry, R., Alperovitch, A., et al. (1991). Le programme de recherche PAQUID sur l'épidémiologie de la démence: Méthodologie et résultats initiaux [The PAQUID research program on the epidemiology of dementia: Methods and initial results]. *Revue Neurologique (Paris), 147*(3), 225–230.

Davidson, A. (1997). *Alzheimer's: A love story.* Seacus, NJ: Carol Publishing Group.

Davidson, A. (2001). An odd quartet: Maintaining intimacy and connection in advanced Alzheimer's. *Alzheimer's Care Quarterly, 2*(4),1–3.

DeBaggio, T. (2000, July). Presentation at the preconference panel of persons with Alzheimer's disease of the World Alzheimer's Congress, Washington, DC.

Diamond, M., & Hopson, J. (1999). *Magic trees of the mind.* New York: Dutton.

Dodee, R. (2000, July). Timing and duration of current therapies. Paper presented at *Alzheimer's disease: A debate defining the value of treatment.* Preconference symposium sponsored by Baylor College of Medicine, World Alzheimer's Congress, Washington, DC.

Eastwood, R., Nobbs, H., Lindsay, J., & McDowell, I. (1992). Canadían study of health and aging. *Dementia, 3*, 209–212.

Eaton, M., Mitchell-Bonair, I., & Friedman, E. (1986). The effect of touch on nutritional intake of chronic organic brain syndrome patients. *Journal of Gerontology, 41*, 611–616.

Emery, O., & Oxman, T. (Eds.). (2003). *Dementia: Presentations, differential diagnosis, and nosology.* Baltimore: The Johns Hopkins University Press.

Englehart, M., Ruitenberg, A., Swieten, J., Witteman, J., Hofman, A., & Breteler, M. (2000). Dietary anti-oxidants and the risk of dementia. The Rotterdam Study. In P. Coleman (Ed.), *Neurobiology of aging: Abstracts from the 7th International Conference on Alzheimer's Disease and Related Disorders* (abstract no. 922). New York: Elsevier.

Evans, D., Funkenstein, H., Albert, M., Scherr, P., Cook, N., Chown, M., Hennekens, C., & Taylor, J. (1989). Prevelance of Alzheimer's disease in a community population of older persons. *Journal of American Medical Association, 262*, 2551–2556.

Evans, D.A., Hebert, L., Beckett, L., Scherr, P., Albert, M., Chown, M., Pilgrim, D., & Taylor, O. (1997). Education and other measures of socio-economic status and risk of incident Alzheimer's disease in a defined population of older persons. *Archives of Neurology, 54*, 1399–1405.

Fazio, S., Seman, D., & Stansell, J. (1999). *Rethinking Alzheimer's care.* Baltimore: Health Professions Press.

Fiatarone, M.A., Marks, E.C., Ryan, N.D., Meredith, C.N., Lipsitz, L.A., & Evans, W.J. (1990). High-intensity strength training in nonagenarians. Effects on skeletal muscle. *Journal of the American Medical Association, 263*, 3029–3034.

Gauthier, S. (Ed.). (1999). *Clinical diagnosis and management of Alzheimer's disease.* London: Martin Dunitz.

Gauthier, S., McDowell, I., & Hill, G. (1990). Canadian study of health and aging (CSHA). *Psychiatric Journal of the University of Ottawa, 15*(4), 227–229.

Gill, T., Williams, C., & Tinetti M. (2000). Environmental hazards and the risk of nonsyncopal falls in the homes of community-living older persons. *Medical Care, 38*(12), 1174–1183.

Gillick, M. (1997). *Tangled minds: Understanding Alzheimer's and other dementias.* New York: Dutton.

Griffin, R., & Vitro, E. (1998). An overview of therapeutic touch and its application to patients with Alzheimer's disease. *American Journal of Alzheimer's Disease, 13*(4), 211–216.

Gross, D. (1990). Communication and the elderly. *Physical and Occupational Therapy in Geriatrics, 9,* 49–64.

Gwyther, L. (1995). *You are one of us: Successful clergy/church connections to Alzheimer's families.* Durham, NC: Duke University Medical Center.

Gwyther, L. (1997). *Home is where I remember things.* Durham, NC: Duke University Medical Center.

Gwyther, L. (2001). Family caregivers and long-term care: Caring together. *Alzheimer's Care Quarterly, 2*(1), 64–71.

Haldeman Martz, S. (Ed.). (1992). *If I had my life to live over I would pick more daisies.* Watsonville, CA: Papier Mache Press.

Henderson, C., & Andrews, N. (1998). *Partial view: An Alzheimer's journal.* Dallas: Southern Methodist University Press.

Hewson, M. (1994). *Horticultural therapy.* Guelph, Ontario: Homewood Psychiatric Hospital.

Holstein, M. (2001). To inhabit a livable moral world: Mrs. Dodge and her caregivers. *Alzheimer's Care Quarterly, 2*(1), 56–63.

Huang, L., Cartwright, W., & Hu, T. (1988). The economic cost of senile dementia in the United States, 1985. *Public Health Reports, 103,* 3–7.

Huang, J., Svenson, L., & Lindsay, J. (1994). Alzheimer's disease: Senile dementia of the Alzheimer's type [Monograph]. *Chronic Diseases in Canada, 15*(2), 59–76.

Huss, J. (1976). Touch with care or a caring touch? *American Journal of Occupational Therapy, 31,* 11–18.

Judd, M. (1983). *Keep in touch.* Winnipeg, Manitoba: Author.

Keating, N. (1997, April). *How families care.* Paper presented at the pre-conference forum on caregiving, Alzheimer Canada National Conference, St. John's, Newfoundland, Canada.

Killick, J., & Cordonnier, C. (2000). *Openings: Dementia poems and photographs.* London: Hawker Publications.

Kitwood, T. (1997). *Dementia reconsidered.* Buckingham, England: Open University Press.

Kitwood, T., & Benson, S. (Eds.). (1995). *The new culture of dementia care.* London: Hawker Publications.

Kolb, B., & Whishaw, I. (1990). *Fundamentals of human neuropsychology.* New York: W.H. Freeman.

Krieger, D. (1979). *The therapeutic touch: How to use your hands to help or heal.* Upper Saddle River, NJ: Prentice Hall.

Kübler-Ross, E. (1969). *On death and dying.* New York: McMillan.

Kuhn, D. (2001). Living with loss in Alzheimer's disease. *Alzheimer's Care Quarterly, 2*(1), 12–22.

Lawton, M.P., & Maddox, G. (Eds.). (1985). *Annual review of gerontology and geriatrics: Vol. 5.* New York: Springer-Verlag.

Lindsay, J. (1994a). The Canadian Study of Health and Aging: Risk factors for Alzheimer's disease in Canada. *Neurology, 44,* 2073–2080.

Lindsay, J. (1994b). Patterns of caring for people with dementia in Canada. *Canadian Journal on Aging, 13*(4), 470–487.

McDowell, I. (1994). Canadian Study of Health and Aging: Study methods and prevalence of dementia. *Canadian Medical Association Journal, 150*(6), 899–913.

Metcalfe, W. (1996, July). *Humor and caregiving.* Keynote address at the American Alzheimer's Association National Conference, Chicago.

Mohr, E., Feldman, H., & Gauthier, S. (1995). Canadian guidelines for the development of antidementia therapies: A conceptual summary. *The Canadian Journal of Neurological Sciences, 22,* 62–71.

Namazi, K., & Johnson, B. (1992). Pertinent autonomy for residents with dementias: Modification of the physical environment to enhance independence. *American Journal of Alzheimer's Care and Related Disorders and Research, 7*(1), 16–21.

Nhat Hanh, T. (1995). *Living Buddha, Living Christ.* New York: Riverhead Books.

Nolen, N., & Garrard, J. (1988). Predicting dependent feeding behaviours in the institutionalized elderly. *Journal of Nutrition for the Elderly, 7,* 17–25.

Perrin, T., & May, H. (2000). *Well being in dementia: An occupational approach for therapists and carers.* London: Churchill Livingstone.

Peterson, R., Mohs, R., Carli, C., & Galasko, D. (2000, July). *Diagnosis of dementia: Diagnostic criteria and early detection.* Proceedings of the Bridging Research and Care Symposium of the World Alzheimer's Congress, Washington, DC.

Petot, G., Cook, T., Chen, C., Tatiana, M., Debanne, S., Koss, E., Lerner, A., & Friedland, R. (2000). A high-fat diet during adulthood increases risk for Alzheimer's disease for those with ApoE4 allele. In P. Coleman (Ed.), *Neurobiology of aging: Abstracts from the 7th International Conference on Alzheimer's Disease and Related Disorders* (abstract no. 1124). New York: Elsevier.

Pillemer, K. (1996). *Solving the frontline crisis in long-term care: A practical guide to finding and keeping quality nursing assistants.* Cambridge, MA: Frontline Publishing.

Post, S. (2001a). Anti-dementia compounds, hope and quality of lives. *Alzheimer's Care Quarterly, 2*(4): 75–77.

Post, S. (2001b). An ethics of love for persons with Alzheimer's disease. *Alzheimer's Care Quarterly, 2*(2), 23–30.

Rader, J., & Barrick, A.L. (2000). Ways that work: Bathing without a battle. *Alzheimer's Care Quarterly, 1*(4), 35–49.

Richards, K., Lambert, C., & Beck, C. (2000). Deriving interventions for challenging behaviors from the need-driven, dementia-compromised behavioral model. *Alzheimer's Care Quarterly, 1*(4), 62–76.

Rose, L. (1996). *Show me the way to go home.* Forest Knolls, CA: Elder Books.

Sacks, O. (1990, March). *Seeing voices* (public lecture). University of California, Berkeley.

Sanbourne, B. (1995, July). *Behavior management of persons with Alzheimer's disease.* Paper presented at the fourth National Alzheimer's Disease Education Conference, Chicago.

Simpson, R., & Simpson, A. (1999). *Through the wilderness of Alzheimer's: A guide in two voices.* Minneapolis, MN: Augsburg Fortress Publishers.

Snowdon, D. (1997). Aging and Alzheimer's disease: Lessons from the Nun Study. *The Gerontologist, 37*, 150–156.

Snowdon, D. (2001). *Aging with grace.* New York: Bantam Books.

Snyder, L. (1999). *Speaking our minds: Personal reflections from individuals with Alzheimer's disease.* New York: W.H. Freeman.

St. George-Hyslop, P.H. (2000, December). Piecing together Alzheimer's. *Scientific American,* 52–59.

Stair, N. (1992). If I had my life to live over I would pick more daisies. In S. Haldeman Martz (Ed.), *If I had my life to live over I would pick more daisies.* Watsonville, CA: Papier Mache Press.

Stern Y., Gurland, B., Tatemichi, T.K., Tang, M.X., Wilder, D., & Mayeux, R. (1994). Influence of education and occupation on the incidence of Alzheimer's disease. *The Journal of the American Medical Association, 271*, 1004–1010.

Stone, J. (1992). Laugh. *In Health, 5*(7), 52–55.

Swanberg, M., & Cummings, J. (2001). Therapeutic approaches to Alzheimer's disease. *Alzheimer's Care Quarterly, 2*(4), 8–16.

Taaffe, D., Duret, C., Wheeler, S., & Marcus, R. (1999). Once-weekly resistance exercise improves muscle strength and neuromuscular performance in older adults. *Journal of the American Geriatrics Society, 47,* 1208–1214.

Talerico, K., & Evans, L. (2000). Making sense of aggressive/protective behaviors in persons with dementia. *Alzheimer's Care Quarterly, 1*(4), 77–88.

Thornbury, J. (1993). The use of Piaget's theory in Alzheimer's disease. *The American Journal of Alzheimer's Care and Related Disorders & Research, 8*(4), 16–21.

Truscott, M. (2004). Adapting leisure and creative activities for people with early stage dementias. *Alzheimer's Care Quarterly, 52,* 92–102.

Tuokko, H., Kristjansson, E., & Miller, J. (1995). Neuropsychological detection of dementia: An overview of the neuropsychological component of the Canadian Study of Health and Aging. *Journal of Clinical and Experimental Neuropsychology, 17*(3), 352–373.

Volicer, L., & Bloom-Charette, L. (1999). *Enhancing the quality of life in advanced dementia.* New York: Brunner/Routledge.

Volicer, L., Fabiszewski, K., Rheaume, Y., & Lasch, K. (1988). *Clinical management of Alzheimer's disease.* New York: Aspen Publishers.

Volicer, L., Seltzer, B., Rheaume, Y., Fabiszewski, K., Herz, L., Shapiro, R., & Innis, P. (1987). Progression of Alzheimer-type dementia in institutionalized patients: A cross-sectional study. *The Journal of Applied Gerontology, 6,* 83–94.

Warner, M. (2000). *The complete guide to Alzheimer's proofing your home.* West Lafayette, IN: Purdue University Press.

Weintraub, S. (2003, July). *Atypical dementia syndromes: Four neuropsychological profiles of dementia: Clinical, anatomical, and management aspects.* Handout from the preconference workshop at the Alzheimer's Association Annual Education Conference, Chicago.

White L., Katzman, R., Losonczy, K., Salive, M., Wallace, R., Berkman, L., Taylor, J., Fillenbaum, G., & Havlik, R. (1994). Association of education with incidence of cognitive impairment in three established populations of epidemiologic studies of the elderly. *Journal of Clinical Epidemiology, 47,* 363–374.

Wilcock, G., Bucks, R., & Rockwood, K. (1999). *Diagnosis and management of dementia.* New York: Oxford University Press.

Winblad, B., Wang, H., Zenchao, G., & Fratiglioni, L. (2000). New possibilities for prevention in dementia. In P. Coleman (Ed.), *Neurobiology of aging: Abstracts from the 7th International Conference on Alzheimer's Disease and Related Disorders* (abstract no. 979). New York: Elsevier.

Woods, D., & Diamond, M. (2002). The effect of therapeutic touch on agitated behavior and cortisol in persons with Alzheimer's disease. *Biological Research in Nursing, 4*(2), 104–114.

Zubek, J. (Ed.). (1969). *Sensory deprivation: Fifteen years of research.* New York: Appleton-Century-Crofts.

Permissions

Permission to reprint the following is gratefully acknowledged:

Excerpts from *Speaking Our Minds: Personal Reflections from Individuals with Alzheimer's Disease* by Solomon Snyder. Copyright © 1999 by W.H. Freeman and Company. Reprinted by permission of Henry Holt and Company, LLC.

Quotes from *Through the Wilderness of Alzheimer's: A Guide in Two Voices* by Robert and Anne Simpson, Copyright © 1999 Augsburg Fortress. Used by permission.

Quotes from Callahan, S. (2000). *My Mother's Voice.* Forest Knolls, CA: Elder Books. Copyright © 2000 by Sally Callahan. Used by permission.

Quotes from Christine Boden, *Who Will I Be When I Die?* Copyright © Christine Boden, 1997. With the permission of HarperCollins Publishers (Australia) Pty Limited.

The poem on pp. 27–28 is reprinted with the permission of Papier Mache Press and is from the book *If I Had to My Life to Live Over I Would Pick More Daisies.*

Quote from LIVING BUDDHA, LIVING CHRIST by Thich Nhat Hanh, Copyright © 1995 by Thich Nhat Hanh. Used by permission of Riverhead Books, an imprint of the Penguin Group (USA) Inc.

Appendix A

All About Me

As discussed throughout this book, and as care partners appreciate better than anyone else, caregiving is about people, not a disease or a disability. This form gives persons with dementia and the people who care about and for them a place to share their story with other caregivers. It is vital to begin as early as possible to complete the following form. The earlier you start, the more the person with dementia will be able to contribute—to let future caregivers know his or her story and the ways in which he or she would like to receive care. In addition, even though the help of other caregivers may not be needed now, you never know when it will be, either due to changes in your own health or that of the person with dementia.

The personal information in this form can help ensure that the person with dementia receives the type of care that he or she wishes and needs. To appreciate the vital importance of this information, it may help to put yourself in the shoes of a person needing care. Imagine that you need help with the very personal activity of bathing and that you cannot tell the person helping you with a bath what you would like. Think of the many things that you would like this person to know about you and your routines; this should help you to record these same sorts of details with and for the person with dementia.

The form has three sections. Section I, Essential Information, is a quick guide that gives new caregivers the most vital information about providing care. Section II, Daily Life Routines, provides a summary guide and then detailed information about the person's routines and daily activities. Section III, My Story, shares the most important things about the person's life, providing caregivers with the information needed to provide care based on a personal relationship. Section III can also be enjoyed with the person as a memory book or life story book. Guidelines for completing these sections follow a list of basic suggestions.

BASIC SUGGESTIONS FOR COMPLETING THE ALL ABOUT ME FORM

- Start immediately.
- Work with the person who has dementia, using communication tips from Chapter 4; be sure to ask opinion-seeking, nonconfrontational questions.
- Make completing the form a fun time of sharing stories, laughter, and snacks.
- Involve all others who are important in the person's life.
- Include as many details as possible about routines, habits, and wishes.
- Work on the form a bit at a time so you don't become overwhelmed.
- Begin with the essential information section.
- Write with pencil in areas where changes may occur (e.g., communication tips, mealtime and daily routines, help needed).
- Update the information regularly.
- Add helpful information from other caregivers.

- Encourage other caregivers to use the communication section.
- Be sure to share the information with all other caregivers (e.g., day program staff, long-term care staff, paid in-home caregivers, visiting family members).
- Make a photocopy of the finished form in case the original is lost.
- Use copies of photographs (if included) so that precious family photos don't get lost.

GUIDELINES FOR COMPLETING EACH SECTION

Guidelines are provided only for sections for which some pertinent information may not be immediately self-evident.

Section I: Essential Information

Other significant people: Include lifelong friends, helpful neighbors, or anyone who now plays a special role in the person's life.

Health issues:

- *Medications:* Detail the names, doses, times, and methods for taking all medications; also note how much help the person needs with properly taking medications.
- *Allergies:* List drugs, foods, environmental, and other substances to which the person has any kind of reaction.
- *Vision:* Include information on the wearing of glasses and the location of spares.
- *Hearing:* If the person wears a hearing aid, include instructions for placement and adjustment.
- *Movement ability:* List any aids used, such as walker or cane, and how much help is needed.

- *Supervision:* Indicate how much supervision is needed and for which activities, such as cuing for help with transfers.

Significant life events: Briefly list the person's most significant life accomplishments (e.g., winning the hockey championship) and other major life events (e.g., serving overseas in World War II, losing a child). This list is intended to alert other caregivers both to sad topics that may come up and things that bring the person satisfaction and pride. Fully detail these events in the Life Story section.

Things that bring pleasure: Provide a brief list of foods, music, topics of conversation, or other activities that the person really enjoys; more details should be written in the Favorites section.

Special skills/strengths: Briefly list the things that the person can do well and enjoys, such as walk the dog, set the table, or fold the laundry.

Special needs: Include routines and details that are important to the person, such as "He always sits in the brown recliner but needs help finding it" or "She always carries a purse."

Things to avoid: List any questions (e.g., "What are we going to have for supper?") or activities (e.g., watching the television news) that may cause the person to become confused or distressed.

Communication tips: List any special phrases the person uses or understands best or other ways the person may communicate, such as walking up and down the hallway and opening doors to indicate a need to find the bathroom.

Section II: Daily Life Routines

A calendar page for the weekly routine is key to helping you share the person's lifestyle preferences with others. As needs and abilities change, changes may need to be made to this page. I suggest that you make a few copies of these blank pages (enlarged as necessary) that you can share with others or can use to make changes to as time goes on. In addition, it is a good idea to use pencil, so that changes can be made easily. Fill in the pre-retirement routine to remind yourself and other caregivers that the person may revert to these habits as more recently acquired habits fade. In the portion about daily life habits, it is essential to share as much detail as possible. Even though both you and the person you are caring for may be able to make these choices and share these preferences now, there will come a time when either one or both of you will not be able to do so. Work together now, when you can, to list every possible detail for future caregivers who otherwise would not know that the person always takes his or her coffee black and lukewarm or that the person always bathes at night and does not wear pajamas. The following types of information, in as much detail as possible, should be included. This information should be updated often, including things that other care-givers have discovered. The following categories have been included to help you think about these details.

Specific Activity Routines

Usual Habits: Provide a detailed outline of the person's usual way of doing each daily activity. For example, the getting-up routine should include when the person gets up, how he or she likes to be awakened (e.g., alarm clock, telephone call, wake up naturally), whether the person likes to lie in bed for awhile before rising or prefers to leap out bed. Then, continue to list what comes next, such as using the toilet, showering, eating breakfast, and so forth.

Favorites: List the favorites associated with this particular daily activity. For example, when completing the dressing information, list the person's favorite type of clothing (e.g., casual sport clothes, shirt and tie) as well as favorite items.

Suggestions/tips: As dementia progresses, the person will have increasing difficulty with maintaining his or her lifelong routines and with doing daily activities. This is very embarrassing, and it can be difficult for caregivers to help. Caregivers often discover unique ways to provide help and to get the person started on an activity. In this part, include tips such as looking at family photos while sitting on the toilet or having the person hold a razor while he is being shaved. Write in pencil so that these tips can be updated often.

Can do: Describe the parts of the activity that the person can do—for example, the person can put on socks if he or she is handed the socks one at a time.

Help needed: Describe the parts of the activity that the person needs help with—for example, he or she can put on shoes but needs help with tying the laces.

Steps: Especially for activities in which the person's routine may have changed, it is important that caregivers follow the same exact steps and use the same language every time. For example, the person may have decreased physical ability and need to be reminded how to use his or her arms to stand up from a chair. For other activities, such as washing, dressing, or eating, memory loss may mean that the person forgets how to move from one step to the next. For instance, the person may need to be told the steps for each body area to be washed (dip the cloth in the water, wring it out, rub on soap, wash your face, and so forth). Caregivers can help the person to succeed by using the same steps and verbal directions every time. These can be written on a small card and kept where the activity is usually done.

Things to avoid: Caregivers also may have discovered statements or methods that start the activity off on the wrong foot or cause the person distress. For example, the person may always resist getting dressed if caregivers picked out his or her clothes.

Section III: My Story

This section takes a narrative format. In many cases, the portions to be completed are self-explanatory. For places requiring guidelines, however, directions are found in the narrative section. Sections I and II aim to provide a succinct, clear outline of vital information without cluttering the pages with directions or overwhelming the person who needs a quick reference. However, the purpose of Section III is rather different, and keeping the directions in Section III prevents the caregiver from having to break up the narrative flow by having to look back to get directions. In addition, having the descriptive guidelines in the My Story text may be helpful for the person with dementia if he or she enjoys using it as a memory book.

SECTION I
ESSENTIAL INFORMATION

Full name: _____

My long-time friends call me: _____

My new friends call me: _____

My grandchildren call me: _____

Current age:_____ Date of birth: _____

Place of birth: _____

Spouse's/partner's name: _____

Children

Name	Spouse's/partner's name	Place of residence

Other Significant People

Name	Relationship to person

Emergency Contact Information

Ambulance: _____

Police: _____   Fire: _____

Doctor's name: _____

Doctor's telephone number: _____

Family Members or Others to Contact in an Emergency

Name	Relationship to person	Telephone number

Health Issues

Medications

Medication	Dose/amount	Time of day taken	Reminder needed for when or how to take this medication?

Allergies: _____
_____

Vision: _____
_____

Hearing: _____
_____

Communication tips: _____
_____
_____
_____
_____
_____

Movement ability: _____
_____

Previous occupation(s): _____
_____

Significant life events: _____
_____
_____
_____
_____

Things that bring pleasure:_____

_____

_____

Special skills/strengths:_____

_____

_____

Special needs:_____

_____

_____

Things to avoid: _____

_____

_____

SECTION II
DAILY LIFE ROUTINES

Preretirement Daily Routine

	Sunday	Monday	Tuesday	Wednesday	Thursday	Friday	Saturday
6:00 A.M.– 7:00 A.M.							
7:00 A.M.– 9:00 A.M.							
9:00 A.M.– 11:00 A.M.							
11:00 A.M.– 1:00 P.M.							

	Sunday	Monday	Tuesday	Wednesday	Thursday	Friday	Saturday
1:00 P.M.–3:00 P.M							
3:00 P.M.–5:00 P.M							
5:00 P.M.–7:00 P.M.							
7:00 P.M.–11:00 P.M.							
11:00 P.M.–6:00 A.M.							

Present Daily Routine

	Sunday	Monday	Tuesday	Wednesday	Thursday	Friday	Saturday
6:00 A.M.– 7:00 A.M.							
7:00 A.M.– 9:00 A.M.							
9:00 A.M.– 11:00 A.M.							
11:00 A.M.– 1:00 P.M.							

	Sunday	Monday	Tuesday	Wednesday	Thursday	Friday	Saturday
1:00 P.M.–3:00 P.M							
3:00 P.M.–5:00 P.M							
5:00 P.M.–7:00 P.M.							
7:00 P.M.–11:00 P.M.							
11:00 P.M.–6:00 A.M.							

Specific Activity Routines

Getting Up

Usual habits: _____

_____

Favorites: _____

_____

Suggestions/tips: _____

_____

Can do: _____

_____

Help needed: _____

_____

Steps: _____

_____

Things to avoid: _____

_____

Bedtime Routine

Usual habits: _____

_____

Favorites: _____

_____

Suggestions/tips: _____

_____

Can do: _____

_____

Help needed: _____

_____

Steps: _____

_____

Things to avoid: _____

_____

If the person wakes in the night, try the following: _____

_____

_____

Bathing

Usual habits: _____

_____

Favorites: _____

_____

Suggestions/tips: _____

_____

Can do: _____

_____

Help needed: _____

_____

Steps: _____

_____

Things to avoid: _____

_____

_____

Dressing

Usual habits: _____

_____

Favorites: _____

_____

Suggestions/tips: _____

_____

Can do: _____

_____

Help needed: _____

_____

Steps: _____

_____

Things to avoid: _____

_____

Toileting

Usual habits: _____

_____

Favorites: _____

_____

Suggestions/tips: _____

_____

Can do: _____

_____

_____

Help needed: _____

_____

Steps:_____

_____

Things to avoid: _____

_____

Grooming

Usual habits: _____

_____

Favorites: _____

_____

Suggestions/tips: _____

_____

Can do: _____

_____

Help needed: _____

_____

Steps:_____

_____

Things to avoid: _____

_____

Meals

Breakfast
Usual habits: _____

_____

Favorites: _____

_____

Suggestions/tips: _____

_____

Can do: _____

_____

Help needed: _____

_____

Steps: _____

_____

Things to avoid: _____

_____

Lunch/Dinner

Usual habits: _____

_____

Favorites: _____

_____

Suggestions/tips: _____

_____

Can do: _____

_____

Help needed: _____

_____

Steps: _____

_____

Things to avoid: _____

_____

Supper/Dinner
Usual habits: _____

_____

Favorites: _____

_____

Suggestions/tips: _____

_____

Can do: _____

_____

Help needed: _____

_____

Steps: _____

_____

Things to avoid: _____

_____

Snacks
Usual habits: _____

_____

Favorites: _____

_____

Suggestions/tips: _____

_____

Can do: _____

_____

Help needed: _____

_____

Steps: _____

_____

Things to avoid: _____

_____

Housekeeping

Usual habits: _____

_____

Favorites: _____

_____

Suggestions/tips: _____

_____

Can do: _____

_____

Help needed: _____

_____

Steps: _____

_____

Things to avoid: _____

_____

SECTION III
MY STORY

I, _____ , was born

at _____ on _____ .

I grew up in _____

and went to school at _____ .

During all of these years, many wonderful things happened in

my life. Some of the best were: _____

_____

_____

_____

_____

There were also hard times. Some of the worst were: _____

_____

_____

_____

_____

_____

People and/or things helped me to get through these hard

times. Some of the most important were: _____

_____

_____

_____

When I look back over my life, I feel pleased and proud that:

_____

_____

_____

_____

_____

Family and Friends

These are the people who mean the most. Although names may be forgotten, recalling the person and special times spent together can help the person with memory loss to still be in the company of these special people. As you think about these people, recall as many things about them as possible—for example, nicknames, eye color, favorite stories, occupation, favorite sayings, and so forth. Photographs can help with recollections, and you may wish to copy favorite photographs to put them right on the page.

Spouse(s)/Partner(s)

Name	
Date of birth	
Birthplace	
Eye color	
Favorite expressions	
Favorite foods	
Occupation(s)	
Special memories of this person	

Name	
Date of birth	
Birthplace	
Eye color	
Favorite expressions	
Favorite foods	
Occupation(s)	
Special memories of this person	

Name	
Date of birth	
Birthplace	
Eye color	
Favorite expressions	
Favorite foods	
Occupation(s)	
Special memories of this person	

Name	
Date of birth	
Birthplace	
Eye color	
Favorite expressions	
Favorite foods	
Occupation(s)	

Special memories of this person	

Children

Name	
Spouse's name	
Date of birth	
Birthplace	
Eye color	
Favorite expressions	
Favorite foods	
Occupation(s)	
Special memories of this person	

Name	
Spouse's name	
Date of birth	
Birthplace	
Eye color	
Favorite expressions	
Favorite foods	
Occupation(s)	
Special memories of this person	

Name	
Spouse's name	
Date of birth	
Birthplace	
Eye color	
Favorite expressions	
Favorite foods	
Occupation(s)	
Special memories of this person	

Name	
Spouse's name	
Date of birth	
Birthplace	
Eye color	
Favorite expressions	
Favorite foods	
Occupation(s)	
Special memories of this person	

Name	
Spouse's name	
Date of birth	
Birthplace	
Eye color	
Favorite expressions	

Favorite foods	
Occupation(s)	
Special memories of this person	

Name	
Spouse's name	
Date of birth	
Birthplace	
Eye color	
Favorite expressions	
Favorite foods	
Occupation(s)	
Special memories of this person	

Mother

Name	
Date of birth	
Birthplace	
Eye color	
Favorite expressions	
Favorite foods	
Occupation(s)	
Special memories of this person	

Father

Name	
Date of birth	
Birthplace	
Eye color	
Favorite expressions	
Favorite foods	
Occupation(s)	
Special memories of this person	

Grandmother (maternal)

Name	
Date of birth	
Birthplace	
Eye color	
Favorite expressions	
Favorite foods	
Occupation(s)	
Special memories of this person	

Grandmother (paternal)

Name	
Date of birth	
Birthplace	
Eye color	

Eye color	
Favorite expressions	
Favorite foods	
Occupation(s)	
Special memories of this person	

Grandfather (maternal)

Name	
Date of birth	
Birthplace	
Eye color	
Favorite expressions	
Favorite foods	
Occupation(s)	
Special memories of this person	

Grandfather (paternal)

Name	
Date of birth	
Birthplace	
Eye color	
Favorite expressions	
Favorite foods	

Special memories of this person	

Siblings

Name	
Spouse's name	
Current residence	
Date of birth	
Birthplace	
Eye color	
Favorite expressions	
Favorite foods	
Occupation(s)	
Special memories of this person	

Name	
Spouse's name	
Current residence	
Date of birth	
Birthplace	
Eye color	
Favorite expressions	
Favorite foods	
Occupation(s)	

Special memories of this person	

Name	
Spouse's name	
Current residence	
Date of birth	
Birthplace	
Eye color	
Favorite expressions	
Favorite foods	
Occupation(s)	
Special memories of this person	

Name	
Spouse's name	
Current residence	
Date of birth	
Birthplace	
Eye color	
Favorite expressions	
Favorite foods	
Occupation(s)	
Special memories of this person	

Name	
Spouse's name	
Current residence	
Date of birth	
Birthplace	
Eye color	
Favorite expressions	
Favorite foods	
Occupation(s)	
Special memories of this person	

Name	
Spouse's name	
Current residence	
Date of birth	
Birthplace	
Eye color	
Favorite expressions	
Favorite foods	
Occupation(s)	
Special memories of this person	

Grandchildren

Name	
Spouse's name	

Current residence	
Date of birth	
Birthplace	
Eye color	
Favorite expressions	
Favorite foods	
Occupation(s)	
Special memories of this person	

Name	
Spouse's name	
Current residence	
Date of birth	
Birthplace	
Eye color	
Favorite expressions	
Favorite foods	
Occupation(s)	
Special memories of this person	

Name	
Spouse's name	
Current residence	
Date of birth	
Birthplace	
Eye color	

Favorite expressions	
Favorite foods	
Occupation(s)	
Special memories of this person	

Name	
Spouse's name	
Current residence	
Date of birth	
Birthplace	
Eye color	
Favorite expressions	
Favorite foods	
Occupation(s)	
Special memories of this person	

Name	
Spouse's name	
Current residence	
Date of birth	
Birthplace	
Eye color	
Favorite expressions	
Favorite foods	
Occupation(s)	
Special memories of this person	

Name	
Spouse's name	
Current residence	
Date of birth	
Birthplace	
Eye color	
Favorite expressions	
Favorite foods	
Occupation(s)	
Special memories of this person	

Great-Grandchildren

Name	
Date of birth	
Birthplace	
Eye color	
Favorite expressions	
Favorite foods	
Occupation(s)	
Special memories of this person	

Name	
Date of birth	
Birthplace	
Eye color	
Favorite expressions	

Favorite foods	
Occupation(s)	
Special memories of this person	

Name	
Date of birth	
Birthplace	
Eye color	
Favorite expressions	
Favorite foods	
Occupation(s)	
Special memories of this person	

Name	
Date of birth	
Birthplace	
Eye color	
Favorite expressions	
Favorite foods	
Occupation(s)	
Special memories of this person	

Name	
Date of birth	
Birthplace	

Eye color	
Favorite expressions	
Favorite foods	
Occupation(s)	
Special memories of this person	

Name	
Date of birth	
Birthplace	
Eye color	
Favorite expressions	
Favorite foods	
Occupation(s)	
Special memories of this person	

Name	
Date of birth	
Birthplace	
Eye color	
Favorite expressions	
Favorite foods	
Occupation(s)	
Special memories of this person	

Other special relatives (e.g., aunts, uncles, cousins)

Name	
Spouse's name	
Current residence	
Date of birth	
Birthplace	
Eye color	
Favorite expressions	
Favorite foods	
Occupation(s)	
Special memories of this person	

Name	
Spouse's name	
Current residence	
Date of birth	
Birthplace	
Eye color	
Favorite expressions	
Favorite foods	
Occupation(s)	
Special memories of this person	

Name	
Spouse's name	

Current residence	
Date of birth	
Birthplace	
Eye color	
Favorite expressions	
Favorite foods	
Occupation(s)	
Special memories of this person	

Name	
Spouse's name	
Current residence	
Date of birth	
Birthplace	
Eye color	
Favorite expressions	
Favorite foods	
Occupation(s)	
Special memories of this person	

Name	
Spouse's name	
Current residence	
Date of birth	
Birthplace	
Eye color	

Favorite expressions	
Favorite foods	
Occupation(s)	
Special memories of this person	

Name	
Spouse's name	
Current residence	
Date of birth	
Birthplace	
Eye color	
Favorite expressions	
Favorite foods	
Occupation(s)	
Special memories of this person	

Are there or were there family gatherings? If so, where were they held? Who came? What was done on these occasions?

_____

_____

_____

_____

_____

_____

_____

Friends

List the person's current and past friends. Questions to consider for this section include: Who was the person's best friend growing up? What did the person do with this friend? Are there any funny stories or unique experiences in connection with this friend?

Name	
Spouse's name	
Current residence	
Date of birth	
Birthplace	
Eye color	
Favorite expressions	
Favorite foods	
Occupation(s)	
Special memories of this person	

Name	
Spouse's name	
Current residence	
Date of birth	
Birthplace	
Eye color	
Favorite expressions	

Favorite foods	
Occupation(s)	
Special memories of this person	

Name	
Spouse's name	
Current residence	
Date of birth	
Birthplace	
Eye color	
Favorite expressions	
Favorite foods	
Occupation(s)	
Special memories of this person	

Name	
Spouse's name	
Current residence	
Date of birth	
Birthplace	
Eye color	
Favorite expressions	
Favorite foods	
Occupation(s)	
Special memories of this person	

Name	
Spouse's name	
Current residence	
Date of birth	
Birthplace	
Eye color	
Favorite expressions	
Favorite foods	
Occupation(s)	
Special memories of this person	

Name	
Spouse's name	
Current residence	
Date of birth	
Birthplace	
Eye color	
Favorite expressions	
Favorite foods	
Occupation(s)	
Special memories of this person	

Name	
Spouse's name	
Current residence	
Date of birth	

Birthplace	
Eye color	
Favorite expressions	
Favorite foods	
Occupation(s)	
Special memories of this person	

Homes and Houses

Include not only the address but also anything special and unique about that place and the house. Ask the following questions: Who were the neighbors? Which special friends lived nearby? What special activities occurred in this location? Get as many details as possible: What color was the outside of the house? Where was the person's bedroom? What was the house like? Who shared the house? Was it one story or more? Was there a garden or a yard? What special events happened in the house? What was the town like? In which community activities was the person involved? As you complete this section, remember that information about the person's childhood home is especially important, as these memories are likely to be the most deeply ingrained and also have rich emotional associations that bring comfort.

Current home: _____

_____

_____

_____

_____

Navigating the Alzheimer's Journey: A Compass for Caregiving by Carol Bowlby Sifton
© 2004 Health Professions Press, Inc. All rights reserved.

Childhood home(s): _____

_____

_____

_____

_____

_____

Adult home(s): _____

_____

_____

_____

_____

Life Work

Not all sections of the following narrative pieces will be applicable. Write "not applicable" in portions that do not apply so it is obvious that these portions were not merely skipped.

My main work was as a homemaker/mother. It was a busy life but I feel satisfied when I think about _____

_____

_____

_____.

On the other hand I always found it frustrating when _____

_____

_____.

My funniest memory of those times was when _____

_____

_____ .

My happiest memories of those times are _____

_____

_____ .

My favorite recipes were for _____

_____

_____ .

My first job was_____

at _____ .

My boss was named _____ ,

and I also worked with _____ .

My wages were _____ , which in those days would

buy_____

_____ .

I worked there for _____ years, and then I moved on

because _____

_____ .

I also worked for _____

as a _____ .

I worked with _____ ,

and _____ was our boss. I worked there for

years and then moved on because _____

_____ .

Navigating the Alzheimer's Journey: A Compass for Caregiving by Carol Bowlby Sifton
© 2004 Health Professions Press, Inc. All rights reserved.

I also worked for _____
as a_____ .
I worked with _____ ,
and_____was our boss. I worked there for
years and then moved on because_____
_____ .

I also worked for _____
as a_____ .
I worked with _____ ,
and_____was our boss. I worked there for
years and then moved on because_____
_____ .

The job that I liked the most was _____
because _____
_____ .

The job that I liked the least was _____
because _____
_____ .

The things that I am most pleased with from my working life
are _____
_____
_____
_____
_____ .

Navigating the Alzheimer's Journey: A Compass for Caregiving by Carol Bowlby Sifton

Spiritual Life

In my life, I have been most inspired by _____
_____
_____ .

In my life, I have been most comforted by _____
_____
_____ .

I grew up in the _____ religious tradition.
My fondest memories of this tradition are _____
_____
_____ .

As an adult I belonged to _____ .
In these communities I served as _____
_____ .

My richest memories of these times are _____
_____
_____ .

My favorite sacred music is _____
_____
_____ .

My favorite sacred/spiritual readings are _____
_____
_____ .

My favorite religious holiday is _____
because _____ .

The spiritual activities which I enjoy most now are _____
_____
_____ .

To participate in these activities, I may need help to _____
_____
_____ .

Hobbies and Interests

Over the years I have enjoyed _____
_____
_____
_____
_____ .

When I think about all of these interests, the times that I have
been happiest were _____
_____
_____
_____ .

When I think about all of these interests, the things I am most
satisfied with were (include any special accomplishments,
such as championships won, offices held, and so forth) _____
_____
_____
_____
_____
_____ .

I still enjoy _____

_____

_____

_____ .

To continue doing this, sometimes I may need help _____

_____

_____

_____

_____ .

Favorites

Activities: _____

_____

_____

_____

_____

_____ .

Books/magazines/newspapers: _____

_____

_____

_____

_____

_____

_____ .

Chair/place to sit: _____

_____

_____

_____

_____

_____ .

Clothing: _____

_____

_____

_____

_____

_____ .

Colors: _____

_____

_____

_____

_____

_____ .

Expressions: _____

_____

_____

_____

_____

_____

_____ .

Foods: _____

_____

_____

_____

_____

_____

_____ .

Jokes: _____

_____

_____

_____

_____

_____ .

Memories: _____

_____

_____

_____

_____

_____ .

Movies: _____

_____

_____

Navigating the Alzheimer's Journey: A Compass for Caregiving by Carol Bowlby Sifton
© 2004 Health Professions Press, Inc. All rights reserved.

_____

_____

_____

_____ .

Music: _____

_____

_____

_____

_____

_____

_____ .

People: _____

_____

_____

_____

_____

_____

_____ .

Pets: _____

_____

_____

_____

_____

_____

_____ .

Plants/flowers: _____

_____

_____

_____

_____

_____

_____ .

Radio stations/programs: _____

_____

_____

_____

_____

_____ .

Relaxing activities: _____

_____

_____

_____

_____

_____ .

Sports:_____

_____

_____

_____

_____

_____

_____ .

Stories: _____

_____

_____

_____

_____

_____

_____ .

Travel experiences: _____

_____

_____

_____

_____

_____ .

Television programs: _____

_____

_____

_____

_____

_____ .

Unwinding activities: _____

_____

_____

_____

_____

_____

_____ .

Least Favorites

Just as favorite things and experiences bring pleasure and relaxation, certain things and experiences are upsetting. When a person has dementia, he or she may not be able to respond in the usual way to this situation, leading both the person and the caregiver to become distressed. By learning about the person's least favorite things (sometimes called *triggers*) and sharing them with other caregivers, distress can often be avoided.

Activities: _____

_____

_____

_____

_____

_____

_____ .

Books/magazines/newspapers: _____

_____

_____

_____

_____ .

Chair/place to sit: _____

_____

_____

_____

_____

_____

_____ .

Clothing: _____

_____

_____

_____

_____

_____ .

Colors: _____

_____

_____

_____

_____

_____ .

Expressions: _____

_____

_____

_____

_____

_____

_____ .

Foods: _____

_____

_____

_____

_____

_____ .

Jokes: _____

_____

_____

_____

_____

_____ .

Memories: _____

_____

_____

_____

_____

_____ .

Movies: _____

_____

_____

_____

_____

_____

_____ .

Music: _____

_____

_____

_____

_____

_____ .

People: _____

_____

_____

_____

_____ .

Pets: _____

_____

_____

_____

_____

_____ .

Plants/flowers: _____

_____

_____

_____

_____

_____ .

Radio stations/programs: _____

_____

_____

_____

_____

_____ .

Relaxing activities: _____

_____

_____

_____

_____

_____ .

Sports: _____

_____

_____

_____

_____

_____

_____ .

Stories: _____

_____

_____

_____

_____ .

Travel experiences: _____

_____

_____

_____

_____ .

Television programs: _____

_____

_____

_____

_____ .

Unwinding activities: _____

_____

_____

_____

_____

_____

_____ .

Appendix B

Resources

MAJOR ALZHEIMER'S DISEASE/DEMENTIA
ORGANIZATIONS REFERENCED IN THIS BOOK

Alzheimer's Association

225 North Michigan Avenue, Floor 17, Chicago, IL 60601
800-272-3900 (toll free in the United States) or 312-335-8700
http://www.alz.org

The Alzheimer's Association is a voluntary organization based in Chicago, Illinois, that publishes a wealth of educational materials (much of it free for caregivers), funds research, and serves as an advocacy body. Many U.S. educational and program initiatives have been sponsored by the Alzheimer's Association. It coordinates the work of more than 200 local chapters in the United States, each of which operates a unique range of educational and support programs for caregivers and persons with Alzheimer's disease. Contact your local chapter for more details. The national organization can provide contact information and a catalog of educational materials.

Alzheimer Society of Canada

20 Eglinton Avenue West, Suite 1200, Toronto, Ontario M4R 1K8
Canada • 800-616-8816 (toll free in Canada) or 416-488-8722
http://www.alzheimer.ca

The Alzheimer Society is a voluntary organization with a small office staff, which coordinates the work of the provincial organizations; develops educational materials and Canadian pilot programs; sponsors a yearly conference; and raises funds to support the three-fold focus of the organization: support, education, and research.

Each provincial chapter offers a unique variety of services: support groups for persons with Alzheimer's disease and/or their caregivers; resources such as videotapes, books, and journals; education sessions; referral and/or counseling services; and, in some cases, direct services such as day programs. Contact your provincial chapter for more details on services in your area.

OTHER ORGANIZATIONS AND GOVERNMENT AGENCIES

The Alzheimer's Disease Education and Referral Center (ADEAR)

Post Office Box 8250, Silver Spring, MD 20907-8250
800-438-4380 • http://www.alzheimers.org • adear@alzheimers.org

ADEAR is funded by the U.S. National Institutes of Health and serves as an information clearinghouse on educational materials, research, drug trials, and information on Alzheimer's disease. Informational pamphlets, a newsletter and numerous other free publications, abstracts of articles, research reports, and information on drug testing can be requested by mail or viewed on line.

ADEAR also lists Alzheimer's Disease Research Centers that receive federal funding from the U.S. National Institute on Aging to operate memory disorder clinics, offer educational programs for family and professional caregivers, and conduct research. To learn about possible Alzheimer's Disease Research Centers in your area, go to http://www .alzheimers.org/adcdir.htm or contact ADEAR via telephone or e-mail.

Note: If you find out that do not live near an Alzheimer's Disease Research Center, contact the one closest to your region for referral to a clinic in your area. Some states also fund memory disorder clinics, so contact your state department of health for information. Your local Alzheimer's Association or Alzheimer Society chapter can also provide information about other local memory disorder clinics and local clinicians who have expertise in Alzheimer's disease and dementia.

American Association of Retired Persons (AARP)

601 East Street NW, Washington, DC 20049
888-687-2277 • http://www.aarp.org

The AARP publishes a number of practical guides on care planning, financial, and tax matters. It also provides information on reminiscence and other therapeutic activities.

**National Center for Complementary and
Alternative Medicine (NCCAM) Clearinghouse**

Post Office Box 7923, Gaithersburg, MD 20898
888-644-6226 • http://nccam.nih.gov

NCCAM is a division of the U.S. National Institutes of Health. It publishes a variety of facts sheets on complementary and alternative medical practices.

Professional Organizations Offering
Information and Referrals for Specific Issues

American Dietetic Association

120 South Riverside Plaza, Suite 2000, Chicago, IL 60606-6995
800-877-1600 • http://www.eatright.org

American Occupational Therapy Association

4720 Montgomery Lane, Post Office Box 31220
Bethesda, MD 20824-1220 • 301-652-2682 • http://www.aota.org

American Physical Therapy Association

1111 North Fairfax Street, Alexandria, VA 22314-1488
703-684-2782 • http://www.apta.org

American Speech-Language-Hearing Association

10801 Rockville Pike, Rockville, MD 20852
800-638-8255 • http://www.asha.org

Canadian Association of Occupational Therapists

CTTC Building, Suite 3400, 1125 Colonel By Drive
Ottawa, ON K1S 5R1 Canada • 800-434-2268 • http://www.caot.ca

**Canadian Association of
Speech-Language Pathologists and Audiologists**

401-200 Elgin Street, Ottawa, ON K2P 1L5 Canada
613-567-9968 • http://www.caslpa.ca

Canadian Pysiotherapy Association

2345 Yonge Street, Suite 410, Toronto, ON M4P 2ES Canada
416-932-1888 • http://www.physiotherapy.ca

Dieticians of Canada

480 University Avenue, Suite 604, Toronto, ON M5G 1V2 Canada
416-596-0857 • http://www.dieticians.ca

CATALOG AND PRODUCT INFORMATION

The Alzheimer's Store (at Ageless Design)

12633 159th Court North, Jupiter, FL 33478 • 561-745-0210
http://www.alzstore.com • http://www.agelessdesign.com

The Alzheimer's Store carries helpful products for home care. It is part of
Ageless Design, a web site that offers a free monthly newsletter for caregivers, current news on Alzheimer's disease, and a free caregiver question-
and-answer service.

Cross Creek Recreational Products

Post Office Box 289, Millbrook, NY 12545 • 800-645-5816

Cross Creek Recreational Products offers a catalog with more than 30
interesting activity products for persons with moderate and advanced
dementia. Activities include puzzles, self-directed materials, musical supplies, activity aprons, and games.

Eldergames

1710 Hunters Lane, Rockville, MD 20852

Eldergames carries a variety of materials for various functional levels, memory games, trivia questions, and fabric books for stimulation.

ERP Group

3232 autoroute Laval ouest, Laval, PQ H7T 2H6 Canada
450-687-0780 • http://www.erp.ca

ERP Group is a distributor for Nottingham Rehabilitation Equipment. In addition to standard rehabilitation equipment, the company carries an interesting selection of adaptive equipment. See the "Solutions for Daily Living" portion of ERP Group's web site.

Geriatric Resources

Post Office Box 239, Radium Springs, New Mexico 88054
800-359-0390 or 505-524-0250
http://www.geriatric-resources.com

Geriatric Resources is a private company run by Mary Lucero, an educator and former nursing facility administrator. The company offers educational programs and carries a line of helpful products and resources in three catalogs: Alzheimer's Comfort Care Video Training (home videotape training materials), Alzheimer's Education and Training Resources (publications about Alzheimer's disease), and Alzheimer's Sensory Stimulation Products (contains more than 400 interactive products for behavioral interventions).

BOOKS, ARTICLES, AND OTHER RESOURCES

General

For Caregivers

Alzheimer Society of Canada. (1991). *Alzheimer disease: A handbook for care*. Toronto: Author.

This handbook is intended for family members and presents basic information on Alzheimer's disease and caregiving.

Alzheimer Society of Canada. (1992). *Guidelines for care*. Toronto: Author.

This booklet sets out the goals and values that achieve an optimum level of care for a person with Alzheimer's disease.

Alzheimer Society of Canada. (1993). *A personal care book*. Toronto: Author.

This book about the person with Alzheimer's disease is completed by the person who knows him or her best. Filled with information about the person's likes, dislikes, routines, and history, the booklet helps provide continuity of care.

Alzheimer Society of Canada. (2002). *Daily living*. Toronto: Author.

Daily Living is a series of information sheets on how to deal with practical day-to-day issues. Available topics include bathing, communication, meal time, personal care, and toileting.

Ballard, E., & Poer, C. (1999). *Lessons learned: Shared experiences in coping*. Durham, NC: Duke University Medical Center.

This well-done booklet contains brief guidelines for caregivers and moving quotes from other caregivers.

Gwyther, L. (1995). *You are one of us: Successful clergy/church connections to Alzheimer's families*. Durham, NC: Duke University Medical Center.

Despite the title, this excellent booklet has applications for a broader audience, helping others learn how to relate to and visit with persons who have dementia.

For Persons Diagnosed with Alzheimer's Disease

Alzheimer Society of Canada. (2002). *Shared experiences: Suggestions for those with Alzheimer disease*. Toronto: Author.

This resource is for persons recently diagnosed with Alzheimer's disease and explains what that person may be experiencing and offers suggestions on how to make life easier. It is available as a printed booklet or an audiotape, both of which are available free of charge while quantities last. Or see the Alzheimer Society's web site for information on downloading the booklet in print or audio form.

As Related to this Book's Chapters

Chapter 1

Alzheimer Society of British Columbia. (n.d.). *Memory problems?* Vancouver: Author.

This excellent 15-page booklet was written by persons with Alzheimer's disease. It shares insightful comments about how Alzheimer's disease affects their daily lives and tips for caregivers from the point of view of persons with Alzheimer's disease. It is available for a small fee from the Alzheimer Society of British Columbia (604-681-6530; http://www .alzheimerbc.org).

Ballard, E. (1993). *Managing grief and bereavement: A guide for families and professionals caring for memory impaired adults and other chronically ill persons.* Durham, NC: Duke University Medical Center.

Davidson, A. (1997). *Alzheimer's: A love story.* Secaucus, NJ: Birch Lane Press.

Innovative Caregiving Resources. (n.d.). *Video respite* [videotapes]. Salt Lake City, UT: Producer.

Video Respite is a collection of 13 videotapes designed to engage persons with mid- to late-stage dementia. It addresses a variety of topics (e.g., music, reminiscence) from different cultural traditions (e.g., African American, Jewish, Canadian). The narrator talks directly to the viewer and seeks his or her involvement. Caregivers should preview the videotapes first: Some people with dementia may find them comforting and interesting for brief periods; others may find them too condescending or confusing. Some Alzheimer's organizations chapters loan out these videotapes; they are also available from Innovative Caregiving Resources (801-272-9806 or 800-249-5600; http://www.videorespite.com).

Kuhn, D. (2003). *Alzheimer's early stages: First steps for family, friends and caregivers* (2nd ed.). Alameda, CA: Hunter House Publishers.

This book provides an excellent overview of the diagnosis of dementia as well as other background information. It also gives suggestions and resources for issues that arise during the early stages.

Lustbader, W. (1997). *Prescription for caregivers: Take care of yourself* [video-tape]. Chicago: Terra Nova Films.

Noyes, L.E. (2000). *Caregiving at a glance: Fingertip help for families taking care of people with Alzheimer's type illnesses.* Falls Church, VA: Family Respite Center.

This resource offers help for families taking care of people with Alzheimer's disease or dementia. This excellent, manageable resource is in a flip-chart format that presents background information and possible solutions in many areas, such as communication, activities of daily living, wandering, and so forth. It is available from the Family Respite Center (703-532-8899).

Media One Health Video. (n.d.). *Dementia with dignity* [videotape]. Producer.

Dementia with Dignity is an excellent 60-minute videotape on caring for a person with dementia. Although family caregiving is included, the primary focus is on long-term care. However, the principles can be universally applied. The videotape covers the topics of enhancing quality of life, continuing a familiar lifestyle, communicating, and responding to challenging behaviors. It is an excellent teaching or in-service tool because the content is based on actual interactions between staff and residents. The videotape is available from Customflix (978-626-0061; http://www.customflix.com); Terra Nova Films (800-779-8491; http://www.terranova.org); and the Training and Resource Centre for Residential Aged Care (TARCRAC), Queensland University of Technology, Post Office Box 284, Zillmere, QLD 4034 Australia.

Oliver, R., & Bock, F. (1989). *Coping with Alzheimer's: A caregiver's emotional survival guide.* North Hollywood, CA: Wilshire Book Company.

Ronch, J. (1991). *Alzheimer's disease: A practical guide for families and other caregivers.* New York: Continuum Publishing.

Simpson, R., & Simpson, A. (1999). *Through the wilderness of Alzheimer's: A guide in two voices.* Minneapolis, MN: Augsburg Fortress Publishers.

ALZwell Caregiver Support

Prism Innovations, 50 Amuxen Court, Islip, NY 11751
http://www.alzwell.com

ALZwell Caregiver Support is a volunteer group dedicated to helping dementia caregivers find understanding, wisdom, and support on the caregiving journey. It offers an on-line newsletter, a dementia care library, and on-line store for caregiver education booklets.

Caregiver Network

561 Avenue Road, Suite 606, Toronto, ON M4V 2J8 Canada
http://www.caregiver.on.ca • http//www.howtocare.com

The Caregiver Network is a private company focusing on support and training for family caregivers. It offers a quarterly newsletter, two caregiver information web sites, caregiver training, and resources such as videotapes and a Personal Care Binder. The emphasis is on caregiving in general, but issues that are specific to dementia care are sometimes addressed.

Duke Family Support Program

Box 3600 DUMC, Durham NC 27710 • 919-660-7510
http://www.dukefamilysupport.org

This innovative center publishes helpful guidebooks and carries videotapes and other information materials.

Family Caregiver Alliance

690 Market Street, Suite 600, San Francisco, CA 94104
800-445-8106 or 415-434-3388
http://www.caregiver.org/index.html

The Family Caregiver Alliance is a not-for-profit organization dedicated to addressing the needs of home caregivers for older adults and people with chronic illnesses or disabilities. As well as publishing a newsletter and maintaining a web site, the organization provides various local support services.

National Family Caregivers Alliance

10400 Connecticut Avenue #500, Kensington, MD 20895
800-896-3650 • http://www.nfcacares.org

The National Family Caregivers Alliance is a national not-for-profit advocacy and educational organization for families that provide care. The organizations publishes a quarterly newsletter that is free to U.S. residents (and is available for a fee to Canadian residents) and maintains a web site on caregiving issues. U.S. caregivers can receive a free caregiver survival kit, which includes videotapes and other educational materials.

National Institute on Aging

NIA Information Center, Post Office Box 8057
Gaithersburg, MD 20898 • http://www.nia.nih.gov

For a fee, the U.S. National Institute on Aging offers a set (7-minute videotape and 100-page book) that provides home exercises for older adults. Go to http://www.niapublications.org/exercisevideo/index.asp for information on this resource.

Chapter 2

Alzheimer Society of British Columbia. (n.d.). *Memory problems?* Vancouver: Author.

Please refer to the information for this item under the Chapter 1 listings.

Davis, R. (1989). *My journey into Alzheimer's disease.* Wheaton, IL: Tyndale House Publishers.

This book is a good resource because it was written by a person with Alzheimer's disease.

Yeh, C., Truscott, T., & Snyder, L. (2001). The benefits of a support group for persons with Alzheimer's disease. *Alzheimer's Care Quarterly, 2*(4), 42–46.

This article covers the importance of support groups.

Dementia Advocacy and Support Network

http://www.dasninternational.org

This site was developed by a group of people with Alzheimer's disease and other dementias to exchange information and to advocate for treatment and for care that recognizes the dignity and personhood of those affected. The site links to a chat room that can provide on-line support for persons with Alzheimer's disease and other dementias.

Early Alzheimer's: A Forum for Early Stage Dementia Care

c/o Alzheimer's Association of Santa Barbara • 2024 De La Vina Street Santa Barbara, CA 93105 • 805-563-0020

Early Alzheimer's is a quarterly newsletter for persons with Alzheimer's disease and for family and professional caregivers.

I Have Alzheimer Disease

http://www.alzheimer.ca/english/haveAD/intro.htm

This excellent web page, which contains information for and by persons with Alzheimer's disease, is part of the Alzheimer Society web site.

Perspectives: A Newsletter for Individuals Diagnosed with Alzheimer's Disease

c/o Editor • 9800 Gilman Drive, LaJolla, CA 92093 • 691-622-5800

Perspectives is a quarterly publication available for an annual fee.

Chapter 3

Alzheimer's Association. (1997). *Just for teens: Helping you understand Alzheimer's disease*. Chicago: Author.

Alzheimer's Association. (1998). *Just for children: Helping you understand Alzheimer's disease*. Chicago: Author.

These two free fact sheets are available from the Alzheimer's Association (please refer to the contact information given at the beginning of this appendix).

Kuhn, D. (2003). *Alzheimer's early stages: First steps for family, friends and caregivers* (2nd ed.). Alameda, CA: Hunter House Publishers.

Please refer to the information under the Chapter 1 listings.

The Cognitive Neurology and Alzheimer's Disease Center at Northwestern University

http://www.brain.nwu.edu

This site offers information on Alzheimer's disease and atypical dementias as well as information for caregivers.

Dementia Research Group

http://dementia.ion.ucl.ac.uk

Based in London, England, this site is sponsored by numerous researchers and health care professionals. It offers advice and information as well as research findings.

Various **fact sheets** on drugs and testing at research centers and clinics throughout the United States are published by the Alzheimer's Association (please refer to the contact information given at the beginning of this appendix).

Numerous **videotapes** provide an excellent overview of Alzheimer's disease and other dementias. For availability in your area, check with your local Alzheimer's Association or Alzheimer Society chapter or the public library. For example, the pharmaceutical company that makes Aricept (donepezil) produced a good education series for family members. Videotapes of this series were distributed to local Alzheimer's chapters and other care centers.

Chapter 4

Brown, C. (Ed.). (1984). *The many facets of touch*. Skillman, NJ: Johnson & Johnson.

Vortherms, R. (1991). Clinically improving communication through touch. *Journal of Gerontological Nursing, 17*(5), 6–10.

The preceding two items are good resources regarding the effects of touch.

Steps to . . .

The Alzheimer's Association's *Steps to . . .* pamphlet series for front-line caregivers offers many helpful suggestions. The following is recommended as an excellent guide to communication:

Steps to Enhancing Communication: Interacting with Persons with Alzheimer's Disease, http://www.alzoc.org/support/Helplinetopics/comm_enhancing .htm

Chapter 5

Print and Videotape Resources

Calkins, M.P., Nainazi, K.H., Rosner, T.L., Olson, A., & Brabender, B. (1990). *Home modifications: Responding to dementia.* Chardon, OH: Corinne Dolan Center at Heather Hill.

This booklet, based on a caregiver survey, is available for a nominal fee from the Corinne Dolan Center at Heather Hill (440-285-4040; http://www.heatherhill.org).

Canada Mortgage and Housing Corporation. (1990). *At home with Alzheimer's disease: Useful adaptations to the home environment.* Ottawa, ON: Author.

Canada Mortgage and Housing Corporation. (1992). *Maintaining seniors' independence through home adaptations.* Ottawa, ON: Author.

The booklets *At Home with Alzheimer's Disease: Useful Adaptations to the Home Environment* and *Maintaining Seniors' Independence Through Home Adaptations* are free. In addition, a videotape (also titled *Maintaining Seniors' Independence Through Home Adaptations*) is available on free loan from district offices of the Canada Mortgage and Housing Corporation (800-668-2642; http://www.cmhc-schl.gc.ca).

Olsen, R., Ehrenkrantz, E., & Hutchings, B. (1993). *Homes that help: Advice from caregivers for creating a supportive home.* Newark: New Jersey Institute of Technology.

This 77-page book contains illustrations and is available for a fee from CABSR/New Jersey Institute of Technology, Hazell Center, Room 312, 323 Martin Luther King Boulevard, Newark, NJ 07102 (201-596-3097).

Warner, M.L. (2000). *The complete guide to Alzheimer's proofing your home.* West LaFayette, IN: Purdue University Press.

The Complete Guide to Alzheimer's Proofing Your Home, a 477-page book written by architect and gerontologist Mark Warner, is an excellent guide that has dozens of practical suggestions and resources for improving home safety and creating a supportive environment for persons with dementia. The suggestions range from simple and inexpensive additions, such as antiscald devices in faucets, to the very expensive, such as suggestions for renovations and additions. This book may be ordered from Purdue University Press (http://www.thepress.purdue.edu or 800-247-6553), from Ageless Design (please refer to "Catalog and Product Information" for contact information), or through your local bookstore.

Steps to . . .

The following pamphlets in the Alzheimer's Association's *Steps to . . .* series are particularly recommended for more information on wandering (please refer to the contact information provided at the beginning of the appendix or go to http://www.alz.org/resources/factsheets.asp):

Steps to Ensuring Safety: Preventing Wandering and Getting Lost

Steps to Enhancing Your Home: Modifying the Environment

Steps to Understanding Challenging Behaviors: Responding to Persons with Alzheimer's Disease

Steps to Enhancing Communication: Interacting with Persons with Alzheimer's Disease

Resources for Equipment

Many drug stores and department stores carry adaptive equipment. Some stores will provide a temporary loan for assessment purposes and may rent more expensive equipment. Contact a qualified occupational therapist or other health care professional for a specialized assessment and advice on home adaptations and adaptive equipment. The following are a few of the many companies that offer adaptive equipment.

Ableware-Maddak (Pequannock, NJ)	800-443-4926
AdaptAbility (Colchester, CT)	800-288-9941
AliMed (Dedham, MA)	800-225-2610
Alsto's Handy Helpers (Galesburg, IL)	800-447-0048

Easy Living Specialties (Newport RI)	800-406-1338
ERP Group (Laval, PQ)	450-687-0780
Guardian Products (Simi Valley, CA)	800-423-8034
Improvements (Hanover, PA)	800-642-2112
Independent Living Aids (Plainview, NY)	800-537-2118
JCPenney Special Needs (Milwaukee, WI)	800-222-6161
Sammons Preston Rolyan (Bolingbrook, IL)	800-323-5547
Sears Home Healthcare (Garland, TX)	800-326-1750
Sears Canada	800-267-3277

Chapter 6

Alzheimer's Association. (1995). *Activity programming for persons with dementia: A sourcebook.* Chicago: Author.

To get this excellent manual from the Alzheimer's Association, please refer to the contact information provided at the beginning of the appendix.

Geriatric Resources

Please refer to the information provided under the heading "Catalog and Product Information."

Chapter 7

Alzheimer Society of Canada. (1993). *Alzheimer disease: Care at home.* Toronto: Author.

Care at Home is a caregiver training package for frontline workers providing care at home for persons with Alzheimer's disease. The package includes an instructor's guide, a participants' workbook, and 7 videotapes and is designed for both facilitator-led group training and self-directed learning. Topic titles are Aging, The Nature of Alzheimer Disease, Communication Strategies, Working with Families, The Home Environment, Activities of Daily Living, and Challenging Behaviours. This package is available from the Alzheimer Society of Canada or can be obtained on free loan in Canada from local Alzheimer Society chapters (refer to the information provided at the beginning of the appendix).

Ballard, E., & Poer, C. (1993). *Sexuality and Alzheimer's disease.* Durham, NC: Duke University Alzheimer's Disease Center.

This important resource is one of few such guides available on the topic and is available from the Duke Family Support Program at the Center for the Study of Aging and Human Development (919-660-7502).

Crabtree, J., & Crabtree, D. (1993). *Home caregivers guide: Articles for adult daily living.* Tuscon, AZ: Therapy Skill Builders.

Home Caregivers Guide is an excellent, practical, illustrated guide. It is for training caregivers to use adaptive equipment and transfers and provides techniques in helping with the activities of daily living. Special suggestions are given for persons with cognitive impairment. This resource is available from Therapy Skill Builders (602-323-7500).

Hewson, M. (1996). *Horticultural therapy.* Guelph, ON, Canada: Homewood Psychiatric Hospital.

Kuhn, D. (1994). The changing face of sexual intimacy in Alzheimer's disease. *The American Journal of Alzheimer's Disease and Related Disorders and Research, 9*(5), 7–14.

Lustbader, W. (1992). *Counting on kindness: The dilemmas of dependency.* New York: The Free Press.

This book is a resource that covers the importance of independence in activities of daily living (ADLs).

Media One Health Video. (n.d.). *Dementia with dignity* [videotape]. Producer.

Please refer to the information provided under the Chapter 1 listings.

Morris, A., & Hunt, G. (1994). *A part of daily life: Alzheimer's caregivers simplify activities and the home* [videotape]. Bethesda, MD: American Occupational Therapy Association.

A Part of Daily Life is a 16-minute videotape with dementia patients and their families. It demonstrates task breakdown and environmental modifications for dementia care at home. This videotape and its accompanying resource guide are useful for teaching caregivers and are available from the American Occupational Therapy Association (please refer to the information provided under "Professional Organizations that May Offer Information and Referrals for Specific Issues").

Noyes, L.E. (2000). *Caregiving at a glance: Fingertip help for families taking care of people with Alzheimer's type illnesses.* Falls Church, VA: Family Respite Center.

Please refer to the information provided under the Chapter 1 subheading.

Vanden Bosch, J.A. (1995). *A thousand tomorrows: Intimacy, sexuality and Alzheimer's* [videotape]. Chicago: Terra Nova Films.

This sensitive, well-done videotape helps caregivers discuss these challenging issues. Part Two, *More than a Thousand Tomorrows* (2004), is also available from Terra Nova Films (800-779-8491; http://www.terranova .org).

Yeomans, K. (1992). *The able gardener: Overcoming barriers of age and physical limitations.* Pownal, VT: Storey Communications.

American Alliance for Health, Physical Education, Recreation and Dance

1900 Association Drive, Reston, VA 20191 • 800-213-7193
http://www.aahperd.org

The American Alliance for Health, Physical Education, Recreation and Dance has numerous publications on exercises for older adults.

Laughing Matters

c/o The Humour Project, Subscriptions Department
480 Broadway, Suite 210, Saratoga Springs, NY 12866
518-587-8770 • http://www.HumorProject.com

The magazine *Laughing Matters* is published four times per year by Dr. Joel Goodman, who is well known for his humor seminars. The magazine includes suggestions on using humor to lighten the life of caregivers (personally and professionally) as well as ways to use humor therapeutically.

Chapter 9

Robinson, A., Spencer, B., & White, L. (1991). *Understanding difficult behaviors.* Ypsilanti: Eastern Michigan University.

This excellent, practical book is available from the Alzheimer's Education Program at Eastern Michigan University (734-487-2335; http://www .emich.edu/public/alzheimers/Manual.htm).

Terri, L. (n.d.) *Managing and Understanding Behavior Problems in Alzheimer's Disease and Related Disorders.* Seattle: University of Washington, Alzheimer's Disease Research Center.

This excellent videotape series is a training program for various types of caregivers. For more information, go to http://depts.washington.edu/adrc web/educat.shtml or call the assistant to the director of the University of Washington Alzheimer's Disease Research Center at 206-277-3281.

Tuokko, H., Purves, B., & Baisley, K. (1993). *Understanding dementia: A problem solving approach for caregivers* [videotape]. Vancouver: British Columbia Health Research Foundation, the Alzheimer Society of British Columbia, and the Clinic for Alzheimer's Disease and Related Disorders.

Understanding Dementia is a good teaching tool for caregivers. This resource consists of a half-hour videotape and a small guidebook that take actual caregivers through the problem-solving process. Available from the Alzheimer Society of British Columbia (604-681-6530; http://www .alzheimerbc.org).

Chapter 10

Alzheimer's Association. (1992). *Family guide for Alzheimer care in residential settings.* Chicago: Author.

Alzheimer's Association. (1999). *Residential care: A guide for choosing a new home.* Chicago: Author.

The preceding two brief guidelines are available from the Alzheimer's Association; please refer to the information provided at the beginning of the appendix.

Alzheimer Society of Canada. (1993). *Alzheimer disease: Care at home.* Toronto: Author.

Please refer to the Chapter 7 listings for a description of this training package.

Alzheimer Society of Canada. (1997). *Facing the tough issues: Alzheimer ethical guidelines.* Toronto: Author.

This thoughtful document was developed with caregivers, persons with dementia, and professionals to guide ethical decision making. It has since been updated to cover various issues through the following articles: Communicating the Diagnosis, Driving, Living Alone, Decision-Making, Respecting Individual Choices, Quality of Life, Participation in Research, Genetic Testing, Restraints, and Intimacy and Sexuality.

American Bar Association. (1997). *In your hands: The tools for preserving personal autonomy* [videotape]. Chicago: Producer.

This videotape is available for purchase or rental through Terra Nova Films (800-779-8491; http://www.terranova.org).

Ballard, E., & Poer, C. (1999). *Lessons learned: Shared experiences in coping.* Durham, NC: Duke University Medical Center.

For a description of this booklet, please refer to the "General" subheading of the main heading "Books, Articles, and Other Resources."

Greene Burger, S., Fraser, V., Hunt, S., Frank, B., & The National Citizens Coalition for Nursing Home Reform. (1996). *Nursing homes: Getting good care there.* San Luis Obispo, CA: American Source Books.

This is an excellent guide for caregivers on questions to ask when searching for a nursing facility as well as ways to advocate for your loved one.

Kuhn, D. (2003). *Alzheimer's early stages: First steps for family, friends and caregivers* (2nd ed.). Alameda, CA: Hunter House.

Please refer to the Chapter 1 listings for a description of this book.

Taxes and Alzheimer's Disease is a series of short publications from Alzheimer's Association (please refer to the information provided at the beginning of the appendix). The publications cover a variety of tax issues and are periodically updated.